College of Occupational Therapy
(Liverpool) Ltd.
Victoria Road
Huyton, Liverpool, L36 5SB

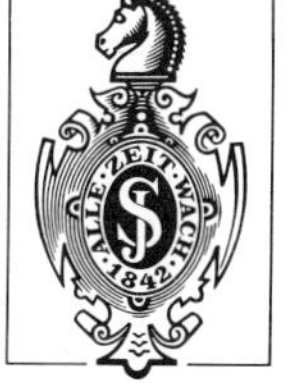

Myocardial Infarction at Young Age

International Symposium
Held in Bad Krozingen
January 30 and 31, 1981

Edited by H. Roskamm

With 83 Figures

Springer-Verlag
Berlin Heidelberg New York 1981

Professor Dr. Helmut Roskamm
Benedikt Kreutz Rehabilitationszentrum
für Herz- und Kreislaufkranke e.V.
Südring 15
D-7812 Bad Krozingen

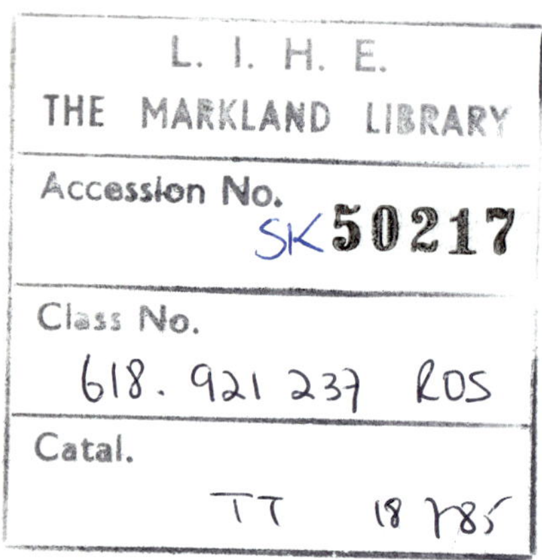

ISBN 3-540-11090-9 Springer-Verlag Berlin Heidelberg New York
ISBN 0-387-11090-9 Springer-Verlag New York Heidelberg Berlin

Library of Congress Cataloging in Publication Data. Myocardial infarction at young age. Papers from the International Symposium on Myocardial Infarction at Young Age sponsored by the European Society of Cardiology and the Pharma Schwarz Co. Includes bibliographical references and index. 1. Heart-Infarction–Age factors–Congresses. 2. Young adults–Diseases–Congresses. I. Roskamm, H. (Helmut), 1933–. II. International Symposium on Myocardial Infarction at Young Age (1981: Bad Krozingen, Germany). III. European Society of Cardiology, IV. Pharma Schwarz Co. [DNLM: 1. Myocardial infarction – In adulthood–Congresses. WG 300 M99735 1981] RC685.I6M895 616.1'237 81–18309 AACR2.

Typesetting, printing and bookbinding: Konrad Triltsch, Graphischer Betrieb, Würzburg
2119/3130-543210

Preface

The papers presented in this book were held at the International Symposium on Myocardial Infarction at Young Age on January 30 and 31, 1981, in Bad Krozingen, FRG.

The symposium was sponsored and supported by the European Society of Cardiology and the Pharma Schwarz Co. The scientific committee was composed of H. Denolin (Bruxelles), F. Loogen (Düsseldorf), E. Nüssel (Heidelberg), J. Widimsky (Prague), M. Schmuziger (Bad Krozingen), and the editor of this book.

To all of these, as well as to my co-workers, many thanks.

Bad Krozingen, October 1981   H. ROSKAMM

Contents

Session 3
Pathology and Pathomechanisms I

Contents   IX

Contributors

You will find the addresses at the beginning of the respective contributions

Amor, M. 78
Balcon, R. 137
Barra, J. 215
Beaune, J. 115
Bergstrand, R. 23, 161
Bertrand, A. 78
Betz, P. 174
Biagini, A. 129
Blessey, R. 196
Blümchen, G. 137
Born, G. V. R. 155
Bourdon, J. L. 78
Breithardt, G. 166
Brodner, G. 187
Broustet, J. P. 108
Brunelli, C. 129
Buchholz, L. 13
Burkart, F. 56
Cabrol, C. 215
Cattell, M. 137
Cherrier, F. 78
Danchin, N. 78
Delahaye, J. P. 115
Delaye, J. 115
Diamond, P. S. 208
Droste, C. 61, 82
Engel, E. 122
Engel, H. J. 122
Farrel, P. W. 29
Fischer, M. 78
Fontaine, G. 215
Frank, R. 215
Gohlke, H. 61, 82
Gold, F. 143
Görnandt, L. 61
Gosse, R. 108
Guern, P. 108
Guiraudon, G. 215
Gunnar, R. M. 208

Gutzwiller, F. 17
Hahn, C. 201
Junod, B. 17
Kaindl, F. 148
Kaliman, J. 148
Karcher, G. 78
Kawalczyk, L. 208
L'Abbate, A. 129
Lamm, G. 5
Langosch, W. 187
Lichtlen, P. R. 122
Lim, Y. J. 47
Marzilli, M. 129
Maseri, A. 129
Mazzei, M. G. 129
McAllister, H. A. jr. 92
Michallik-Herbein, U. 187
Moret, P. 17
Müller, F. 174
Nikkilä, E. E. 38
Nüssel, E. 13
Pachinger, O. 148
Pavie, A. 215
Petersen, J. 82
Pic, A. 108
Pifarre, R. 208
Probst, P. 148
Radtke, H. J. 201
Razavi, M. 47
Rissanen, A. M. 38
Roberts, W. C. 104
Roskamm, H. 1, 61, 82, 174, 201
Rutsch, W. 156
Saliou, B. 108
Salzmann, C. 56
Samek, L. 82, 174
Sanmarco, M. 196
Scharf-Bornhofen, E. 137
Scheidt, R. 13

Introduction

H. ROSKAMM [1]

In preparing the program for this symposium, the following question arose: Is it really necessary to have a specific symposium on myocardial infarction at young age? Are the problems not the same as in older age groups? Our experience has taught us that young postinfarction patients represent a rather heterogeneous group of patients.

The following cases are typical examples of groups that show significant differences in coronary morphology:

1. The first group are patients with usually large infarctions in whom coronary angiography shows normal coronary arteries (Fig. 1). This is a rather frequent finding in young women who are heavy smokers and use oral contraceptives. The same constellation can be found in very young men, sometimes after unusally strenuous physical exercise. Spontaneous lysis of a thrombus is the most likely explanation, and spasm may play a role in triggering the thrombotic event.
2. The most frequent finding seems to be one-vessel disease, which is often a unilocular disease, i.e., one obstruction with the remaining vessels being angiographically normal (Fig. 2). In this category infarctions are also mostly large: Patients have no angina pectoris before or after their infarction. In this group a predominant thrombosis may be expected, and spasm can have been a triggering mechanism.
3. The third group are patients with multivessel disease (Fig. 3). This is, as we all know, the common situation in older age groups of postinfarction patients. In these cases, coronary arteriosclerosis is the most significant underlying process. Thrombosis may or may not play an important role in triggering myocardial infarction. If we had only this type of patient, a symposium specifically dealing with young patients would not be necessary.
4. In a small group of patients, very diffuse coronary arteriosclerosis can be found (Fig. 4). These patients usually have very significant risk factors, for example, hypercholesterolemia as a family disease, or severe hypertension.

What is the prognosis for patients with these different types of coronary morphology?

Do postinfarction patients with normal coronary arteries have an excellent prognosis as far as coronary artery disease is concerned?

In unilocular disease (one obstruction or stenosis with the remaining vessels being angiographically normal), we have learned that regression of the coronary angiographic finding is quite frequent, especially if the patients are very young

---

1 Rehabilitationszentrum, Südring 15, 7812 Bad Krozingen, FRG

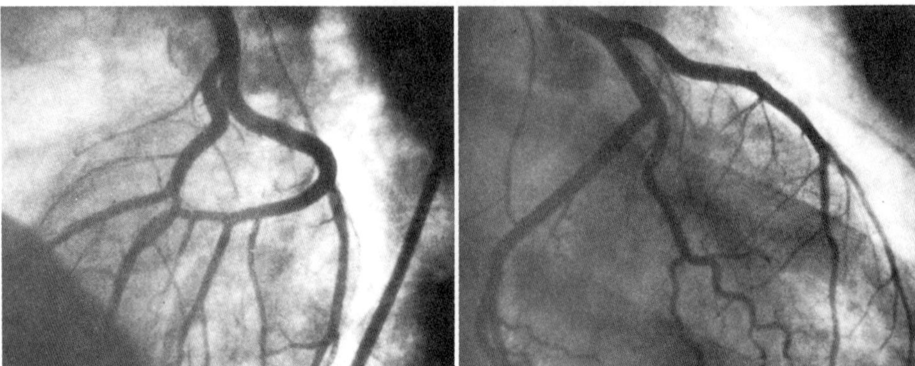

Fig. 1. Angiogram of the left coronary artery in LAO-hemiaxial and RAO position of a 22-year-old woman 2 months after having suffered a large anteroseptal infarction. The predominant left coronary artery and a rudimentary (not shown) right coronary artery were angiographically normal. The patient was a heavy smoker and used oral contraceptives. Lysis of the thrombus should be discussed

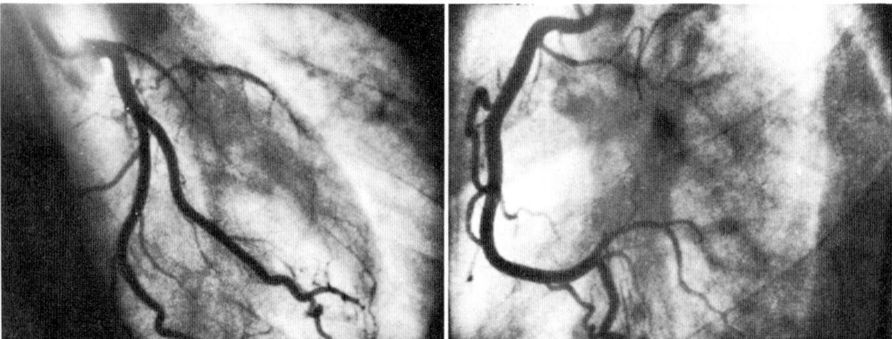

Fig. 2. Angiogram of the left coronary artery in RAO position and of the right coronary artery in LAO position of a 37-year-old man 3 months after having suffered a large anteroseptal infarction. The left anterior descending artery was found to be totally occluded and the remaining arteries were angiographically normal. This constellation is frequent in young patients. This patient had none of the accepted risk factors

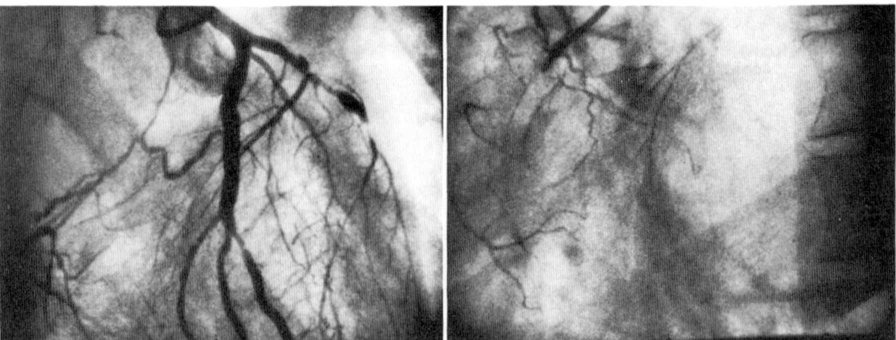

Fig. 3. Angiogram of the left coronary artery in RAO position and of the right coronary artery in LAO position of a 38-year-old man with an anteroseptal infarction. The LAD, which is the infarction-related vessel, is totally occluded. In addition, the right coronary artery is totally occluded and the circumflex artery shows a medium degree of stenosis. In young patients a multivessel disease constellation like this is far less common than in older patients

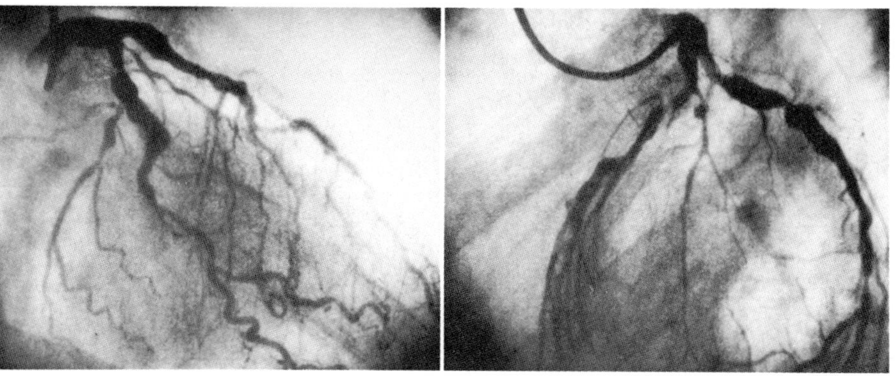

Fig. 4. Angiogram of the left coronary artery in RAO and LAO position of a 36-year-old man 2 months after an acute event with severe pain and elevation of serum enzymes. Left and right (not shown) coronary arteries show a diffuse type of coronary artery sclerosis. The patient had a risk factor constellation as follows: His father had died at age 48 years and his mother at age 58 years, both from myocardial infarction. There was also significant hypercholesterolemia, hyperuricemia, and hypertension present

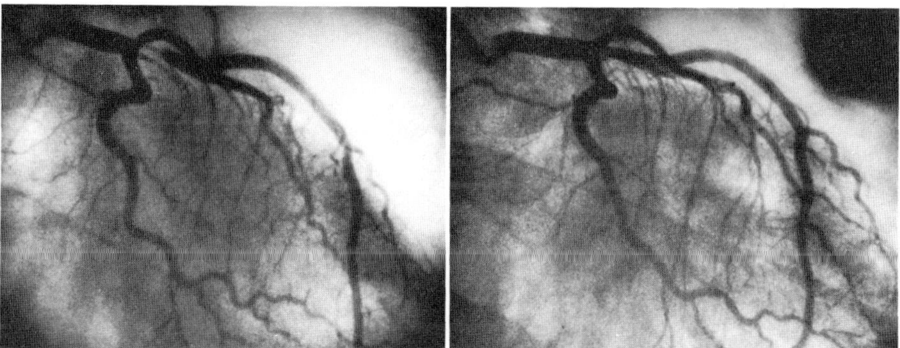

Fig. 5. Angiogram of the left coronary artery in RAO position 8 weeks (*left panel*) and 4 years (*right panel*) after anteroseptal infarction in a 39-year-old man. Both angiograms were performed after nitroglycerine. Regression of a 95%–99% stenosis to a 25%–50% stenosis is clearly seen. Here, recanalization and organization of a thrombus is the most likely explanation

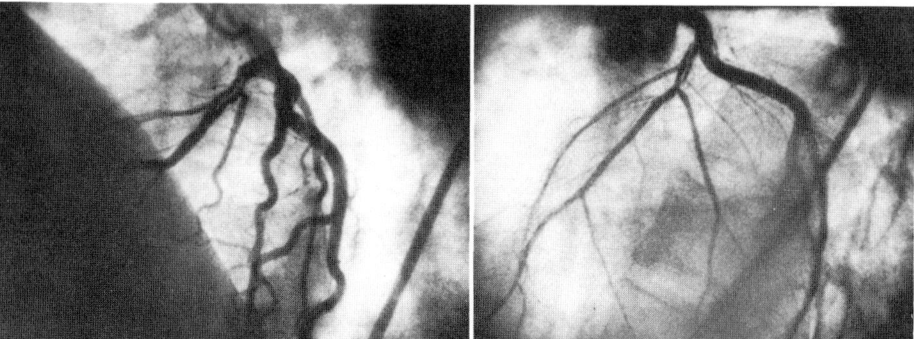

Fig. 6. Angiograms of the left coronary artery in LAO hemiaxial position of a 35-year-old man (*left panel*) and a 28-year-old woman (*right panel*) 3 months and 4 months, respectively, after anteroseptal myocardial infarction. In both patients, two streaks of contrast medium in the proximal left anterior descending artery are seen, indicating recanalization of a thrombus

(Fig. 5). The most likely explanation of this kind of regression is recanalization and organization of a thrombus.

If two streaks of contrast medium can be seen in the proximal part of the left anterior descending (LAD), as Fig. 6 shows for two patients, recanalization of a thrombus is obvious. Progression on the other hand seems to be very frequent in multilocular disease and, in that group of patients, regression is very rare.

What is the future of the ventricle, especially in those patients with very large scars, even if coronary morphology does not change?

What is the future of the overloaded residual myocardium? Is there a place for early scar-ectomy?

I think we all agree that the angiographic findings in patients with myocardial infarction at young age can be very variable. Does this mean that etiology and pathogenesis is totally different? Might there even be two different diseases: Predominantly coronary arteriosclerosis and predominant thrombosis without significant primary affection of the vessel wall possibly triggered by spasm.

I hope the studies presented at this symposium will provide a better understanding of myocardial infarction at young age, not at last because of the tremendous impact on the patient's family and the patient's own abilities and productivity.

The Epidemiology of Acute Myocardial Infarction in Young Age Groups

G. Lamm [1]

The steady increase of mortality due to coronary heart disease (CHD) in the 1940s and 1950s was followed by a declining trend in the United States, Australia, New Zealand, and several European countries since the late 1960s. During the period of increase, a menacing shift of coronary mortality towards younger age groups and a diminishing male/female ratio were also observed. These were slowly corroborated by clinical morbidity data, showing more and more frequently the occurrence of acute myocardial infarction (AMI) in young males and even females.

Now, when we are hopefully nearing the end of the tidal wave of the coronary epidemy, at least in some countries (but definitely not in many others), it would be of special interest lo learn how far these changes are affecting the younger age groups. One cannot simply assume that, in countries where CHD is still low, the trend will go upwards, and vice versa; This is true for all age groups. A glance at the mortality trends in Europe illustrates this (Table 1).

Table 1. Six top-ranking countries in male CHD mortality

All ages (1975)	35 – 44 years old (1975)	Increase 1968 – 1976 (35 – 44 years old)
Sweden	Northern Ireland	Poland
Scotland	Finland	Sweden
Denmark	Scotland	Hungary
England and Wales	Hungary	Denmark
Northern Ireland	Ireland	Ireland
Ireland	England and Wales	Northern Ireland

For the sake of brevity, the all-ages ranking, which to a large extent reflects the age composition of the population can be disregarded. From the countries with high mortality in the young age group (35–44 years old), Northern Ireland, Hungary, and Ireland also show a steep increase in the same age group (Table 1). Finland, Scotland, England and Wales, while in the high-mortality bracket, are not of high rank in 8-year increase (note the decrease in Finland), while medium-ranking Sweden and Denmark and low-ranking Poland belong to the six countries with the steepest mortality increase in this age group.

The fact that no easy prediction is at hand from age and sex-specific mortality figures is, among other things, an additional impetus to directly study the morbidity due to AMI in younger age groups.

---

1 Regional Officer for Chronic Diseases, World Health Organization, 8, Scherfigsvej, DK-2100 Kopenhagen, Denmark

Background

The three best indices of the spread and evolution of a disease are prevalence, incidence, and mortality: Only the latter is available for analysis in CHD among the young. Cross-sectional (prevalence) and prospective (incidence) epidemiological studies almost exclusively focus on the age group of 40–65 years because of numbers. The relatively low prevalence and incidence below 40 years old would dictate sample sizes too large for study, and this was felt impracticable in most cases. Thus, scrutiny of the published epidemiological studies leaves us with practically no clue to the incidence and time trends of CHD in the young.

As a compromise, one must be satisfied with morbidity data on AMI, although even these are scanty. The fact that the so-called apparent morbidity is always lower than the true incidence (as subclinical and silent cases are, by definition, missed) is the lesser evil. The impossibility of relating premorbidity characteristics to events is the major drawback. We are left in the dark as to the problem of risk factors for AMI in the young: Are they the same as for the older age groups and, if yes, do they have the same, lesser, or stronger influence? Well-conducted case-control studies might shed some light on the problems, but no attempt will be made here to go into this kind of epidemiological analysis. We will simply review available morbidity data on AMI in the young from the last 10 years. Conforming with the definition of this symposium, "young" are men below 40 and women below 50 years of age.

Material Reviewed

The richest source of information on the morbidity of AMI in Europe is still the WHO AMI Community Register Study from 1971 [1]. In 16 centers covering a total population of approximately 3 million, 10 121 AMI cases were rigorously registered and followed up for 1 year. The lowest age limit of registration was 20 years and the highest was 64 years in both sexes. Morbidity (attack rates) were presented in 5-year age- and sex-specific groups and for the whole sample (20–64 years old) for males and females. Various diagnostic categories were used in this study but, for the present analysis, AMI is defined as the sum of definite and possible myocardial infarction. For details of the definition, we refer to the original publication [1].

Some of the 16 AMI Registers continued their activity after the official termination of the WHO study, and a few up to the present. These still-active centers, together with some newly established ones, have been approached by the author, requesting their most recent available data on the "young" to establish some time trends. I am greatly indebted to all the directors of these centres for their invaluable contributions.

Finally, published material was screened for any possible information related to the morbidity due to AMI in the young. The list of reviewed papers [2–8] is conspicuously short. The explanation of this is easy: Although many more papers dealt with the problem of AMI in the last decade, only very few contained sufficient information on the population sampled or studied, to allow calculation of age- und sex-specific morbidity rates. In the majority of papers there is no description of the population from which the patients are derived, of diagnostic criteria, period of sampling, etc. Use of available data is further restricted by discrepancies in data presentation: some papers do not separate male and female morbidity; in others 10-year age groups are used starting at 25 years, etc. It is extremely rare to find tables where, in addition to rate, number of cases, and the relevant denominators (i.e., number of population in the corresponding age-sex bracket) are indicated.

These were factors limiting the number of utilizable information sources. Caution should, however, be expressed as to the quality of data as well. Although it was attempted to always use broadly similar data for any comparison, strictly standard criteria could not be applied to the sampling, the diagnostic criteria, or the validity of the data in general. The broad general conclusions made here seem to be permissible even within these limitations.

Findings

AMI Community Register Study (1971)

There is fortunately a great deal of information published on young ages in this study. The main findings are presented in Table 2 for males and Table 3 for females. In men, the range between the lowest center (Sofia) and the highest (Helsinki) is from 1.4–7.3/1000 in the age group 20–64 years, while for the young it is 0.1–0.6/1000. In women the corresponding ranges are from 0.2 (Sofia) to 1.6 (Helsinki), while in the young it is from 0.04 (Sofia) to 0.45 (London). For the sake of comparison, the data on the subgroup of young women in the age group 20–39 are also included in Table 3. The range here extends from 0.0 to 0.1/1000.

Table 4 gives a simplified overview of the concordance in geographical distribution of AMI between all ages up to 64 years and the young in males. The range within each category was arbitrarily divided into low, medium, and high subclasses. Centers which fall under different subclasses from one age category to another are indicated in the respective brackets. All others maintaining their subgroup are omitted; e.g., Sofia ranks in the low subgroup in the 20–64-year age category, but in the medium one in the young category.

Table 2. Ranking of AMI Community Registers for 1971 (15 Centers): males (incidence/1000/year)

Age (years)					
20–64 (range 1.4–7.3)	< 2.0 Bucharest, Erfurt, Sofia	< 3.0 Göteborg, Berlin, Budapest, Lublin, Heidelberg, Innsbruck, Kaunas, Pasewalk	< 4.0 Prague, Warsaw, Tel Aviv	< 5.0 Dublin, London, Nijmegen	< 8.0 Helsinki, Tampere
20–39 (range 0.1–0.6)	< 0.1 Göteborg, Bucharest, Erfurt	< 0.2 Tampere, Innsbruck, Sofia, Tel Aviv, Berlin, Lublin	< 0.3 Prague, Budapest, Heidelberg, Warsaw, Nijmegen, Kaunas, Pasewalk	< 0.4 Dublin, Helsinki	< 0.6 London

Table 3. Ranking of AMI Community Registers for 1971 (15 Centers): females (incidence/1000/year)

Age (years)					
20 – 64 (range 0.2 – 1.6)	0.5 Erfurt, Heidelberg, Lublin, Innsbruck, Kaunas, Sofia, Pasewalk	0.7 Göteborg, Prague	0.9 Warsaw, Berlin, Budapest	1.2 London, Nijmegen, Tampere	1.6 Dublin, Helsinki, Tel Aviv
20 – 49 (range 0.04 – 0.45)	0.1 Sofia, Innsbruck, Heidelberg	0.2 Göteborg, Prague Bucharest, Tampere, Lublin	0.3 Budapest, Nijmegen, Warsaw	0.4 Helsinki	0.5 Dublin London
20 – 39 (range 0.01 – 0.1)	0.01 Prague, Tampere, Sofia, Kaunas, Pasewalk, Berlin	0.02	0.03 Göteborg, Dublin, Warsaw, London, Lublin, Tel Aviv, Erfurt	0.04 Innsbruck	0.1 Budapest, Helsinki, Nijmegen

Table 4. AMI Community Registers for 1971: concordance of geographical distribution in young males (incidence/1000/year). Four centers of 19 fall under a different category in the "young" age group (three decrease, one increases)

Age group (years)	Incidence		
	Low	Medium	High
20 – 64	< 2.0 Sofia	2.0 – 3.9 Göteborg	4.0 – 7.3 Nijmegen, Tampere
20 – 39	0.1 Göteborg	0.2 – 0.3 Nijmegen, Tampere, Sofia	0.4 – 0.6

Only four centers of 19 change their relative position in the young category; three of them shift to a lower subgroup (Nijmegen, Tampere, and Göteborg) and one (Sofia) to a higher. Table 5 shows the same concordance along similar lines for females. It is easy to see that, moving to increasingly younger age groups, the number of centers shifting from one subgroup to another increases. In contrast to men, where the shift was always to one of the near subgroups (e.g., from high to medium), in women there is often a jump over a subgroup (e.g., from high to low). All these are probably due to the very low number of observed cases in these age groups. One might, therefore, state that there is no conspicuous difference in the geographical distribution of AMI incidence in young males compared to the usually published data on the age group of 20–64 years. In relation to women, not even such a cautious statement can be made. It is probable, however, that the wide variation in women is due to very low numbers.

It is of interest to look at the age gradient of AMI incidence in both sexes: The age group 20–39 years was compared with that of 50–54 years for this purpose. In men the incidence is approximately 25-times higher in the latter group, thus the gradient is very steep. In women this gradient is smaller (around 15), though the scatter around this mean for all centers is much larger.

Table 5. AMI Community Registers for 1971: concordance of geographical distribution in young females (incidence/1000/year). The younger the age group considered, the larger the difference in distribution of young women

Age group (years)	Incidence			
	Low	Medium	High	Number of Shifted centers
20 – 64	0.2 – 0.5	0.6 – 0.9	1.0 – 1.6	
45 – 49	<0.6	0.7 – 1.1	1.2 – 1.8	4 ↓ 1 ↑
40 – 44	0 – 0.1	0.2 – 0.3	0.4 – 1.1	3 ↓ 5 ↑
20 39	0 0 – 0.02	0.03 – 0.04	0.1	6 ↓ 4 ↑

When we are working in the clinic we usually do not think in terms of rates, but in proportions. We have an interest in, and an impression of what proportion of our AMI patients are young. Analyzing the AMI Register data from this aspect, one finds that roughly 5% of males and 16% of females qualify as "young" of the total number of AMI patients up to age 65 years. The "true" proportion of young cases among all our AMI patients will be still lower, since approximately the same total number of infarctions occur above the age 65 as below in a given population.

Incidence of AMI in the Young (1972–1980)

As mentioned earlier, sources of these data were partly personal communications from some of the still active registers, and partly published papers.

The empty boxes in the tables reflect the discrepancies in data presentation. Table 6 for males shows that the range of incidence in the "young" is practically the same as in the AMI Register study (Table 2). The single exception is North Karelia with an incidence of 0.9/1000, but this is hardly surprising. The wide variation within Finland might need some comment, but again the low number of events in any single center, taking the denominator (the size of population followed) also into account, makes interpretation hazardous. Table 7 presents the same for women.

Table 6. Incidence of AMI/1000/Year in young males (1972 – 1980)

	Age group (years)				
	20 – 24	25 – 29	30 – 34	35 – 39	20 – 39
France					0.10
Kaunas		0.2	0.6	1.1	
North Karelia	0.19		0.9	1.4	0.9
Helsinki					0.46
Turku					0.26
Tampere					0.25
Finland					0.47
Göteborg			0.08	0.3	
London		0.4			
Edinburgh					0.6
Denmark					0.2
Budapest			0.3	1.3	0.4
Oslo			0.3	0.6	

Again, there seems to be no difference in the range from the AMI Register study. The scarcity of data for the hole young (20–49 years) group is conspicuous, and explained by the same reasons as above. Even the three indicated figures (last column) might be biased, as it was impossible to establish whether calculations were based on the whole population in that age group or only those 25–49 years old, or even on age groups where events were found at all. Exceptions to this limitation are the data from Budapest, as indicated. This bias might be small in centers with small populations becoming larger with increasing population size. The last row in both Tables 6 and 7 gives the available figures from the classical study of Westlund from Oslo in 1965 [8]. This is used partly as a reference and partly as a broad indicator, but def-

Table 7. Incidence/1000/year in young (< 50 years) females (1972 – 1980)

	Age group (years)					
	25 – 29	30 – 34	35 – 39	40 – 44	45 – 49	25 – 49
France						0.06
Kaunas		0.07	0.07	0.2	0.4	
North Karelia		0.3	0.3	0.9	1.6	0.4
Helsinki		0.07		0.4	1.6	
Turku		0.00		0.0	0.6	
Tampere		0.00		0.0	0.4	
Finland		0.04		0.3	1.2	
Göteborg		0.00		0.08	0.3	
London		0.00	0.4			
Edinburgh		0.14		1.41		
Budapest		0.1	0.2	0.8	0.8	0.3[a]
Oslo		0.04	0.07	0.17	0.35	

[a] 25 – 49 years

initely not a basis for comparison. The methodological, geographical, and time differences are too large to allow this. A very cautious statement might be attempted, however, by saying that rates seem to have increased a bit in the last 10 years and perhaps more so in women than in men.

The question whether incidence in the young has changed in the last 10 years can be answered with some confidence only by relying on centers where registration was going on continuously, in the same population, and with the same methods and criteria. Information was received only from six such centers and their experience is condensed in Table 8. An upward trend is observed in centers with low and medium

Table 8. Local time trends

Trend	Males	Females
↑	Montpellier, Rouen, Kaunas, Budapest	Kaunas
=	Copenhagen	Budapest, Montpellier, Rouen, Copenhagen
↓	North Karelia	North Karelia

levels of incidence, while in North Karelia, where the level was the highest (at least in men), there is a decline. It is also noteworthy that data on males and females tend to behave similarly in this respect. There are, however, to few centers analyzed here to allow generalization from these findings.

In turning from epidemiological facts to their meaning as they affect clinical practice, as shown earlier, about 4% of all AMI cases will occur in the young. Transforming age- and sex-specific incidence rates into frequency of AMI in a whole population, one has to know not only these rates, but also the age structure of the population. Using gross average rates and a mean standard population one can calculate that in a city like New York or a country like Hungary (populations approximately 10 million), around 900 "young" people will suffer from AMI in 1 year. An average general practitioner serves roughly 3000 persons in Europe. On the grounds of the AMI Register data, he/she is likely to have about 15 AMI cases in a year, though he/she will not necessarily "see" them all, as a fair proportion will die before reaching medical assistance. The same general practitioner, in contrast, will meet a "young" AMI only every third year. Using the WHO recommendations for the establishment of coronary care units (CCU) [2] (and assuming that this is evenly applied throughout Europe), one can also make assumptions on the load of "young" AMI patients on these units. Taking ten beds for a population of 250 000 one arrives at a figure of approximately 20 "young" patients admitted yearly to an average CCU of eight to ten beds.

Of course, these practical examples are merely gross generalizations, and a general practitioner with cardiological interests and reputation will have many more cases. Similarly, some one working in a CCU in a specialized hospital may feel that this indicative figure is unacceptably low. In spite of these limitations, such examples help to put the problem in the proper perspective.

Summary

1. Data on AMI in the young are scarce and poorly presented (i.e., age brackets, denominators, etc.).
2. Existing evidence does not hint at a different geographical distribution in young AMI patients compared to older cases.
3. Clinical studies of the special features of AMI in the young promise to be more rewarding.
4. Such studies can efficiently be undertaken only in big centers, so as to allow sufficient number of cases.
5. The two main questions, whether AMI in the young is on the increase and whether it is influenced in the same way and by the same risk factors, remain unanswered.
6. More knowledge can be gathered only by concentrated international studies with standardized protocols.

Acknowledgments. Appreciation is expressed to the following Register Directors for their kind assistance: J. N. Bloozhas (Kaunas), F. Dienstl (Innsbruck), I. Gyarfas (Budapest), O. Horwitz (Copenhagen), P. Puska (North Karelia), and J. L. Richard (French Registers).

References

1. World Health Organization (1976) AMI Community Registers. Public Health in Europe, No. 5, Copenhagen
2. Armstrong A, Duncan B, Oliver MF et al. (1972) Natural history of acute coronary heart attacks: A community study. Br Heart 34:67–80
3. Puska P, Mustaneimi H (1975) Incidence and presentation of myocardial infarction in North Karelia, Finland. Acta Med Scand 197:211–216
4. Pohjola S, Siltanen P, Romo M et al. (1980) Duodecim 96:18–31
5. Elmfeldt D, Wilhelmsen L, Tibblin G et al. (1975) J Chronic Dis 28:173–186
6. Tunstall-Pedoe H (1977) Dissertation, University of London
7. Bergstrand L (1980) Dissertation, University of Gothenburg
8. Westlund K (1965) Further observations on the indidence of myocardial infarction in Oslo. Oslo City Hosp 15:201–231

Myocardial Infarction in Young Men in the Heidelberg Register Area

E. NÜSSEL, L. BUCHHOLZ, and R. SCHEIDT[1]

According to the data collected during 1971 in the Heidelberg myocardial infarction (MI) register area, MI in young people amounts to 7% in men and 14% in women below the age of less than 65 years. Within the last 10 years, we have closely observed 126 young men with MI for at least 2-year period.

From these 126 patients, 73% were residents of the register area, and 27% received medical treatment because they suffered from an acute infarction during a short stay in the register area. We call these patients "visitors". There was no appreciable difference between the residents and the visitors as far as the survival rate and the incidence of risk factors are concerned. This backs the hypothesis that our young MI patients living in the register area are representative of large parts of the Federal Republic of Germany. We will report results of the residents and vistors as a whole.

One hour after the onset of an acute infarction 90% of the patients were alive, after 8 and 24 h this number dropped to 82%.

From days 2 to 5 after the onset of infarction, another 3% of the patients died. No patients died from day 5 to day 28 after the onset of infarction. After 6 months the survival rate was 78%, after 12 months it was 75%, and after 24 months 74% (Fig. 1). Therefore, 26% of the patients having suffered from MI died within the course of 2 years.

We were able to watch 44 patients closely for 8 years. From these, 61% were still alive after this time (Fig. 2).

Risk Factors. Of the 126 young patients with MI, 3% showed none of the seven classical risk factors of coronary heart disease, and if the factor overweight is not included, 6% of patients show no risk factors at all. Of the 126 MI patients, we have compared the 30–40-year-olds with patients of the same age group out of a total investigation of 30–40-year-old men of two provincial towns. In Fig. 3 the left column refers to men with MI, the right column to a control group of the same age, i.e., men without MI out of the normal population of both provincial towns. Of the persons in the MI group, 45% were overweight, while the same applied to 21% in the control group.

In the MI group 74% were smokers and, in the control group this rate was 44%. There was no appreciable difference as to the rate of ex-smokers. Hypertension in the MI group was found in 20% and, in the control group, in 13%. Hypercholesterinemia in the MI group amounted to 63%, in the control group to 17%. Hypertriglyceridemia in the MI group was at 56%, compared to the control group with 17%. Hyperuricemia in the MI group was at 29%, compared to 6% for the control group.

1 Klinikum der Universität Heidelberg, Klinische Sozialmedizin, Bergheimer Straße 58, 6900 Heidelberg, FRG

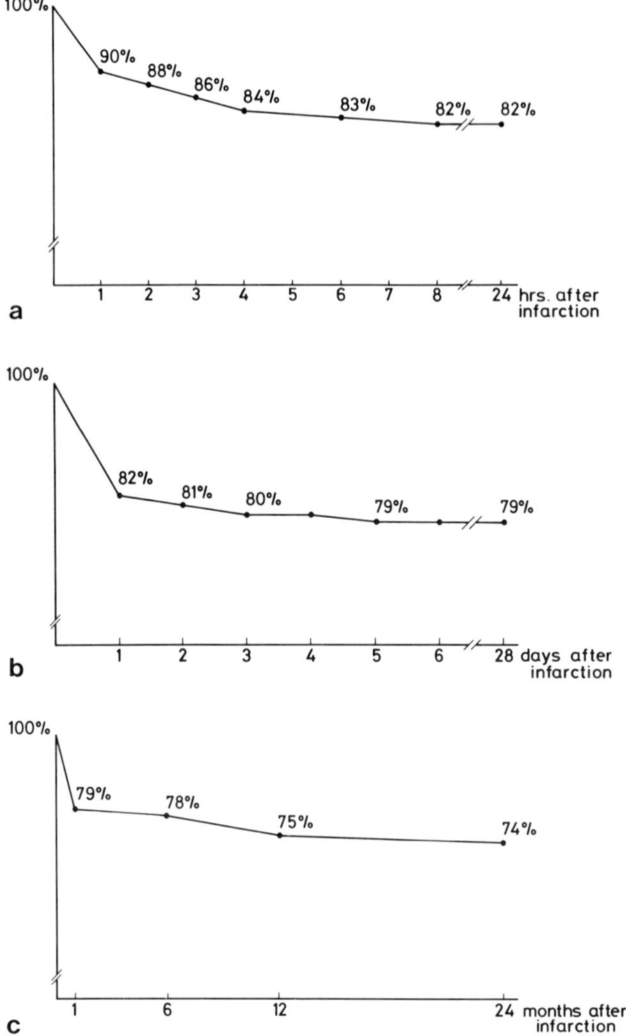

Fig. 1a–c. Survival rate after MI among men ($N = 126$) 40 years old or less at **a** 1–24 h, **b** 1–28 days and **c** 1–24 months after MI. WHO Project, Heidelberg, January 81. (After E. Nüssel)

Diabetes, with 10% in the MI group, was found in 3% persons in the control group. Of the MI group, 3% showed none of these seven risk factors, while the control group showed tenfold this figure (Fig. 4). Sixty-four percent of MI patients and 8% of the control group showed three risk factors or more. Upon comparison of the MI and control group, the MI group shows three and more risk factors eight-fold more frequently.

From individual histories we found, that 37% of the young men with MI had suffered angina pectoris, and 73% of these did not give up smoking, in spite of the pains they had to endure, until they were finally afflicted with MI. The percentage

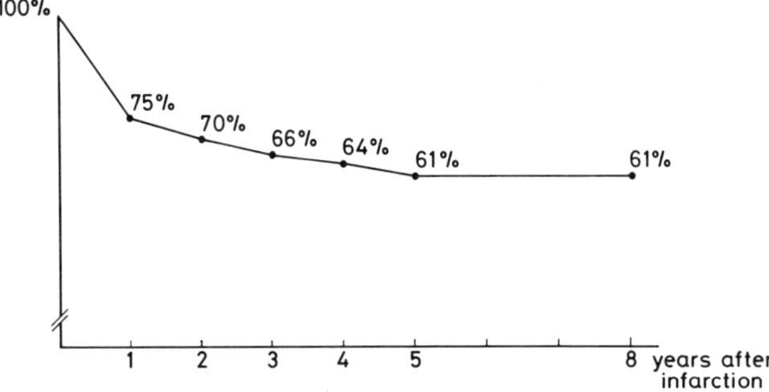

Fig. 2. Survival rate after MI among men ($N=44$) 40 years old or less at 1–8 years after MI. WHO Project, Heidelberg, January 81. (After E. Nüssel)

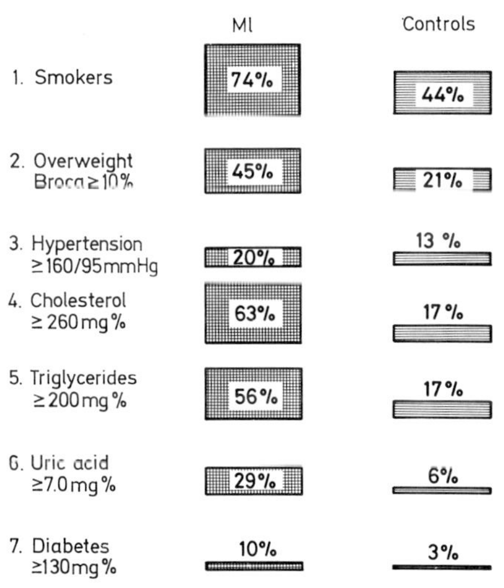

Fig. 3. Risk factors and MI among men 30–40 years of age. N (MI, controls) = *1*, 107/95; *2*, 103/95; *3*, 99/95; *4*, 100/190; *5*, 99/95; *6*, 94/95; *7*, 107/95. WHO Project, Heidelberg, January 81. (After E. Nüssel)

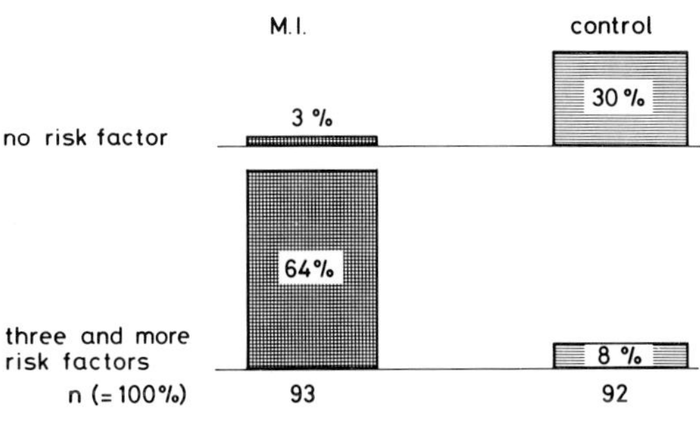

Fig. 4. Summarized risk factors among men 30–40 years old in the MI ($N=93$) and control ($N=92$) groups. WHO Project, Heidelberg, January 81. (After E. Nüssel)

of smokers among patients with no history of angina pectoris is 75%. After having survived the acute MI, about 50% of the patients started smoking again, and 46% showed a Broca index of more than 10%.

The results for young women with MI are very similar.

In summary, the reduction of the classical risk factors of coronary heart disease form an essential part of primary and secondary prevention.

According to the data collected in the Heidelberg Register during 1970 to 1971, about 3000 young male and 1500 young female patients with MI per year are to be expected in the Federal Republic of Germany. These figures emphasize the importance of prevention.

Coronary Artery Disease in Young Adults
Under 35 Years Old:
Risk Factors (Swiss Survey)

P. Moret[1], F. Gutzwiller[2], and B. Junod[2]

The importance of the most common risk factors in patients under 35 years old, who have had clinical syndromes of ischemic heart disease, such as angina pectoris and/or myocardial infarction (MI) and/or intermediary syndrome, and in whom coronary angiography has been performed, has been reviewed in a retrospective study made under the auspices of the Swiss Cardiac Society (SCS). The results of this survey are compared with those of a national control population study (PNR) carried out in four cities in Switzerland (Nyon, Vevey, Aarau, Soluthurn) on a population of about the same age group (25–40 years).

In this paper, we first compare the prevalence of risk factors in the two groups (SCS and PNR). We then analyzed in the SCS group the correlations between the risk factors and the importance of coronary lesions and the long-term prognosis.

Patients and Methods

For the SCS group with ischemic heart disease, the clinical data with the hemodynamic investigations including coronary angiography and ventriculography were collected by a questionnaire from the university centers (Basel, Bern, Geneva, Lausanne, and Zurich) and a few cases from Lugano. Postcoronarographic medical history was obtained directly from the patient or from the physician. The retrospective study dates, for Zurich, to 1965, and to 1970 for the other centers. A sample of 185 patients (174 men and 11 woman; 94% and 6%, respectively) was collected. Among these patients, 118 were married, 38 single, 9 divorced, and 20 were of unknown marital status; 57 (7%) were blue-collar workers, 82 (44%) white-collar workers, and 13 (7%) were self-employed. These figures do not differ from the general population distribution. It should be noted that in this retrospective survey, the patients who died before or during hospitalization were not included in this study.

The PNR control population study carried out in four different cities includes 1078 men and 1102 woman of the age group 25–40 years.

The exposure to risk factors was defined as follows: cigarettes (cig) smoking habits of more than 8 cig/day in the PNR study and more than 10 cig/day in the SCS study; hyperlipidemia (including hypercholesterolemia and/or hypertriglyceridemia) values well above those of normal subjects for each center, usually cholesterol of more than 250 mg/100 ml; hypertension values of more than 160/95 mmHg;

---

1 Center of Cardiology, Hôpital Cantonal Universitaire, Geneva, Switzerland
2 Project-Director of the Swiss National Research Program Study Group (PNR)

overweight as indicated by Broca index over 15%; and family history of systemic hypertension (HTA), of MI, or cerebrovascular accident (CVA) in first-degree relatives.

Results

The prevalence of risk factors in the two groups (SCS group with ischemic heart diesease and PNR control population group) are reported in Table 1. Differences between SCS and PNR groups are striking. Cigarette smoking is the first and the most important risk factor, followed by obesity, hyperlipidemia (especially hypercholesterolemia), and family history. It should be noted that the prevalence of CVA was higher in the PNR control than in the SCS group. Hypertension, in spite of the fact that it is less frequent than in the 20–40-year age group, was encountered more often in the SCS than in the PNR group. No values are yet available for exercise, diabetes, uric acid, or for use of oral contraceptives in the PNR group. For the 11 women in the SCS survey, 64% were taking oral contraceptives. All female patients except one were also smokers.

In Fig. 1, we compared exposure to no risk factor, or to one, two, and three main or major factors (e.g., cigarette smoking, hypercholesterolemia, hypertension) in the PNR study and the SCS survey, but included only the patients with MI (139 men and 10 women). The differences between the two groups are evident. In the group of men there are only 10% of 139 patients who have none of the three main risk factors, compared to 44.9% in the PNR study, and 38.8% had two risk factors in the

Table 1. Prevalence of various risk factors in the SCS group (185 patients with ischemic heart disease) and the PNR group (control population study). Values taken from Stähelin (1976)

	SCS ($\leqq$ 35 years)	PNR (20 – 40 years)
Cigarette smoking	78.5%	47% ***
Hyperlipidemia	41.0%	
Hypercholesterolemia	34.6%	12% ***
Hypertension (HTA)	13.5%	5% ***
Family history		
Infarction (INF)	30.3%	16% ***
CVA	4%	12% **
INF + CVA + HTA	38.0%	
Obesity	52.9%	30% ***
Diabetes	9.2%	
Uric acid	7.6%	
Exercise		
None	21.1%	
Regularly	26.5%	
Contraceptives (11 women)	63.6%	

** $P < 0.01$ *** $P < 0.001$

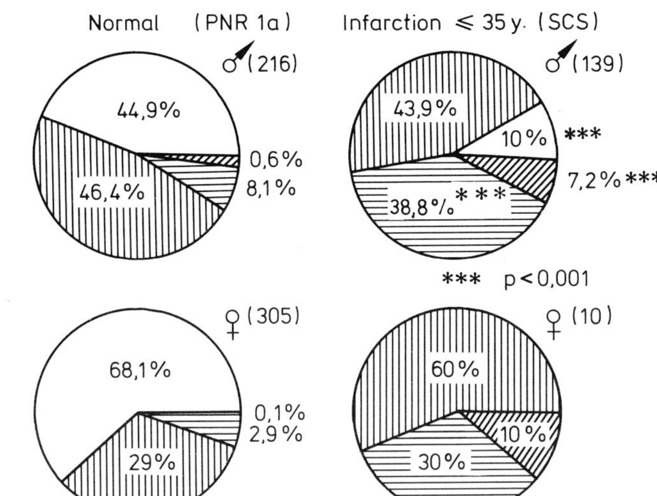

Fig. 1. Exposure to none, one, two, and three risk factors (tobacco, cholesterol, and hypertension) in the SCS group of 139 males and 10 females with MI and in the PNR group (control population study) of 216 males and 305 females

SCS survey, compared to only 8.1% in the PNR study. Only 0.6% had three risk factors in the PNR group, against 7.2% in the SCS group. Differences are also obvious in the women. No statistical analysis has been made, the SCS group being too small (only 10 women).

The relationships between risk factors and coronary lesions are reported in Tables 2 und 3. We considered only the 139 men with infarction, the group of women being too small. At the time of the coronary angiography 24 patients (17.2%) had normal coronary vessels or stenosis of less than 50%, and 115 (82.8%) had definite coronary lesions. As can be seen on the left side of Table 2, the prevalence of the various risk factors is almost identical among the groups with normal or abnormal vessels. Statistical differences are present only for hyperlipidemia. On the right side of Table 2 are the numbers of risk factors per patient (RF/P). If only the first three risk factors are considered (cigarette smoking, hyperlipidemia, and hypertension), there is no difference between the groups with normal coronary vessels and abnormal ones (1.08 RF/P with normal vessels and 1.42 RF/P with abnormal vessels). If the first five risk factors listed on Table 2 are taken into account together, the differences become statistical significant; 1.12 RF/P with normal vessels and 1.63 RF/P ($P < 0.05$) with abnormal vessels. The differences become more significant if six or all risk factors are considered.

Among the 115 male patients with infarction and definite coronary lesions, 72 (62.6%) had one-vessel disease, 27 (23.5%) had two-vessel disease, and 16 (13.9%)

Table 2. Relation between various risk factors and coronary lesions in 139 male patients with MI: Normal and abnormal vessels

	Normal vessels	Abnormal vessels	No. risk factors per patient				
Tobacco (> 10 cig/day)	75.0%	80.8%	1.08				
Hyperlipidemia	29.2%	49.6%	1.42				
Hypertension	25.0%	31.3%		1.12			
Diabetes	0%	10.0%		1.63 *			
Hyperuricemia	4.2%	7.8%			1.37		
					2.31 ***		
Family history	25.0%	42.5%				1.95	
						2.85 **	
Obesity	58.3%	55.6%					
No. patients	24	115					
Age (years)	30.4	31.8					

* $P < 0.05$ ** $P < 0.01$ *** $P < 0.001$

had three-vessel disease. As shown in Table 3, hyperlipidemia, hypertension, and hyperuricemia are more frequent in the group of patients with three-vessel disease. If one considers, as for Table 2, the number of risk factors per patient, there is a striking difference between the two groups of patients whatever the number of risk factors taken into consideration. There are, for instance, 2.5 risk factors per patient for the patients with three-vessel disease against 1.3 ($P < 0.001$) for the patients with one-vessel disease if smoking habits, hyperlipidemia, and hypertension are considered.

The long-term prognosis of 139 men who had an infarction has been analyzed regarding the presence or absence of risk factors prior to the infarction. During the follow-up period after the infarction, 53 (38.1%) patients had neither angina pectoris

Table 3. Relation between various risk factors and coronary lesions in 115 male patients with MI: One- and three-vessel disease

	One vessel	Three vessels	No. risk factors per patient				
Tobacco (> 10 cig/day)	80.5%	87.0%	1.3				
Hyperlipidemia	38.9%	93.7% ***	2.5 ***				
Hypertension	8.3%	25.0% *		1.4			
Diabetes	6.9%	12.5%		3.0 ***			
Hyperuricemia	5.5%	25.0% **			1.8		
					2.9 ***		
Family history	44.0%	56.0%				2.3	
						3.5 **	
Obesity	51.0%	62.5%					
No. patients	72	16					

* $P < 0.05$ ** $P < 0.01$ *** $P < 0.001$

Table 4. Relation between various risk factors and long-term prognosis in 139 male patients with MI: 53 patients without postinfarction angina or recurrent infarction and 59 patients with either postinfarction angina or recurrent infarction

	No angina or recurrent infarction	With angina or recurrent infarction	No. risk factors per patient
Tobacco (> 10 cig/day)	77.3%	78.5%	1.26
Hyperlipidemia	37.7%	61.3% **	2.0 *
Hypertension	11.0%	13.4%	1.39
Diabetes	9.9%	11.2%	2.25 *
Hyperuricemia	3.7%	8.3% *	1.79
			2.75 *
Family history	39.0%	41.0%	2.13
			3.37 ***
Obesity	58.9%	56.8%	
No. patients	53	59	

* *P* < 0.05   ** *P* < 0.01   *** *P* < 0.001

Table 5. Relation between various risk factors in 139 male patients with MI: 53 patients without postinfarction angina or recurrence of infarction and 14 patients who died after hospital discharge (1 – 12 years)

	No angina or recurrent infarction	Patients died	No. risk factors per patient
Tobacco (> 10 cig/day)	77.3%	57.0%	1.26 NS
Hyperlipidemia	37.7%	42.8%	1.35
Hypertension	11.0%	14.2%	1.39 NS
Diabetes	9.9%	0%	1.57
Hyperuricemia	3.7%	21.4%	1.79 NS
			1.92
Family history	39.0%	35.7%	2.13 NS
			2.28
Obesity	58.9%	35.7%	
No. patients	53	14	

nor recurrence of infarction, 47 (33.8%) had residual or recurrence of angina pectoris, and 12 (8.6%) had a recurrence of infarction (Table 4). Eight had both angina and recurrent infarction. Hyperlipidemia and hyperuricemia were more frequent in the group of 59 patients with postinfarction complications. The number of risk factors per patient was also greater than in the group without complications.

Of 139 men with infarction, 14 (10%) patients died during the follow-up period. As seen in Table 5, there are no differences between this group of 14 patients and the group of 53 patients who had no complications after their infarction: No difference in the prevalence of the various risk factors or in the number of RF/P.

Summary

During a period of about 10 years, 185 patients under 35 years of age with clinical syndromes of ischemic heart disease, in whom coronary angiography had been performed, have been studied in Switzerland. From this retrospective study, it clearly appears that the risk factors cigarette smoking, hyperlipidemia, hypercholesterolemia, obesity, hypertension, and family history are more frequent in this patient group than in a control population group of same age. Diabetes, hyperuricemia, and physical exercise were also factors present in the group with ischemic heart disease, but values for the control population are not yet available. Of patients with MI, 17% had normal coronary vessels or a stenosis of less than 50%. Patients with infarction and severe coronary disease (three-vessel disease) have a higher prevalence of hyperlipidemia, hypertension, and hyperuricemia, and greater number of RF/P (over 2.5). Patients with postinfarction complications (angina 34%, recurrent infarction 9%) have higher prevalence of hyperlipidemia and hyperuricemia, and a greater number of RF/P (over 2.25). Ten percent of patients with MI died during the follow-up period. There was no difference in the prevalence of the various risk factors or in the number of risk factors per patient with the survivors who had no complication, angina, or recurrent infarction.

In summary, it can be said that in young adults under 35 years with ischemic heart disease, the most common risk factors are cigarette smoking of more than 10 cig/ day (80%), followed by obesity (53%), hyperlipidemia (41%), and family history of MI, hypertension, or CVA (38%). Twenty-one percent of patients had low physical exercise. The prevalence of hypertension, diabetes, and uric acid was low, respectively 13%, 9%, and 8%. Of women, 64% were taking oral contraceptives. Patients who had more than three risk factors, including abuse of tobacco, hypercholesterolemia, have a high probability for severe coronary disease and poor long-term prognosis with higher risk of having postinfarction angina or recurrence of infarction.

This study suggests that the pathogeny of infarction at young age (less than 35 years) is probably different than in the older age group. Tobacco may be responsible for the primary lesion of coronary vessels with formation of thrombi, sometimes occluding the artery and secondary lysis leaving a normal or "normalized" vessel. The passage of time and lipid disturbances, associated with other risk factors, lead to formation of arteriosclerotic plaques and severe stenosis.

Acknowledgements. We are very grateful to the Swiss National Research Program 1A Study Group (PNR), especially to Prof. W. Schweizer, Basel (director of the program), and to Prof. F. H. Epstein, Zurich (Scientific Expert of the program).

Reference

Stähelin HB (1976) Epidemiologie der Adipositas. Ther Umsch 33:717–722

Myocardial Infarction Among Men Below Age 40 in Göteborg

R. Bergstrand, A. Vedin, C. Wilhelmsson, and L. Wilhelmsen [1]

From January 1, 1968, and onwards, all cases of acute myocardial infarction (MI) occurring in the population of Göteborg in certain age groups have been registered in the special Infarction Register. This register comprises more than 90% of all diagnosed cases of MI in this city. All survivors have been systematically cared for after the acute phase of the infarction at a special post MI clinic. During follow-up, deaths and reinfarctions were registered in the Infarction Register (Elmfeldt et al., 1975 a, b).

The purpose of the present study was to define incidence and prognosis as well as to describe socioeconomic and risk factor patterns among men with MI below age 40 in a demographically and geographically defined area.

Materials and Methods

Incidence figures were calculated on all cases of MI among men below age 40 from 1968 to 1978, and were compared with the total population figures. The prognosis among survivors was compared with males in the age groups 40–49 years and 50–59 years who suffered nonfatal MI during the same period.

The socioeconomic variables, place of birth, number of days of sickness benefit, annual income, and alcohol abuse, were compared between all cases of MI among men below age 40 from 1970 to 1977 and a random sample of 536 men from the general population in the age group 30–39 years. The socioeconomic variables were collected from public registers. The risk factors (smoking, serum cholesterol, and blood pressure) were compared between surviving patients and the general population sample.

Results

During the 11-year period (1968–1978), 61 cases of MI below age 40 were registered. Eleven men (18%) died outside the hospital and four (7%) during the hospital stay. The average age was 35.6 years and the age distribution can be seen in Fig. 1. The annual incidence of a first MI per 100000 males was in the age group 25–29 years, 1.7; 30–34 years, 6.1; and 35–39 years, 29.4 (Table 1). There was a significantly lower incidence among men of Swedish origin than among men of Finnish origin ($P < 0.01$), while no difference was noticed between men of Swedish and foreign

---

1 Department of Medicine, Östra Hospital, S-41685 Göteborg, Sweden

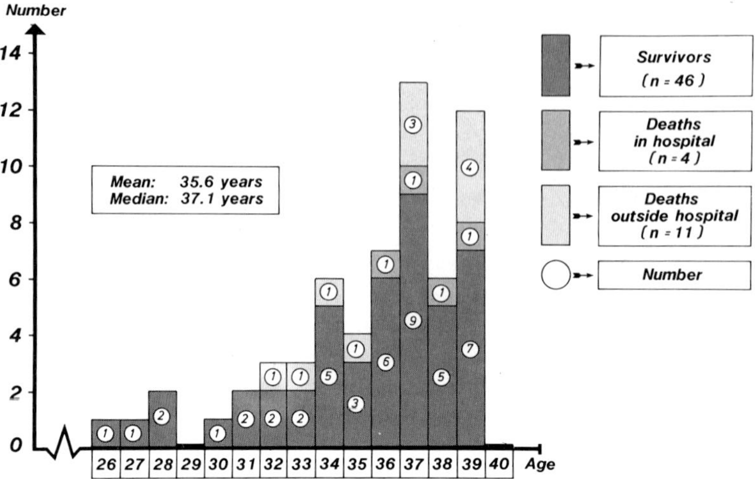

Fig. 1. Age distribution among men with MI below age 40 in Göteborg (1968–1978)

non-Finnish origin. Among men of foreign origin the Finns tended to have a higher incidence than other immigrants ($P = 0.10$). The annual number of MI cases was too low to expose any time trends.

The survival rate during the follow-up was higher among younger patients ($P < 0.05$, Fig. 2).

During the follow-up, 14 of the 46 younger patients suffered a nonfatal reinfarction which was as frequent as in older age groups (Fig. 3). There were no differences between patients with and without nonfatal reinfarctions with respect to the variables cholesterol, blood pressure, and smoking habits.

The annual income among men with MI was lower than among the population ($P < 0.05$). The accumulated number of days of sickness benefit 2 years prior to MI was significantly higher among the MI cases than that among the total population

Table 1. Incidence of MI among men below age 40 in Göteborg, Sweden

Age (years)	Annual incidence per 100 000			
	Sweden	Finland	Foreign, except Finland	Total
30 – 34	6.5	23.6	7.2	6.1
35 – 39	24.2	72.6	34.5	29.4
30 – 39	13.7	44.7	20.4	16.8

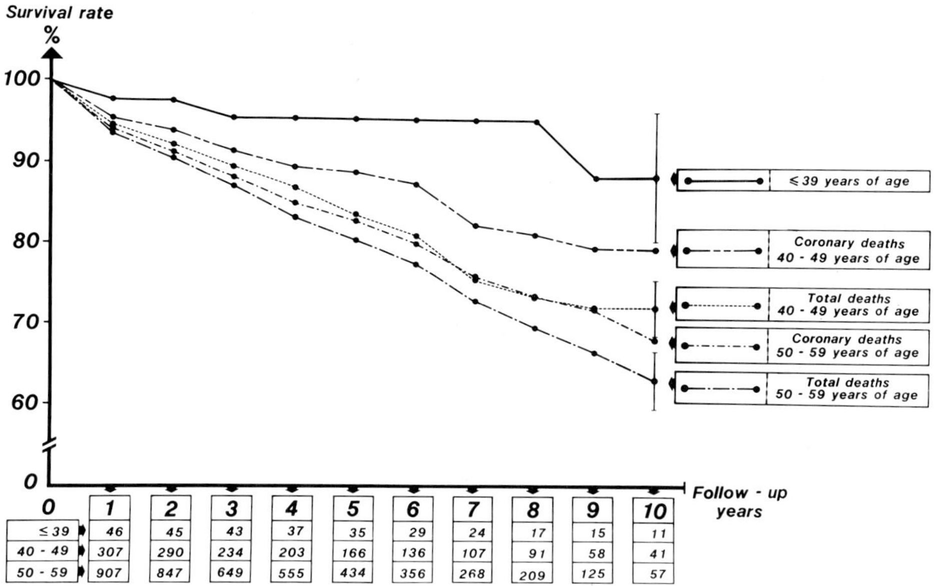

Fig. 2. Survival rate among men discharged from the hospital after a first MI

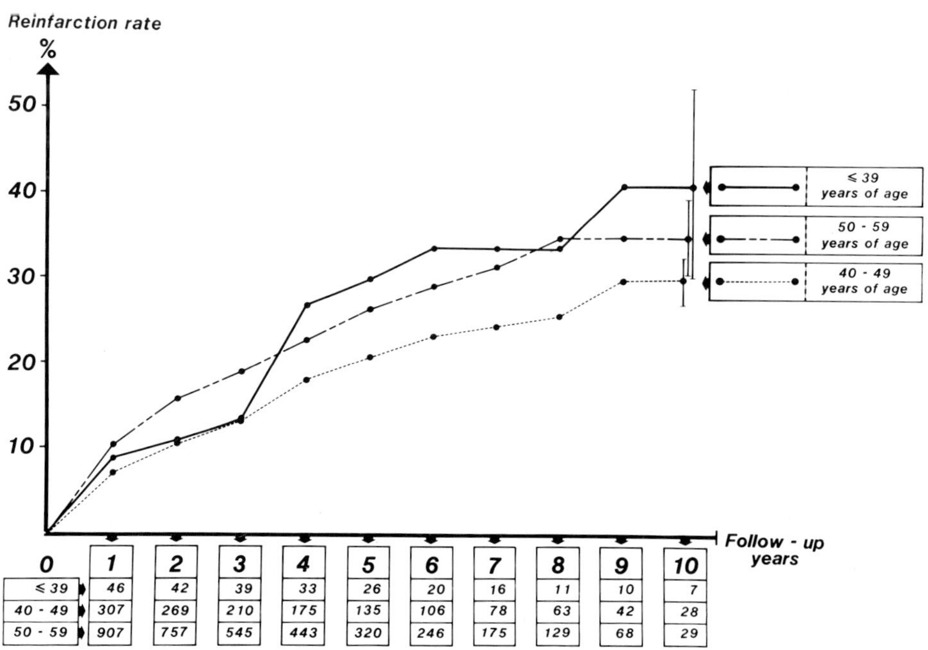

Fig. 3. Rate of nonfatal reinfarctions among men discharged from the hospital after a first MI

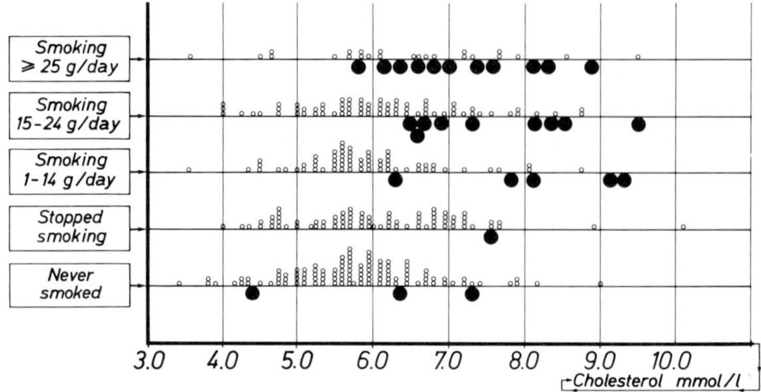

Fig. 4. Combination of the risk factors smoking and cholesterol in men with MI (●) and individuals in the general population sample (○)

sample ($P < 0.001$). The MI cases were more often registered at the Temperance Board for alcohol abuse compared with the population sample ($P < 0.01$, Table 2).

Of 33 MI survivors, 28 were smokers, compared with 46% of the population sample ($P < 0.01$, Fig. 4). The serum cholesterol value of the survivors 3 months after MI was significantly higher than in the population sample ($P < 0.01$, Fig. 4). Systolic, as well as diastolic blood pressure was higher among the survivors 3 months after MI than in the population sample, but only the difference between the diastolic pressures was significant ($P < 0.05$). The combination of the two risk factors smoking and serum cholesterol among the survivors and the population sample is presented in Fig. 4. The combination of heavy smoking and a high serum cholesterol value discriminated most of the survivors from the individuals in the population sample.

Table 2. Alcohol abuse among young men with MI in Göteborg, according to origin

Case of MI	Registered at Temperance Board
Origin	(%)
Swedish ($n = 28$)	39
Finnish ($n = 10$)	70
Foreign, except Finnish ($n = 8$)	0
Total ($n = 46$)	39
General population sample ($n = 536$)	20

Discussion

More than 90% of all MI cases are registered in the Infarction Register in Göteborg (Elmfeldt et al. 1975 a). The Infarct Register and the special Postmyocardial Infarction Clinic (Elmfeldt et al. 1975 b) are well known to doctors in Göteborg and young patients who have suffered a MI outside the city are always sent to the Postmyocardial Infarction Clinic for follow-up. The patients studied can be regarded as representative for acute MI in patients below 40 years of age. The annual incidence during the studied period was in concordance with the results seen in the WHO study of 1970–1971, where only 2 of 21 centers had the same low incidence as Göteborg (WHO 1976). Most of the other centers had a higher incidence and in Perth, Western Australia, the incidence was 2.5–5-times higher than in Göteborg (Pole et al. 1977). The mortality outside hospital was somewhat lower than among older patients in Göteborg (Elmfeldt et al. 1975 a).

Several studies show a relatively good long-time survival rate among young patients (Kovacsics et al. 1977; Georgiou et al. 1978), as well as a longer survival time than among older patients (Helmers 1974; Pole et al. 1976). However, despite the low absolute mortality, there was a marked relative excess mortality compared to healthy contemporaries (Weinblatt et al. 1968; Vedin et al. 1975; Kjøller 1978; Helmers and Lundman 1979). The high rate of nonfatal reinfarctions suggests severe coronary artery disease.

Men with MI below age 40 seemed to have a lower socioeconomic status than the population. However, the variables studied might be secondary to more complex socioeconomic and psychosocial factors.

The present study supports the previous investigations that cholesterol, smoking habits, and hypertension are major risk factors for acute MI. The difference between serum cholesterol values in the patients and the population was greater in this study than for older age groups in Göteborg (Elmfeldt et al. 1976). High cholesterol levels and heavy smoking discriminate the majority of the patients. Blood pressure-cholesterol or blood pressur-smoking habits did not similarly discriminate the MI patients from the population sample.

Men who suffered a MI at young age have lower socioeconomic status than contemporaries in the population. However, independent of socioeconomic status, these patients were heavily burdened with the risk factors smoking, serum cholesterol, and blood pressure.

References

Elmfeldt D, Wilhelmsen L, Tibblin G et al. (1975 a) Registration of myocardial infarction in the city of Göteborg, Sweden. A community study. J Chronic Dis 28:173–186

Elmfeldt D, Wilhelmsen L, Tibblin G et al. (1975 b) A postmyocardial infarction clinic in Göteborg, Sweden. Acta Med Scand 197:497–502

Elmfeldt D, Wilhelmsson C, Vedin JA et al. (1976) Characteristics of representative male survivors of myocardial infarction compared with representative population samples. Acta Med Scand 199:387–398

Georgiou V, Athanassiades D, Hadjigeorge C et al. (1978) Die Langzeitprognose der koronaren Herzerkrankungen bei jungen hospitalisierten Patienten. Herz Kreisl 10:279–283

Helmers C (1974) Short and long-term prognostic indices in acute myocardial infarction. Acta Med Scand [Suppl] 555

Helmers C, Lundman T (1979) Early and sudden deaths after myocardial infarction. Acta Med Scand 205:3–9

Kjøller E (1978) Long-term prognosis after acute myocardial infarction with special reference to the expected mortality. Dan Med Bull 25:148–155

Kovacsics H, Kovascics A, Petersen I et al. (1977) Langzeitschicksal nach Myokardinfarkt bei Männern unter 40 Jahren. Verh Dtsch Ges Kreislaufforsch 43:280

Pole DJ, Thompson PL, Woodings TL et al. (1976) Acute myocardial infarction: One year follow-up of 1138 cases from the Perth Community Coronary Register. Aust NZ J Med 6:437–440

Pole DJ, McCall MG, Reader R, Woodings T (1977) Incidence and mortality of acute myocardial infarction in Perth, Western Australia. J Chronic Dis 30:19–27

Vedin A, Wilhelmsson C, Elmfeldt D (1975) Deaths and nonfatal reinfarctions during two years follow-up after myocardial infarction. Acta Med Scand 198:353–364

Weinblatt E, Shapiro S, Frank CW, Sager RV (1968) Prognosis of men after first myocardial infarction: Mortality and first recurrence in relation to selected parameters. Am J Public Health 58:1329–1347

World Health Organization, Regional Office for Europe (1976) Myocardial Infarction Community Registers. Public Health in Europe 5, Copenhagen

Myocardial Infarction at Young Age: Risk Factors and Natural History[1]

G. S. Uhl and P. W. Farrel[2]

Ischemic heart disease continues to be the primary cause of death among adults in the United States. There is general agreement on a multifactorial etiology of the disease and that the incidence of disease increases with age. However, coronary heart disease has been recognized in young age groups more frequently in recent years (Davia et al. 1974; Dolder and Oliver 1975; Bergstrand et al. 1978; Gohlke et al. 1980). These individuals with precocious atherosclerosis may be the ideal population to study the relative role of the conventional risk factors.

A sample of young patients with myocardial infarction (MI) was studied on the assumption that predisposing risk factors should be more evident in those with premature coronary heart disease. We evaluated the prevalence of various risk factors in younger patients with MI and compared these to a population of infarction victims older than 40. Early and late morbidity and mortality were also compared.

Materials and Methods

From January, 1973 to December, 1975, all cases of an initial MI who met World Health Organization criteria (chest pain, electrocardiographic changes, and serum enzyme rises) who were admitted to Wilford Hall Medical Center were reviewed. This included 165 patients under 40 years of age (mean 34.5 ± 6.1 years) including 13 under 30, 47 at 30–35, and 105 who were 35–39 years of age. This group was compared to 100 patients who were 40 or older and admitted during the same time, randomly selected as the first three or four patients admitted each month having suffered an initial transmural MI.

Chart review of a standard history and physical form recorded at the time of admission yielded pertinent history and known risk factor data. Prior outpatient records were reviewed for substantiation of historical data and previous laboratory-derived values. All data were stored in a computer for retrieval and data analysis. The baseline data included vital statistics; social history (including smoking habits and physical activity); family history of significant cardiovascular disease in first-degree relatives; knowledge of previous hypertension, glucose intolerance, or hyperlipidemia; previous angina pectoris; and physical activity at the onset of MI. Location of infarction, complications, and other follow-up data was added as collected.

Admission height and weight was used and patients were considered obese if they were 20% overweight from standard tables (Metropolitan Life Insurance Company

---

1 The opinions expressed in this manuscript do not reflect the policies of the United States Air Force, but are solely the responsibility of the authors
2 Wilford Hall USAF Medical Center, Lackland Air Force Base, TX 78236, USA

1959). This index of obesity has been shown to correlate well with obesity defined as relative body weight calculated by Quetelet's rule, which gives an index of body weight easily comparable in adults of varying height (Khosla and Lowe 1967).

Persons were classified as nonsmokers only if they never smoked. Persons who had quit smoking or currently smoked had their tobacco consumption semiquantiated by multiplying the number of packs of 20 cigarettes inhaled per day by the number of years smoked. These were then arbitrarily divided into those above and below 20 pack-years.

Hypertension was considered to be present if the patient was on antihypertensive medication at admission. Evidence of hypertension was sought on review of outpatient records. Evidence of significant hypertension was sought and elevated blood pressure was considered present if systolic pressure was over 160 mmHg or diastolic over 90 mmHg at the time of discharge.

Cholesterol levels in the serum were determined on admission and during weeks 2 and 3 postinfarction after an overnight fast. It was hoped that the effect of the acute stress of the pain would not influence these later values.

The treatment of patients was nonstandardized, as they were all returned to the care of their primary physician. Those that had no prior physician contact were followed up by members of the internal medicine staff or house staff. No attempt was made to recommend certain therapies or restrict these patients from certain medications, such as beta-blockers or long-acting nitrates. All surviving patients were followed up by periodic mailings of questionnaires, telephone communication, and review of recurrent admissions.

Selective coronary angiography and left ventriculography were performed in 81 patients under 40 years (49%) for clinical reasons or to define extent of disease. These were performed at least 3 months after MI using the Judkins technique. The number of patients over 40 years examined angiographically was so small (11%) that these results were not evaluated.

For statistical analyses, the difference of any variable, risk factor, or complication between the patient age group less than 40 and those over 40 was analyzed by Student's nonpaired t-test. The SE of the differences between the proportions in the two samples was determined. The P values were calculated and differences were considered statistically significant if, in a two-tailed test, P was less than 0.05 (Hill 1977).

Results

The two patient groups, those below 40 years (group 1) and those older than 40 years (group 2) were compared as to the presence or absence of each variable (Table 1). In group 1, 53% experienced angina prior to MI, while the remaining 77 denied having any chest pains prior to the infarction (Table 1). Results were similar in group 2, with 46% of these older patients experiencing angina prior to MI.

It has been suggested that extreme physical exertion prior to MI may be more common in younger patients or in those with normal coronary vessels, suggesting coronary spasm as a possible etiology (Gohlke et al. 1980). In group 1, 32% of the younger patients were exerting themselves at the time of MI pain onset, while only 20% of the older patients had onset of their infarction with stress (Table 1).

Table 1. Comparison of variables in groups 1 ($n = 165$) and 2 ($n = 100$)

Mean age (range) at onset of angina (years)	Group 1	Group 2	P
	34.5 ± 6.1	49.9 ± 7.1	
	(22 – 39)	(40 – 59)	
Day of MI	77	54	NS
Prior to MI	88	46	NS
Physical stress with MI	53	20	NS
Positive family history	105	32	< 0.05
Smoking 20 pack-years	102	75	NS
Hyperlipidemia	100	31	< 0.001
Hypertension	48	46	< 0.01
Obesity	95	32	< 0.001
Diabetes mellitus	15	11	NS
Mean number of risk factors present	3.05 ± 1.2	2.03 ± 1.35	

Smoking was the most common risk factor in both age groups with 61% of the younger patients having a smoking history of 20 pack-years or more. This did not differ statistically from the older group in whom the same amount of tobacco con sumption was found (75%). A family history of significant atherosclerosis or risk factors was present in only 32% of patients in the older group, while 69% of the younger patients had a remarkable family history ($P < 0.05$). A family history of atherosclerotic heart disease was defined as any first-degree relative younger than 50 years who had angina pectoris or a MI. Such a history was obtained in 86 patients in the younger group, but only 32 of group 2 patients. Death from a MI in a family member under the age of 50 years was also relatively more common in the younger patients (27%) than in the older group (17%). A family history of hypertension or diabetes mellitus in a first-degree relative was also uncommon in both groups. The incidence of diabetes mellitus was low in both groups, with no difference in either diet-controlled or insulin-dependent diabetes between the groups. A history of hypertension was significantly more common in the older group ($P < 0.01$). Most patients with high blood pressure were taking antihypertensive medication at the time of admission for MI (Table 1).

The indices of relative body weight and obesity were significantly more common in group 1 than group 2 ($P < 0.001$). Of the younger MI patients, 58% were obese, exceeding the upper limits of ideal body weight by 20% or greater. Hypertension, diabetes mellitus, and hyperlipidemia have been associated with obesity. Various combinations of these risk factors were compared between the two groups and are listed in Table 2. Although obesity was very prevalent in the younger patients, obesity *not* associated with any of the other three risk factors was present in 20% of group 1 and 14% in group 2 (NS). The association of obesity with hyperlipidemia was more frequent in the younger group. Conversely, there were 41 patients in group 2 who were not obese or have hyperlipidemia, hypertension, or diabetes while only 18% of the patients in group 1 had none of those risk factors ($P < 0.001$).

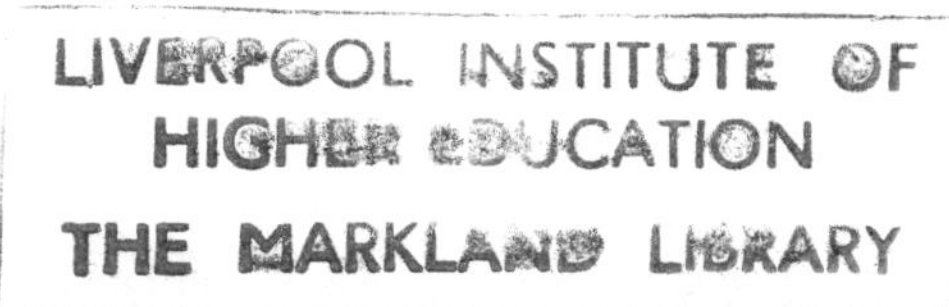

Table 2. Comparison of various combinations of risk factors that may be related to obesity

	Group 1	Group 2	P
Obese only	33	14	NS
Hyperlipidemia (L) only	31	10	<0.05
Hypertension (BP) only	3	8	NS
Obese + L	28	8	<0.05
Obese + BP	13	4	NS
Obese + L + BP	18	0	<0.001
Not obese + L + BP or diabetic	29	41	<0.001

A history of hyperlipidemia before MI or discovered during the hospitalization for MI after the acute stress had subsided was twice as frequent in the younger group (Table 1). In group 1, 100 patients (61%) had hyperlipidemia as a risk factor, while only 31 of the older patients had abnormal lipid values ($P < 0.001$). Hyperlipidemia as the only risk factor present was also more frequent in the younger than the older MI patients (Table 2).

Only one patient in group 1 had none of the conventional risk factors for atherosclerosis. That patient was found to have normal coronaries at catheterization. She was not given ergonovine or a cold pressor test at the time of catheterization. In contrast, six of the older patients had no risk factors. Tabulation of number of risk factors present in each group revealed that the younger MI patients had a larger number of risk factors present (mean 3) than the older patients (mean 2), as shown in Table 1. Of the younger MI patients, 54% had three or more risk factors. The ten young women who suffered a MI had fewer risk factors present (Table 3) than the men, who comprised 94% of group 1. A family history of premature atherosclerosis, hypertension, and hyperlipidemia were the most common risk factors in the young women. Only one was taking oral contraceptives and another was profoundly hypothyroid. None of the young women met the criteria for obesity.

Only 81 of the young MI patients underwent cardiac catheterization, but interesting risk factor data was found in that subgroup as well. Twenty-five had three-vessel disease, 28 had two-vessel disease, 19 had one-vessel disease, and nine were angiographically normal. Only 25 of those catheterized had two or fewer risk factors and of these, 13 (or 52%) had two- or three-vessel disease while 37 of the 47 patients (78%) with three or more risk factors had two- or three-vessel disease. Those 25 patients with three-vessel disease had an average of 3.48 risk factors. That number of risk factors was significantly more than one- or two-vessel disease patients who had 2.8 and 2.9 risk factors, respectively ($P < 0.05$).

Of the nine patients with normal coronary vessels all had suffered an inferior wall MI, with all but two being transmural infarcts. Only one of these patients had no risk factors and the majority had only one or two present (Table 4). None were diabetic, only one was hypertensive, one had a significant smoking history, two had elevated lipid values, and three were obese. However, six had a family history of eith-

Table 3. Description of risk factors in young women with MI

Patient	Age (years)	Conventional risk factors	Other etiologic considerations
A	26	Hypertension	Oral contraceptives for 6 years
B	29	Hypertension, juvenile, juvenile-onset diabetes	None
C	30	Uncle died at age 38 of infarction	Eclampsia during pregnancy
D	30	Hypercholesterolemia, hypertension, sister age 32 with angina	None
E	37	Hypercholesterolemia	Hypothyroidism
F	38	Adult-onset diabetes mellitus, mother died age 40 of infarction	None
G	38	Hypercholesterolemia, 25 pack-year smoker	None
H	39	None	None
I	39	Hypertension, 25 pack-year smoker	None
J	39	Hypertension, 40 pack-year smoker, hypercholesterolemia	None

er premature atherosclerosis or death due to MI at young age in a first-degree relative. These risk factor constellations were distinctly different from the majority of group 1 patients. None of these nine had angina prior to MI and only two were under stress (one emotional, one in athletic competition) at the time of MI.

Subsequent mortality, complications, and morbidity (including angina, reinfarction, and congestive heart failure) were ascertained in both groups (Table 5). There

Table 4. Descriptions of variables in patients with normal coronary vessels

Variable	No. of patients
Smoking:	
None	6
More than 20 pack-years	1
Hyperlipidemia	2
Obesity	4
Hypertension	1
Positive family history:	
None	3
Premature atherosclerosis	4
Death from infarction	2
Recurrent chest pain	5
Transient bundle branch block	2
Death	0

Table 5. Morbidity and mortality in younger versus older MI patients

	Group 1	Group 2	P
Uncomplicated	73	45	NS
Ventricular tachycardia or fibrillation	15	12	NS
Angina (early)	44	12	<0.05
Angina (late)	11	25	NS
Congestive failure	28	17	NS
Reinfarction	24	21	NS
Death (early)	5	17	<0.001
Death (late)	5	24	<0.001
Average annual rat (per year) of			
MI	3%	4.2%	NS
Late mortality	1%	5.0%	<0.01
Angina pectoris	7%	7.5%	NS

were equal percentages of patients in each group who were free of any complications in the first year of follow-up. Of the young infarct patients in group 1, 44 had angina in the immediate postinfarction period, while only 12 of group 2 had immediate postinfarction angina. Angina occurring later had the same occurrence rate in both groups (Table 5). Congestive heart failure was equally prevalent in the young and old MI patients. The presence of ventricular fibrillation or tachycardia was not significantly more common in either age group. Of the older MI patients, 17 died before hospital discharge while only five of the younger patients had early mortality.

On 5-year follow-up, 24 of the younger MI patients had a recurrent infarction as compared to 21 of the older patients. However, the average morbidity rate 1–5 years post-MI was no greater in the older patients (Table 5). The rate of subsequent angina was similar in both groups. Late mortality occurred in the older patients at twice the rate as that in the younger age group.

Discussion

There is a large body of evidence that indicates that one can define the risk factors for MI. Many factors are inter-related and some are age-dependent. This study intended to evaluate the prevalence of risk factors for coronary artery disease in young patients in whom the presence of atherosclerosis may be considered premature. Therefore, the most potent risk factors should be the most common in these patients. The type and number of risk factors in these young patients were compared to a similar, but older population of MI patients to help evaluate this hypothesis.

Among the several risk factors associated with coronary artery disease, hyperlipidemia was one of the most common, especially in the younger patients. It appeared to be a rather potent risk factor, present in 60% of those younger patients, but only 31% of the older patients. Several series of patients with angiographically proven coronary artery disease have found the incidence of hyperlipidemia to range from 54% to 68% (Davia et al. 1974; Falsetti et al. 1968; Heinle et al 1969; Tzagournis et al. 1967; Shekelle et al. 1981). Our data agrees with a study that found that hyperlipidemia in young patients (30–39 years) was a more reliable predictor of subsequent MI than in older groups (Gofman et al. 1966).

Cigarette smoking is firmly established as a risk factor for coronary heart disease by several studies (Doll and Hill 1956; Doyle et al. 1964). However, in our study the prevalence of heavy smoking was higher in older patients than in the younger ones. This may be due in part to the fact that most young patients would have had to smoke at least packs of cigarettes per day to be included in the heavy tobacco-consumer group. Nonetheless, smoking was the second most common risk factor in the younger age group. A previous study actually found smoking to be a stronger risk factor than hypercholesterolemia in young MI patients (Walker and Gregoratos 1967).

The most common risk factor in the younger age group patients was a positive family history of MI at young age or death from MI in first-degree relatives. This was significantly more common in our young group than the older MI patients and was more common in our population than in other series (Dolder and Oliver 1975). This may represent a genetic predisposition to atherosclerosis and is likely to be interrelated to hyperlipidemia and other less well-established metabolic risk factors.

Hypertension is also a conventional risk factor for coronary disease that is firmly established (Doyle et al. 1964; Kannel et al. 1979; Stamler 1978), but appears to be less important in the younger age group than in older patients (Truett et al. 1967). Hypertension prior to MI was more common in our older patients than in the younger, but still more common than has been found in previous studies of young MI patients (Dolder and Oliver 1975; Bergstrand et al. 1978). It is possible that not only the absolute levels of blood pressure elevation, but also the duration of hypertensive disease are of importance in making the risk of MI greater.

Although diabetes mellitus is a well-established risk factor for atherosclerosis (Ostrander et al. 1967; Keen et al. 1965) the prevalence of glucose intolerance was low in both of our groups of MI patients. The probability of a statistical bias against this risk factor may be responsible for its low prevalence, since men with overt diabetes mellitus are excluded from the armed forces.

Previous investigators have suggested that obesity is not a major risk factor for MI (Truett et al. 1967; Tibblin et al. 1975). However, in our population, over half of the younger MI patients were obese while only 32% of the older patients were obese. In addition, obesity was frequently associated with either hyperlipidemia, hypertension, or diabetes mellitus and undoubtedly reflects an interrelationship between these risk factors. Interestingly, 41% of the older patients did not have hyperlipidemia, hypertension, diabetes, or obesity as a combination of risk factors, while only 18% of younger patients were free of all four of these risk factors. Obesity is probably an additive factor in patients with these other risk factors present.

The presence of several of the conventional risk factors appeared to be more common in the younger MI patients. Only one young patient was completely free of all of the accepted risk factors, while six of the older patients had no risk factors. This agrees with some recent reviews (Gohlke et al 1980; Bergstrand et al. 1978), but disagrees with a recent report which found few of the conventional risk factors in patients who suffered MI in the third decade of life (Nixon et al. 1976). Moreover, a recent review suggests that several conditions other than atherogenesis can result in a clinical infarction, especially in young patients (Cheitlin et al. 1975). Of the younger MI patients, 63% had three or more risk factors present while most of the older patients had only one or two risk factors present.

The young women with infarctions represented a subpopulation with few risk factors present. Family history, hypertension, hyperlipidemia, and smoking were the most prevalent in descending order. One patient suffered her MI while eclamptic during pregnancy. Another had insulin-dependent diabetes mellitus with renal failure and hypertension. Yet another was hypothyroid at the time of MI and one other was hypertensive and taking oral contraceptives. Thus, these young women with MI did not have as many conventional risk factors as is described in the literature (Waters et al. 1978) and certainly not as many as the men.

Although this entire population did not undergo cardiac catheterization, there were nine MI patients with normal coronary arteriograms. Only one of these had no risk factors and most of the others only one or two. Obesity and a positive family history of atherosclerosis were the most common risk factors. Unlike other investigators (Gohlke et al. 1980), only one of those who were arteriographically normal was exerting himself at the time of the MI.

Physical exertion at the time of MI was more common in the younger age group and quite possibly played some role in the etiology of these premature MI. Conversely, the presence of angina prior to the MI was present in nearly half of each group, and had little to do with early morbidity or mortality in either group.

Early mortality with MI was significantly more common in the older patients, but signs and symptoms of congestive failure occurred just as frequently in the younger patients as in the older ones. Late complications, such as subsequent infarction or angina, occurred at approximately the same rate in both groups. However, later mortality was less in the younger patients. Thus, MI in younger patients seems to be less lethal than in older victims. The morbidity and mortality in our older patients was similar to recent reports (Kannel et al. 1979). Although this may be due to better overall health status or size of the infarction in the younger patients, it was surprising since it was thought that the older patients may have developed more collateral vessels with time and, thus, be able to survive MI. One classic study (Gertler et al. 1950) found that the long-term prognosis for coronary artery disease is related to the age at the first clinical episode, this does not seem to be the case in our population.

Summary

Younger patients who suffer MI have more conventional risk factors present than older MI victims. In addition to the well-established risk factors of hyperlipidemia, smoking, and family history, obesity was a significant risk both in combination with other risk factors and alone. Young women with MI had fewer conventional risk factors than the young men, but those young patients without coronary arteriosclerosis at catheterization had fewer still. The mortality rate in the younger patients was less, but the incidence of other complications was similar to older patients.

References

Bergstrand R, Vedin A, Wilhelmsson C et al. (1978) Myocardial infarction among men below age 40. Heart J 40:783–788

Cheitlin MD, McAllister HA, de Castro CM (1975) Myocardial infarction without atherosclerosis. JAMA 231:951–959

Davia JE, Hallal FJ, Cheitlin MD et al. (1974) Coronary artery disease in young patients: Arteriographic and clinical review of 40 cases aged 35 and under. Am Heart J 87:689–696

Dolder MA, Oliver MF (1975) Myocardial infarction in young men. Study of risk factors in nine countries. Br Heart J 37:493–503

Doll R, Hill AB (1956) Lung cancer and other causes of death in relation to smoking: second report on mortality of British doctors. Br Med J II:1071–1081

Doyle JT, Dawber TR, Kannel WB et al. (1964) The relationship of cigarette smoking to coronary heart disease. The second report of the combined experience of the Albany, NY and Framingham, Mass., studies. JAMA 190:886–890

Epstein FH (1973) Coronary heart disease epidemiology revisited: Clinical and community aspects. Circulation 48:185–194

Falsetti HL, Schnatz JD, Greene DG (1968) Lipid and carbohydrate studies in coronary artery disease. Circulation 37:184–191

Gertler MM, Gain SM, White PD (1950) Diet, serum cholesterol and coronary artery disease. Circulation 2:696–704

Gofman JW, Young W, Tandy R (1966) Ischemic heart disease, atherosclerosis and longevity. Circulation 34:679–697

Gohlke H, Gohlke-Bärwolf C, Stürzenhofecker P et al. (1980) Myocardial infarction at young age: Correlation of angiographic findings with risk factors and history in 619 patients. Circulation Suppl III 62:39

Heinle RA, Leng RI, Frederickson DS (1969) Lipid and carbohydrate abnormalities in patients with angiographically documented coronary artery disease. Am J Cardiol 24:178–186

Hill AB (1977) A short textbook of medical statistics, 10th edn. Lippincott, Philadelphia Toronto

Kannel WB, Sorlie P, McNamara PM (1979) Prognosis after initial myocardial infarction: The Framingham study. Am J Cardiol 44:53–59

Keen H, Rose G, Pyke DA et al. (1965) Blood sugar and arterial disease. Lancet II:505–508

Khosla T, Lowe CR (1967) Indices of obesity derived from body weight and height. Br J Prev Soc Med 21:122–128

Metropolitan Life Insurance Company (1959) Rise in mortality last year. Stat Bull Metrop Life Insur Co 40:1–32

Nixon JV, Lewis HR, Smitherman TC, Shapiro W (1976) Myocardial infarction in men in the third decade of life. Ann Intern Med 85:759–760

Ostrander LD, Neff BJ, Block WD et al. (1967) Hyperglycemia and hypertriglyceridemia among persons with coronary heart disease. Ann Intern Med 67:34–41

Shekelle RB, Shryock AM, Paul O et al. (1981) Diet, serum cholesterol and death from coronary heart disease: The Western Electric study. N Engl J Med 304:65–70

Stamler J (1978) Lifestyles, major risk factors, proof and public policy. Circulation 58:3–19

Tibblin G, Wilhelmsen L, Werkö L (1975) Risk factors for myocardial infarction and death due to ischemic heart disease and other causes. Am J Cardiol 35:514–522

Truett J, Cornfield J, Kannel W (1967) A multivariate analysis of the risk of coronary heart disease in Framingham. Chron Dis 20:511–524

Tzagournis M, Seidensticker JF, Hamwi GH (1967) Serum insulin, carbohydrate and lipid abnormalities in patients with premature coronary heart disease. Ann Intern Med 67:42–47

Walker WH, Gregoratos G (1967) Myocardial infarction in young men. Am J Cardiol 19:339–343

Waters DD, Halphen C, Theroux P et al. (1978) Coronary artery disease in young women: Clinical and angiographic features and correlation with risk factors. Am J Cardiol 42:41–47

Role of Family History in Coronary Heart Disease at Young Age

A. M. Rissanen and E. E. Nikkilä[1]

Coronary heart disease (CHD) tends to be found in families (Epstein 1976), and this familial component appears to be more conspicuous early in life (Slack and Evans 1966; Phillips et al. 1974). The exact role of familial factors in CHD at different ages is not known, however. We have therefore studied such factors of CHD in relation to age, with special reference to the youngest age groups (Rissanen 1979).

Materials and Methods

Probands. The probands of the study were men under age 56 who suffered a nonfatal or fatal myocardial infarction (MI) between 1972 and 1974 in two industrial communities, or a fatal MI in the adjoining rural district, in two regions of Finland. One of the regions is in the South, and has a moderately high incidence of CHD, the other is in the East (province of North Karelia), and has the world's highest incidence of the disease.

Men with initially nonfatal MI were located by the records of the hospitals admitting patients from the study areas. Cases that proved fatal outside the hospital were located from death certificates obtained from the Central Statistical Office of Finland.

The medical records of all eligible men were carefully reviewed. Only men who met one of the following criteria were included in the study: Unequivocal ECG evidence of a recent MI; diagnostic changes in serum enzyme pattern together with suggestive ECG changes or a history of chest pain; positive postmortem evidence of a recent MI; or sudden death with a history of chest pain together with previous sympotms of CHD or suggestive autopsy findings, such as old MI scars and severely affected coronary arteries. These cirteria were met by 110 men from each of the respective regions.

The living men and the closest relatives of the dead men were asked to participate in the study. Two men in the South refused, and no relatives were located for 15 deceased men. Of the remaining 203 men, 100 were alive at the time of the study. The first definite MI had been diagnosed before age 46 years in 84 of the probands (hereafter referred to as the youngest probands), ages 46–50 in 63 (the middle-aged probands), and the remaining (the oldest probands) were over age 50 at the time of their first MI (Table 1). The age of the probands at the time of the study was 22–55 years (mean 47.6 years).

1 Third Department of Medicine, University of Helsinki, 00290 Helsinki 29, Finland

Table 1. Number of participants

		South				East			
		Age of proband at first MI (years)				Age of proband at first MI (years)			
		< 45	46 – 50	51 – 55	Reference group	< 45	46 – 50	51 – 55	Reference group
Probands	Alive	17	18	15	53	22	15	13	53
	Dead[a]	21	14	13	–	24	16	15	–
Parents	Alive	21	9	4	25	11	10	5	22
	Dead[a]	52	47	50	74	75	47	47	77
Siblings	Alive	107	89	62	122	142	96	88	158
	Dead[a]	14	6	13	11	14	22	32	19
Children	Alive	53	39	49	76	53	73	57	108
All relatives	Alive	181	137	115	223	206	179	150	288
	Dead[a]	66	53	63	85	89	69	79	96

[a] Deceased who survived to age 30 are included

In both study communities, 53 healthy reference men who were 34–55 years old (mean 48.7 years) were selected from the occupational health examinations performed on the employees of local wood and paper companies.

A list of first-degree relatives ages 15 or over was compiled for each proband and reference man, and consent was obtained to contact these relatives and to obtain the death certificates for any deceased family members.

Relatives. Of the relatives, 600 had died and 1660 were reported to be alive. A detailed questionnaire on health was sent to the living relatives. This was completed by 1479 (89.1%), including 107 parents, 864 siblings (mean age 47.7 years), and 508 children (20.7 years) (Table 1). These relatives also visited local medical laboratories where a blood sample was drawn after fasting and height and weight were recorded.

The questionnaires gave information about previously diagnosed diseases as well as symptoms and habits. The diagnoses of cardiovascular diseases reported in the questionnaires were checked against earlier medical records of hospitals and private physicians. The diagnosis of CHD was accepted only when the records revealed an objective basis for the reported diagnosis. This could not be confirmed in five cases. The reported diagnoses of hypertension and diabetes from 450 questionnaires were similarly verified past medical records. Because these diagnoses could invariably be confirmed for the cases in which the treatment was also described, the remaining reports of these disorders were accepted as reported whenever treatment was mentioned.

The death certificates for the dead relatives were located in the Central Statistical Office of Finland, where the primary cause of death was coded according to the 1965 Revision of the International Classification of Diseases, Injuries, and Causes of Death (ICD).

Methods of Data Analysis. Serum cholesterol and triglyceride content from the obtained samples were determined and the lipid values were adjusted to age 45 as described previously (Rissanen and Nikkilä 1977). The criterion for hyperlipemia was set at the 90%-percentile of the age-adjusted values of the reference relatives. The limits were 8.30 mmol/liter for serum cholesterol in both sexes, and 2.15 mmol/liter and 1.70 mmol/liter for serum triglycerides in men and women, respectively.

Life tables were constructed (Cutler and Ederer 1958) for the mortality from all cardiovascular diseases (ICD 400–450), from CHD (ICD 410–414), and for the combined morbidity and mortality from CHD. The differences in the cumulative probabilities of an event between two groups of relatives were evaluated by weighing the life table patterns in their entirety, rather than at isolated points only (Mantel 1966). The effect of multiple (nonindependent) observations within a family was disregarded in all statistical tests used. Hence, the significance tests described should be interpreted as rough measures of strength of association between the variables.

Results

Occurrence of CHD Among Relatives in Relation to the Age of Proband. Among parents of probands, early mortality from cardiovascular diseases was greatest among the fathers of probands whose first MI had been diagnosed before age 46 (the youngest probands) (Table 2). By age 70, the risk of dying from CHD for these fathers was 5.2-times (50%) more than that for reference fathers ($P < 0.001$), for fathers of the middle-aged probands the risk was 3.8-times (32%) that of reference fathers ($P < 0.01$), whereas for fathers of the oldest probands the risk was only slightly greater than for reference fathers. The mortality from all cardiovascular causes, and particularly from CHD, was similarly increased among the mothers of the youngest

Table 2. Cumulative probability of fathers dying from cardiovascular diseases by age 70

| | Probability of dying (%) | | | |
| | Coronary heart disease[a] | | All cardiovascular diseases[a] | |
	South	East	South	East
Age of proband at first MI (years)				
≤45	44.3**	52.3**	55.2**	62.4**
46 – 50	29.5*	35.9*	37.2	58.6*
51 – 55	12.1	20.2*	22.2	31.2
Reference	9.4	7.6	25.2	21.2

[a] International Classification of Diseases Code 410 – 414 (coronary heart disease) and 400 – 450 (all cardiovascular diseases)
* $P < 0.05$ Between proband and reference group
** $P < 0.01$ Between proband and reference group

Table 3. Cumulative probability of mothers dying from cardiovascular diseases by age 70

| | Probability of dying (%) | | | |
| | Coronary heart disease[a] | | All cardiovascular diseases[a] | |
	South	East	South	East
Age of proband at first MI (years)				
≤45	35.8**	24.9*	54.6*	35.0*
46 – 50	14.5	11.3	20.0	14.8
51 – 55	6.7	13.2	21.9	17.5
Reference	10.0	7.4	24.0	19.1

[a] ICD Code 410 – 414 (coronary heart disease) and 400 – 450 (all cardiovascular diseases)
* $P < 0.05$ Between proband and reference group
** $P <$ Between proband and reference group

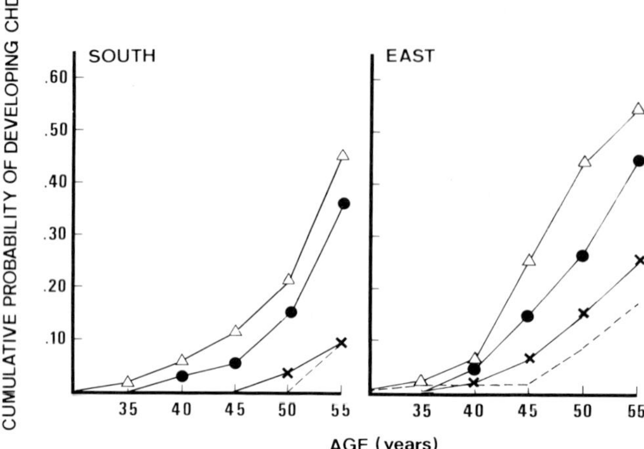

Fig. 1. Cumulative probability of developing fatal or nonfatal coronary heart disease for the brothers of the probands whose first MI was diagnosed before age 46 (–△–), at age 46–50 (–●–), or at age 50–55 (–×–), and for the brothers of reference men (– – –)

probands, but not among those of the probands with the first MI after age 45 (Table 3).

Among siblings of probands, fatal or nonfatal CHD had been diagnosed in one-fifth of the brothers of the probands in the South and in one-third of those in the East: This frequency is four-times that of reference brothers in the respective areas ($P < 0.01$ in both areas). The risk of the disease was greatest for the brothers of the youngest probands (Fig. 1) for whom it was 45% in the South and 54% in the East by age 55, denoting 11.4- and 6.7-fold excesses over the risk in reference brothers in the respective areas ($P < 0.001$ in the South and $P < 0.01$ in the East) (Table 4). The corresponding risks for the brothers of the middle-aged probands were 8.3- and 3.6-times greater than the risks for the Southern and Eastern reference brothers ($P < 0.01$ in both areas). The risks of the brothers of the oldest probands differed

Table 4. Cumulative probability of siblings for developing coronary heart disease by age 55 (%)

	Brothers		Sisters	
	South	East	South	East
Age of proband at first MI (years)				
≦45	45.7***	54.3**	18.6	24.4*
46–50	36.8**	44.7**	6.8	11.2
51–55	9.2	27.7*	–	16.0
Reference	8.9	16.7	6.1	11.5

Between proband and reference group, * $P < 0.05$ ** $P < 0.01$ *** $P < 0.001$

Table 5. Frequency of main coronary risk factors among MI and reference relatives

		South			East		
		Brothers	Sisters	Children	Brothers	Sisters	Children
Hypertension (%)	MI	16.1	17.8	2.8	20.4	26.6	1.6
	Reference	6.0	11.0	–	13.8	20.4	–
Hypercholes-terolemia (%)[a]	MI	32.1**	20.5**	19.1*	38.8	27.1*	19.1
	Rererence	10.0	8.2	6.6	23.1	16.1	10.2
Hypertrigly-ceridemia (%)[a]	MI	21.4	21.1**	12.8	23.1	16.9	7.1
	Reference	14.0	8.2	6.6	13.8	11.8	9.3
Relative weight > 120 (%)	MI	11.6	26.7	4.3	11.6	28.2	2.7
	Reference	6.0	23.3	2.6	10.8	26.9	1.9
Clinical diabetes (%)	MI	2.7	4.1	–	5.4	1.1	–
	Reference	–	4.1	–	–	2.2	–
Regular smoking (%)[b]	MI	42.0	16.4	35.5	46.3	14.6	28.4
	Reference	42.0	13.7	35.5	40.0	14.0	29.5

[a] Serum cholesterol $\geq$ 8.30 mmol/liter; serum triglycerides $\geq$ 2.15 mmol/liter (men) or $\geq$ 1.70 mmol/liter (women). The values are adjusted to age 45

[b] Smoking before the diagnosis of coronary heart disease

* Between proband and reference group

** Between proband and reference group

Table 6. Frequency of main coronary risk factors in relatives according to the age of proband

	Age of Proband at first MI (years)	Hypertensive Observed: expected[b]			Hypercholesterolemia[a] Observed: expected[b]			Hypertriglyceridemia[a] Observed: expected[b]		
		South	East	Both areas	South	East	Both areas	South	East	Both areas
Male	≦45	2.3*	3.2**	2.7**	2.2*	2.9**	2.6**	1.9	1.7	1.8**
Rela-	46–50	1.1	1.0	1.1	2.1*	2.5**	2.3ö**	1.7	1.5	1.6
tives	51–55	1.2	1.4	1.3	2.0	2.2*	2.1*	1.8	1.7	1.7*
Female	≦45	1.2	2.2*	1.8*	2.4**	3.1**	2.8**	2.8	2.2	2.5**
rela-	46–50	0.9	2.2*	1.6	1.6	2.3*	1.9*	1.7	1.5	1.6
tives	51–55	0.8	1.2	1.0	1.4	1.7	1.6	1.2	1.3	1.2

[a] Serum cholesterol ≧8.30 mmol/liter; serum triglycerides ≧2.15 mmol/liter (men) or ≧1.70 mmol/liter (women). The values are adjusted to age 45
[b] Ratio of the observed number of subjects with the abnormality to the expected number calculated from the frequencies among the reference relatives
* $P<0.05$
** $P<0.01$

little from those of reference brothers. Clinical CHD was only slightly more common among the sisters of probands than in reference sisters. The excess risk of the disease was confined to the sisters of the youngest probands, for whom the risks of having developed CHD by age 55 were 2.8-fold (19%) in the South and 3.7-fold (24%) in the East, compared with the risks for reference sisters in the respective areas ($P < 0.05$ in the South and $P < 0.05$ in the East) (Table 4).

Prevalence of Coronary Risk Factors Among Relatives in Relation to the Age of Proband. Of the main coronary risk factors, only hypertension, hypercholesterolemia, and hypertriglyceridemia were more common in the relatives of probands than in reference relatives (Table 5). Alle these abnormalities were most common among the relatives of the youngest probands and declined in frequency with the advancing age of the proband (Table 6).

Discussion

Several studies on the familial occurrence of CHD have suggested a greater familial influence for the disease of early, rather than of late onset (Slack and Evans 1966; Deutscher et al. 1969; Phillips et al. 1974. The strong familial component found in CHD in this study is, therefore, not unexpected. The magnitude of this component in MI of the youngest probands as evidenced by the up to tenfold excess risk of the disease for their sibs is, however, remarkable.

The results of the present study call attention to the value of family history of premature CHD as a predictor of risk. Screening for parental history of coronary death before age 70 would have identified almost one half of the young probands long before the emergence of the clinical disease. By the same procedure, only about one-tenth of reference men would have been identified. A history of early parental death from CHD thus denotes a clearly increased risk of the disease for the offspring. The absence of such a history does not exclude the chance of an excess risk, however. Many young probands with healthy parents had multiple sibs affected by CHD. The sensitivity of screening by family history could, therefore, have been improved considerably if the history of premature CHD in a sibling were also taken into account. By so doing, about three-fourths of the youngest probands would have been identified. Most but probably not all of the familial component in premature CHD is associated with hypertension and hyperlipidemia. The abnormalities were, however, less common among the probands than was positive family history of early CHD (defined as a parental death from CHD before age 70 and/or a sibling affected by the disease before age 56). Among reference men, the reverse was true.

We have had a chance to compare the predictive value of family history with that of the major risk factors in another group of young patients (Liskola and Luomanmäki, unpublished work). They are 128 male and 18 female participants under age 40 in the postcoronary rehabilitation courses arranged in 1974–1980 by the Social Insurance Institution in Finland. Positive family history was given by 62% of the male participants, but hypertension was found in only 45% and hypercholesterolemia in 35%. Of the 18 woman, 15 gave a family history of premature CHD but one or more of the major biometric risk factors were detected in only 11.

Although invaluable in most cases of CHD of early onset, family history may be of limited value in very young patients. Both CHD and its biochemical precursors were extremely scarce in the families of two youngest probands in our study. These men died suddenly and unexpectedly of autopsy-verified MI at ages 22 and 24, respectively. The death in these cases probably was caused by mechanisms other than those of the common atherosclerotic heart disease, as also suggested by the findings of the autopsies of young Finns dying from CHD (Koskenvuo et al. 1978).

The present study strongly suggests that family history of premature CHD has great practical relevance toward identifying persons at highest risk. This risk could probably be substantially reduced if information about the family history were used to identify such persons at an early stage and if they were treated for their correctable risk factors.

Summary

The occurrence of coronary heart disease (CHD) and its main risk factors were assessed in the families of 309 index men. These men included 203 patients with fatal or nonfatal myocardial infarction (MI) and 106 healthy reference men under age 56 from two communities in South and East Finland. Forty percent of the patients and 12% of reference men had at least one first-degree relative affected by CHD before age 56. The younger the patient at the diagnosis of first MI, the more common was CHD in relatives. The risk of having CHD by age 55 was, respectively, 11.4-, 8.3-, and 1.3-times greater in the South and 6.7-, 3.6-, and 1.8-times greater in the East for the brothers of patients than for the brothers of reference men, depending on whether the diagnosis of MI in the patient had been first established before age 46, at age 46–50, or at age 51–55.

Most of the strong familial component in early-onset MI appears to be mediated by familial hyperlipidemia and hypertension. It is suggested that the risk of premature CHD in the persons at highest risk could be substantially reduced if information about family history were used to identify such persons at an early age.

References

Cutler SJ, Ederer F (1958) Maximum utilization of the life table method in analyzing survival. J Chronic Dis 8:699–712

Epstein FH (1976) Genetics of ischemic heart disease. Postgrad Med J 52:477–480

Koskenvuo K, Karvonen MJ, Rissanen V (1978) Death from ischemic heart disease in young Finns aged 15 to 24 years. Am J Cardiol 42:114–118

Mantel N (1966) Evaluation of survival data and two new rank order statistics arising in its consideration. Cancer Treat Rep 50:163–170

Phillips RL, Lilienfeld AM, Diamond EL, Kagan A (1974) Frequency of coronary heart disease and cerebrovascular accidents in parents and sons of coronary heart disease index cases and controls. Am J Epidemiol 100:87–100

Rissanen AM (1979) Familial occurrence of coronary heart disease: Effect of age at diagnosis. Am J Cardiol 44:60–66

Rissanen A, Nikkilä EA (1977) Coronary artery disease and its risk factors in families of young men with angina pectoris and in controls. Br Heart J 39:875–883

Slack J, Evans KA (1966) The increased risk of death from ischemic heart disease in first-degree relatives of 121 men and 96 woman with ischemic heart disease.

Coronary Arteriographic Findings in Younger Survivors of Acute Myocardial Infarction Including Those with Normal Coronary Arteries

W. C. Sheldon, M. Razavi, and Y. J. Lim[1]

Acute myocardial infarction (MI) is often the first indication of the presence of coronary atherosclerosis. In the Framingham study [5], it was the initial manifestation in 42% of men and 21% of women, and 16% of men and 28% of women died during the initial phase after a *recognized* MI: At the end of 1 year 19% of men and 34% of women had died. Including sudden deaths, 35% of men died within 1 year. Subsequent attrition occurs at approximately 5% per year. Recurrent MI afflicts 13% of men and 39% of women within 5 years. Acute MI in younger individuals is of particular concern because of its impact on the family unit, and the potential for disability and diminished productivity.

This report reviews our arteriographic findings and surgical experience in younger survivors of an initial MI studied within 1 year of the event.

Materials and Methods

The data base of the Cleveland Clinic Cardiovascular Information Registry was surveyed for patients who underwent coronary arteriographiy within 1 year of an initial ECG-documented MI. Age at the time of study, sex, and presence or absence of hypertension (blood pressure 160/100 mmHg or higher), diabetes (on pharmacologic treatment or abnormal glucose tolerance test), hypercholesterolemia (300 mg% or higher), smoking, and clinical diagnosis of obesity were identified. Data regarding family history were compiled for patients who were age 40 and younger. Coronary arteriographic findings were tabulated according to the extent of disease in the left main, anterior descending, circumflex, and right coronary arteries and the presence or absence of collaterals was noted in patients with a totally occluded vessel. ECG localization of the infarction was noted, as well as ventriculographic localization of regional myocardial abnormalities.

For each patient treated surgically, the operative procedure was noted, as well as perioperative mortality and morbidity (suspected or definite perioperative infarction). Follow-up was obtained in a subset of patients treated surgically with pure graft procedures from 1971 to 1973. A follow-up survey of medically treated patients is currently in progress.

In a previous study, similar information had been obtained in a series of patients unselected by age, who were studied during 1971 to 1973, also within 1 year after an ECG-documented MI, some of whom were subsequently treated surgically.

The Cleveland Clinic Cardiovascular Information Registry was initiated in 1972 and the data base includes all patients who have had cardiac catheterization and an-

---

1 Department of Cardiology, The Cleveland Clinic Foundation, Cleveland, OH 44106, USA

giography or cardiac surgery since January 1, 1970. Patients prior to 1970 were also included in the Registry if they underwent pure graft revascularization surgery, a repeat cardiac catheterization study, or a reoperation during or after 1970. Currently, the data base includes approximately 60 000 patients.

Results

A total of 236 patients age 40 years and younger were identified as having undergone a coronary arteriographic study within one year after an ECG-documented initial MI (Table 1). During the 1971 to 1973, 1922 patients of all ages were identified as having undergone coronary arteriography within 1 year after an ECG-documented first MI. The median age, sex, and common risk factors of these two groups of patients are compared in Table 1.

The median age of the group unselected by age exceeded that of the younger group by more than 20 years. The proportion of females was smaller in the younger group (6.8% versus 12.6%). Of the younger group, 94% had one or more risk factors present including a positive family history in 57%. Hypertension and diabetes occurred less frequently in the younger group (5.9% versus 23.3% and 2.5% versus 8.1%, respectively), but smoking and hypercholesterolemia were more frequent in the younger groups (83.5% versus 64.6% and 14% versus 8.6%, respectively). Clinical obesity was equally prevalent in both groups.

The extent of coronary atherosclerosis is tabulated in Table 2, which for comparative purposes includes information on extent of disease available from two other series of younger survivors of MI [4, 14], and the Cleveland Clinic series of first MI

Table 1. Survivors of MI. Clinical characteristics and risk factors compared to unselected survivors of MI

	Age $\leq$ 40, all years	All ages, 1971 – 1973 group
No. patients	236	1 922
Median age	37	58
No. males (%)	220 (93.2)	1 679 (87.4)*
No. females (%)	16 (6.8)	243 (12.6)*
No. without risk factors (%)	14 (5.9)	Not available
No. positive family (%)	135 (57.2)	Not available
No. hypertension ($\geq$ 160/100) (%)	14 (5.9)	447 (23.3)**
No. smokers (%)	197 (83.5)	1 241 (64.6)**
No. hypercholesterolemia ($\geq$ 300 mg%) (%)	33 (14.0)	165 (8.6)*
No. diabetes (chemical or abnormal GTT) (%)	6 (2.5)	156 (8.1)*
No. obesity (%)	44 (18.6)	337 (17.5)

* $P < 0.01$
** $P < 0.001$

Table 2. Survivors of MI age 40 and younger: Extent of coronary disease

Series	Age ≤ 40			All ages
	Roskamm, 1973 – 1978	Hamby, 1974 – 1978	CCF, all years	CCF 1971 – 1973 group
Patients	500	51	236	1 922
Significant lesion	$\geq 50\%$	$\geq 50\%$	$\geq 75\%$	$\geq 75\%$
Insignificant or no disease (%)	33 (6.6)	0	45 (19.1)	217 (11.3)
Significant disease (%)	467 (93.4)	51 (100)	191 (80.9)	705 (89.7)
One-vessel (%)	281 (60.2)	(50)	121 (63.3)*	783 (45.9)
Two-vessel (%)	101 (21.6)	(28)	53 (27.7)	572 (33.5)
Three-vessel (%)	85 (18.2)	(21)	16 (8.4)*	318 (18.7)
Left main (%)	(included)	NS	1 (0.5)	32 (1.9)

* $P < 0.001$ (CCF age ≤ 40 versus all ages)

Table 3. First infarction survivors: Extent of disease and severity of occlusion. (LAD = left anterior descending artery; RCA = right coronary artery; LCx = left circumflex artery; LM = left main artery)

	Age ≤ 40, all years				All ages, 1971 – 1973 group			
	Percent narrowing				Percent narrowing			
Vessel, % of patients	< 50	50 – 74	75 – 99	100	< 50	50 – 74	75 – 99	100
LAD	17.4	23.7	37.7	25.4	17.0	19.9	41.8	24.8
RCA	22.9	17.4	24.1	31.3	20.9	16.9	27.7	29.0
LCx	26.7	17.4	17.8	7.6	17.1	15.2	29.6	15.1
LM	5.1	0.8	0.4	0	4.1	1.3	1.4	0.2

survivors of all ages. The presence or absence of significant disease depends upon the definition of a significant lesion. Since surgical candidacy usually requires a lesion of 75% or more, this was the criterion for significance in the Cleveland Clinic series: The cutoff point was 50% for significant lesions in the Roskamm [14] and Hamby [4] series. Of all our younger patients, 19% had lesions less than 75% and 7% of the Roskamm series had lesions less than 50%. It should be noted that the Hamby series excluded patients without significant disease. Of our younger patients, 63% had significant one-vessel disease, 28% two-vessel, 8% three-vessel, and only one patient in this series had a significant left main lesion. The prevalence of multivessel disease (37%) was lower among our younger patients than in the series unselected by age, in which 54% had multivessel disease. The extent of disease in our younger patients is similar to that in the Roskamm series, while in the Hamby series equal proportions of patients had single- and multivessel disease.

The extent of disease in each of the major coronary arteries is presented in Table 3. Twenty-five percent of patients had a totally occluded anterior descending artery, 31% had an occluded right coronary artery, and 8% an occluded left circum-

Table 4. First infarction survivors: Severity of occlusion. Percent of patients with 75% – 100% occlusion

	Age $\leqq$ 40, all years Percent	All ages, 1971 – 1973 group Percent
LAD	63.1	66.6
RCA	55.5	56.7
LCx	25.4	44.7*

* $P < 0.001$

Table 5. ECG abnormalities in survivors of MI

ECG infarction	Age $\leqq$ 40, all years Patients (%)	All ages, 1971 – 1973 group Patients (%)
Anterior	129 (53.3)	503 (48.4)
Inferior	102 (42.1)	478 (46.0)
Lateral	11 (4.5)	57 (5.5)

Table 6. Left ventricle (LV) wall motion abnormalities in survivors of MI

LV regional abnormality	Age $\leqq$ 40, all years Patients (%)	All ages, 1971 – 1973 group Patients (%)
Mild or no dysfunction	28 (11.9)	817 (42.5)
Moderate or severe dysfunction	206 (88.1)	1 060 (57.5)
Anterior	84 (40.7)	386 (36.4)
Inferior	89 (43.2)	512 (48.3)
Lateral	33 (16.0)	162 (15.2)

Table 7. Survivors of MI age 40 or less: Surgical treatment

No surgical treatment (%)	166 (70.3)
Surgical (%)	70 (29.7)
One-graft patients	17
Two-graft patients	23
Three-graft patients	15
Other	15
Hospital mortality	0
Perioperative MI	2
Percent graft patency	95.0

flex. Eighty-five percent of the totally occluded anterior descending arteries, 95% of the right coronary arteries, and 72% of the circumflex vessels received collateral flow. Significant lesions (75% or more) occurred with similar frequency in the anterior descending and right coronary arteries in both series, i.e., younger patients as well as those unselected by age, but with slightly higher frequency in the circumflex and left main coronary arteries in the group unselected by age (Table 4). Eight patients in the younger series had normal coronary arteries.

Among 149 patients with significant disease in the anterior descending artery, 129 showed ECG evidence of anterior infarction at the time of angiography (others had previous ECGs showing infarction), and 84 showed moderate to severe anterior dysfunction on left ventriculography. Of 138 patients age 40 or younger with significant obstructive lesions involving the right coronary artery, 102 had concurrent ECG evidence of inferior MI and 89 had moderate or severe left ventricular dysfunction on left ventriculography. Of 60 patients with significant obstructive lesions involving the circumflex, 11 had ECG evidence indicative of infarction involving the lateral regions of the left ventricle, and 33 showed moderate or severe lateral wall dysfunction on ventriculography. Similar findings were observed in the 1971–1973 series unselected by age (Tables 5, 6).

Seventy patients age 40 and under (29.7%) underwent surgical treatment (Table 7). Fifty-five had only graft operations (17 single, 23 double, and 15 three or more grafts), and 15 underwent ventricular aneurysm resections or complex procedures. One patient who had a single graft had another single graft at reoperation. There were no in-hospital deaths. Two patients sustained a perioperative infarction (none of the patients with only grafts). Only 12 patients subsequently had postoperative arteriography among whom only 1 of 20 grafts were occluded. Thirteen patients who were treated surgically from 1971 to 1973 were followed up for 5 or more years and only one late death occurred: The 5-year survival calculated by the life table technique was 85.7%.

Discussion

This study does not distinguish between patients studied during the early post-MI phase and survivors studied later during convalescence. These latter patients were studied within 1 year after an ECG-documented MI. Many were asymptomatic at the time of the study, not having tested their tolerance for physical exercise, and some were fully active. It is possible that those studied in the early postinfarction phase (within 1–3 months) might have exhibited different arteriographic and ventriculographic findings. Patients studied early after MI are less likely to show complete occlusion of the offending artery [1].

Proudfit et al. [12] reported ECG findings of MI to be a highly reliable indicator of significant coronary artery disease. Ninety-nine percent of patients had at least one vessel containing a lesion-obstructing lumen by 50% or more, and 60% of patients had at least one totally occluded artery. The finding of completely normal coronary arteries in patients with ECG evidence of infarction is rare. Cardiomyopathy is the explanation for this in some patients.

The majority of patients age 40 or under in this study had single-vessel disease, as observed by others [14, 10]. Most patients (94%) had one or more risk factors, and younger patients were more likely to have hypercholesterolemia or a history of smoking than patients in the larger series unselected by age. The latter group, however, in which the median age was greater by more than 20 years, had a greater incidence of hypertension and diabetes. The significance of this disparate distribution of risk factors is not clear, but suggests that consequences of hypercholesterolemia and smoking may emerge earlier in life and they may be associated with a more rapidly progressing form of atherosclerosis, if not the premature complication of acute MI. An even higher incidence of hyperlipidemia has been observed in other studies of young survivors of acute MI [3].

Kramer et al. [7] and Marchandise et al. [9] analyzed factors related to progression of disease and noted a tendency for more rapid progression in patients who were younger at the time of initial study.

Although single-vessel involvement was more frequent in younger survivors of acute MI, there was no predilection for a specific vessel. Others have observed a higher incidence of multivessel than single-vessel disease in survivors of inferior MI [2, 4, 10, 11], and a higher incidence of single-vessel disease in survivors of anterior MI in series unselected by age [4], as well as in younger survivors (under age 35) of MI [10]. It is possible that anterior descending disease may occur earlier in the clinical course of coronary heart disease. Alternatively, it is possible that anterior MI is less likely to escape detection and such patients are more likely to be studied early in the natural history of their disease process. Studies of the correlation between ECG evidence of infarction and regional wall motion abnormalities on left ventriculography have shown a better correlation between ECG and left ventriculographic signs of anterior infarction than inferior infarction [15]. Inferior MI may either occur later in the natural history of the disease or is more likely to escape detection until a later stage, when multivessel disease is more likely to be present.

Table 8. Survivors of MI age 40 or less: Subgroups with normal coronary arteries

	Age $\leqq 40$	All ages
Patients	19	41
Age, median years	32	43
Males	10	19
Females	9	22
Risk factors present	18	36
Family history	6	14
Hypertension	2	8
Smoking	13	25
Hyperlipidemia	5	14
Diabetes	1	2
Oral contraceptive use	8	10
Postpartum	1	2
Pregnancy	1	1
History of infarction event	16	36
Documented by ECG	10	19

Table 9. Survivors of MI age 40 or less: Follow-up of subgroups with normal coronary arteries

	Age ≦ 40	All ages
Patients	19	41
Follow-up		
Range	7 – 98 months	7 – 109 months
Median	51.1 months	50.2 months
Status at follow-up		
Asymptomatic	12	23
Angina pectoris	2	3
Atypical pain	1	11
MI	2	2
Arrhythmia	0	1
Died	1	3

Anterior descending disease and the ECG pattern of anterior MI occurred slightly more frequently than inferior or lateral infarction in both younger and older series of patients. Although all patients had a history of a documented MI, ECG findings sometimes regressed to become nondiagnostic by the time of the arteriographic study. A somewhat smaller proportion of patients showed corresponding wall motion abnormalities which usually paralleled the ECG findings.

Seventy patients age 40 or younger underwent surgical treatment. Indications for surgery included persistent anginal symptoms or myocardial jeopardy due to noncollateralized vessels with significant stenotic lesions. Fifteen patients underwent resection of a ventricular aneurysm alone or in combination with other procedures. The absence of hospital mortality, the perioperative infarction rate of 3%, and graft patency rate of 95% in the series of younger MI survivors compares favorably with other surgical series unselected by age. Complete follow-up was available only for patients operated upon during 1971 to 1973, among whom there was only one late death (during the fifth year).

Lim et al. [8] followed up 116 young men (age 40 years or less) with significant (lesions 50% or more) coronary artery disease without surgical treatment. Fifty had ECG evidence of infarction at the time of study, of whom 21 (42%) died within 5 years. Of 66 patients without ECG evidence of infarction, only 13 (17%) died during this interval. The 5-year survival for the total group of young men was 66.8%.

An interesting subgroup is that of MI survivors with angiographically normal or nearly normal coronary arteries. A series of 41 patients who survived an acute MI, but were found to have no perceptible abnormalities of the coronary arteries by angiography, was collected by Razavi [13]. These patients were studied between 1968 and 1978. Among this group, 19 patients were identified who were age 40 years or younger at the time of the arteriographic study. A previous MI was ECG-documented or documented by left ventriculography in all patients. A higher proportion of women was observed in this select group with normal coronary arteries than in other MI survivors, age 40 or younger, as well as those not selected by age. Again, the majority of these patients had one or more risk factors present, but the frequency of sex-related factors, including the use of oral contraceptives, pregnancy and the postpartum state, was noteworthy (Table 8).

After follow-up intervals of 7–109 months for postinfarction patients with normal coronary arteries, and 7–98 months for the subgroup age 40 and under, most patients were asymptomatic at the time of follow-up. Only one late death occurred; a 28-year-old man who had an acute MI 1 year before angiographic study and a recurrent MI 2 years later. Following this, he developed congestive heart failure and died 6 months later. Postmortem examination demonstrated severe intimal fibroplasia involving the coronary, pulmonary, and intrarenal arteries. The coronary arteries also showed scattered histologic changes resembling atherosclerosis [6] (Table 9).

Summary and Conclusions

Myocardial infarction at a young age is associated with significant coronary atherosclerosis in most instances. Nearly all have lesions of 50% or more in one or more coronary arteries, and 81% have lesions of 75% or more in one or more coronary arteries. Sixty-four percent of patients have one or more totally occluded vessels. The majority of patients have single-vessel involvement, but 40%–45% of patients have multivessel involvement and this is more likely to be found in younger survivors of inferior infarction. Left main coronary artery disease is uncommon. As compared to first infarction survivors unselected by age, younger survivors were more likely to be male smokers with hyperlipidemia.

A small subgroup of patients exists who have angiographically normal coronary arteries despite a documented previous MI. The proportion of women is higher in this subgroup, many of whom used oral contraceptives or experienced infarction in relation to pregnancy or the postpartum state.

This study does not address the prognosis of first infarction survivors with nonsurgical treatment. The finding of normal coronary arteries implies a favorable prognosis, but may not exclude other conditions. For example, one patient was postmortem histologically proven to have intimal fibroplasia involving the coronary, pulmonary, and intrarenal arteries, in addition to scattered lesions resembling atherosclerosis in the coronary circulation that had not been recognized angiographically.

Younger MI survivors may be candidates for surgical treatment if they have persistent symptoms or evidence of jeopardized myocardium. The risk of operation appears to be low in such patients and the late results are comparable to larger surgical series not selected by age.

References

1. Begg FR, Koonos MA, Magovern GJ et al. (1969) The hemodynamic and coronary arteriography patterns during acute myocardial infarction. J Thorac Cardiovasc Surg 58:640–645
2. Chaitman BR, Waters DD, Cohara F, Bourassa MG (1978) Prediction of multivessel disease after inferior myocardial infarction. Circulation 57:1085–1090

3. Gohlke H, Gohlke-Bärwolf C, Stürzenhofecker P et al. (1980) Myocardial infarction at young age: correlation of angiographic findings with risk factors and history in 619 patients. (Abstract) Circulation 62/III:39

4. Hamby RI, Katz S, Hoffman I (1980) Arteriography of coronary disease at clinical onset. Chest 78:686–693

5. Kannel WB, Sorlie P, McNamara PM (1979) Prognosis after initial myocardial infarction: The Framingham study. Am J Cardiol 44:53–59

6. Kramer JR (1981) Acute myocardial infarction with arteriographically normal coronary arteries. In: Vidt DG (ed) Cardiovas Clin, F. A. Davis Co., Philadelphia

7. Kramer JR, Matsuda Y, Mulligan JC et al. (1981) Progression of coronary atherosclerosis. Circulation 63:519

8. Lim YJ, Proudfit WL, Sones FM Jr (1974) Selective coronary arteriography in young men. Circulation 49:1122–1126

9. Marchandise B, Bourassa MG, Chaitman BR, Lesperance J (1978) Angiographic evaluation of the natural history of normal coronary arteries and mild coronary atherosclerosis. Am J Cardiol 41:216–220

10. McMartin DC, Masden RR, Sohi GS, Flowers NC (1979) Patient profile and follow-up in medically and surgically treated young adults with myocardial infarction. Clin Cardiol 2:281–285

11. Miller RR, DeMaria AN, Vismara LA et al. (1977) Chronic stable inferior myocardial infarction: Unsuspected harbinger of high-risk proximal left coronary arterial obstructions amenable to surgical revascularization. Am J Cardiol 39:954–960

12. Proudfit WL, Shirey EK Sones FM Jr (1966) Selective cinecoronary arteriography: Correlation with clinical findings in 1000 patients. Circulation 33:901–910

13. Razavi M (1980) Myocardial infarction with normal coronary arteries. Cleve Clin Q 47:253–254

14. Roskamm H, Sturzenhofecker P, Görnandt I et al. (1980) Progression and regression of coronary artery disease in postinfarction patients less than 40 years of age. Cleve Clin Q 47:192–194

15. Welch CC, Proudfit WL, Sones FM Jr et al. (1970) Cinecoronary arteriography in young men. Circulation 42:647–652

Angiographic Findings in Postinfarction Patients Under the Age of 35

F. BURKART and C. SALZMANN [1]

In Europe the number of patients with myocardial infarction (MI) is still increasing, especially for those with clinical symptoms at relatively young age. We were asked by the Swiss Society of Cardiology, under the sponsorship of the Swiss Foundation of Cardiology, to retrospectively analyze young patients with coronary artery disease for risk factors, clinical course, and angiographic findings, which are possibly different compared to older patients. In the five Swiss university centers, data of all patients were collected who had suffered from angina pectoris or MI at an age of 35 years or younger and in whom selective angiography was performed. At a round table discussion problems of risk factors, clinical course, angiographic findings, operative treatment, and prognosis were presented at the annual session of our society (Burkart et al. 1980). Moret has presented the risk factors of these patients (pp. 17 ff.), therefore, the angiographic findings together with a short description of the clinical course shall be discussed in this paper.

Materials and Methods

Patients. A sample of 185 angiographically documented cases were collected covering an approximately 10-year period. In the Basel study the incidence of coronary artery disease in 25–35-year-old people was 13% (Widmer et al. 1981): This figure includes the asymptomatic patients with diagnostic ST-T changes, however. With the given mortality rate for this age group and assuming a 40% early mortality of MI, the incidence of symptomatic diseases for this young patient group is approximately 10 per 100000 (Junod et al. 1980). The total figure for the 10-year period for Switzerland would then be 400. The presented data therefore covered about half of the diseased people in Switzerland with clinical symptoms (Burkart et al. 1980). In 36 of the 185 patients only angina pectoris was present, in 149 (80.5%) MI had developed.

Clinical Course. Transmural infarction was found in 131 patients and nontransmural infarction in 18. In 86 cases anterior infarction was present, in 61 inferior, and in two patients there was extensive infarction in both areas.

About half of the patients showed angina pectoris prior to MI. In 35 patients the interval between onset of ischemic pain and MI was less than 1 week and in 35 patients it lasted more than 4 weeks. Of these patients, 80% had been hospitalized dur-

---

1 Cardiologic Divisions of the University Clinics, Kantonsspital Basel and Inselspital Bern, Switzerland

ing the acute illness. The following rhythm disturbances were treated as follows: eight ventricular tachycardias; five ventricular fibrillations; five severe conduction defects. In 11 patients clinically important left heart failure was present, in three patients there was pulmonary oedema, and in one patient cardiogenic shock. During the hospital phase there were no deaths, mainly due to the fact that patients who died in the early phase had not been investigated angiographically and were not included in the present study.

Interpretation of Angiographic Findings. In every coronary angiogram the left anterior descending, the right coronary artery, and the circumflex branch were assessed. Stenoses of less than 50% were estimated as insignificant. The significant stenoses were divided into 50%–75% and 76%–90% subtotal stenosis and occlusions, respectively. For the ventriculogram we differentiated hypokinesia, akinesia, and dyskinesia in the anterolateral, the inferior, and the posterior area. The calculated total ejection fraction finally was taken as a figure for the global function of the left ventricle.

Results

As is shown in Fig. 1, in 13 patients coronary arteries were totally normal, and in eight other patients no hemodynamically significant stenosis could be found. Thus, a total of 14% showed no hemodynamic relevant coronary artery disease. More than half of all investigated patients presented one-vessel disease, 23% two-vessel disease, and 35% three-vessel disease. This distribution shows the importance of one-vessel disease in these patients.

In Fig. 2 the 202 diseased vessels were divided according to the severity of stenosis. In 14% the stenosis was moderate to severe (51%–75%), in 32% stenosis was 76%–90%, in 22% of the patients subtotal stenosis, and in 32% total occlusion was found. The left anterior descending was diseased in more than half of the cases, the right coronary artery in 33%, and the circumflex branch in 17% of all hemodynamically relevant stenoses.

In 112 patients one area, in ten patients two, and in one patient all three areas were found to be contracting abnormally. In 19 patients wall motion was thought to

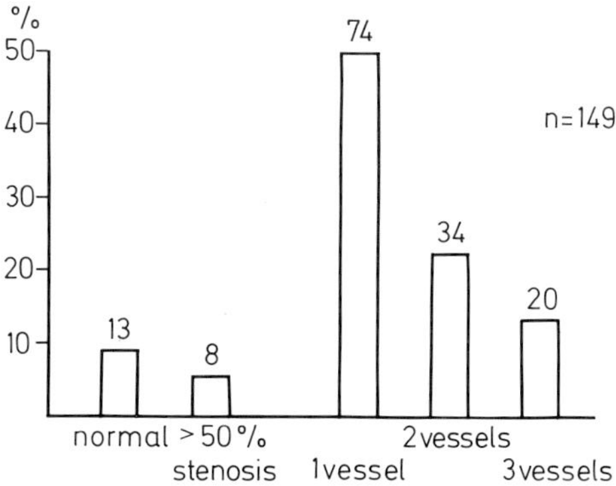

Fig. 1. Severity of coronary artery disease of the 149 patients with a clinical diagnosis of MI

be completely normal and in an additional seven angiograms no classification was possible. The most common finding observed was hypokinesia, as shown in Fig. 3, though 32% of the patients showed akinesia, and the abnormal function was described as dyskinesia in 27 patients. More than for the coronary angiograms, there was a predominance of the anterolateral area which was affected in 60%, followed by the inferior wall.

The ejection fraction was high in one-third of the patients (70% or more). In another 18%, ejection fraction was normal with more than 60% (Fig. 4). In 35%, global

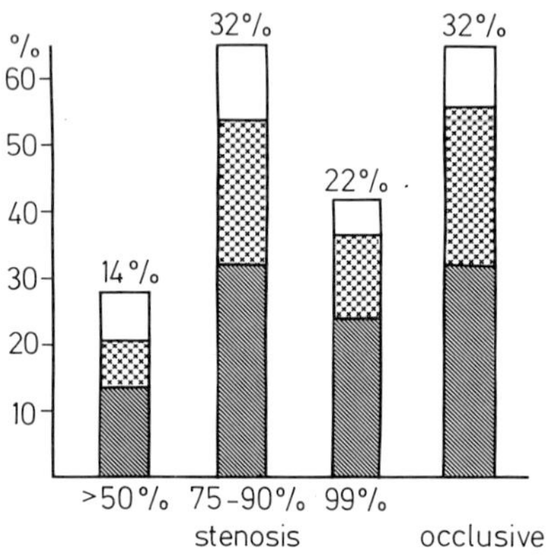

Fig. 2. The degree of stenosis in 202 vessels with hemodynamically significant stenosis. In addition the localization in the left anterior descending (LAD), the right coronary artery (RCA) and the left circumflex (LCX) is shown

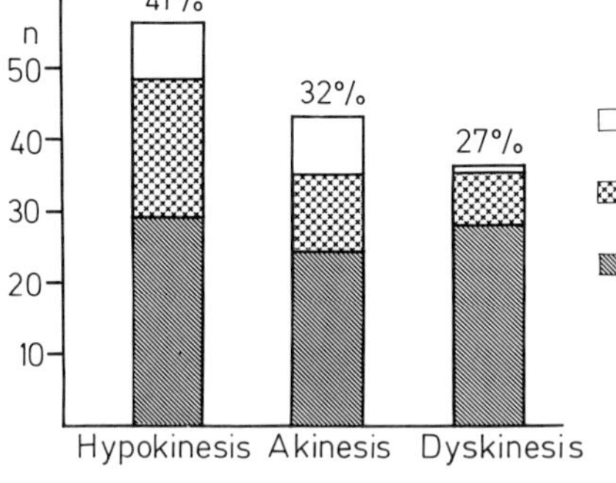

Fig. 3. Abnormal wall motion is divided in hypokinesia, akinesia, and dyskinesia in the anterolateral, inferior, and the posterior areas

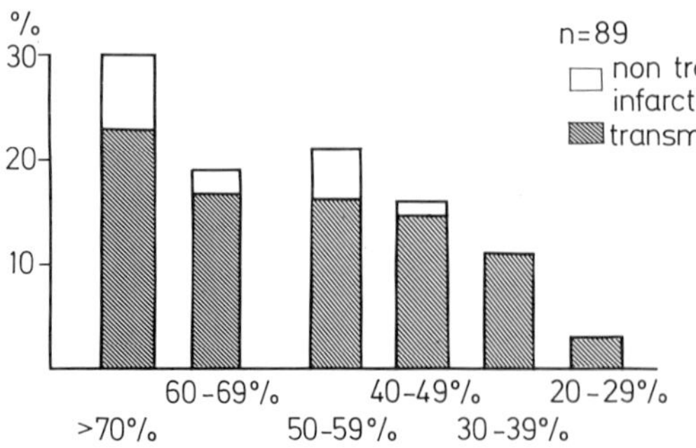

Fig. 4. The calculated ejection fraction from 89 patients. Patients with nontransmural infarctions ($N = 18$) are shown *open columns* and with transmural infarctions ($N = 71$) *hatched columns* are shown

ventricular function was slightly decreased and in 13% there was severe dysfunction of the left ventricle with an ejection fraction of less than 40%. All 18 patients with nontransmural infarction had normal or only slightly decreased ejection fractions.

For the diagnosis, as well as for the prognosis, patients with normal coronary arteriograms and/or normal ventricular wall motion are an important group. We therefore separately analyzed the 21 patients with normal coronary arteries or only insignificant stenosis and the 19 patients with normal ventricular wall motion after MI. Only four patients with nonsignificant stenoses also had a normal ventriculogram: In another nine hypokinesia, in five akinesia, and in three dyskinesia was found. On the other hand, patients with normal ventricular wall motions showed moderate to severe stenoses in four patients, subtotal stenosis in seven, and coronary occlusion in three. Thus, only in four patients with a clinical diagnosis of MI the coronary angiogram and the ventriculogram detected no abnormality.

Discussion

Also the proportion of MI patients with normal coronary arteries at investigation is high compared to a group not corrected for age. As Gohlke and co-workers showed that the percentage of patients with normal coronary arteries decreases with age by 31% in the patients under the age of 30 and 6% in the age group 35–40 years (see p. 61). In these patients coronary spasms, as described by Maseri et al. (1975), or acute thrombosis must be discussed as the cause of acute AMI. If a normal ventriculogram ist present, the correct clinical diagnosis must be discussed. Especially in nontransmural infarction with normal QRS complexes, diagnosis may be incorrect despite elevated enzyme levels and the typical pain. On the other hand, we have found normal ventricular wall motion in 15 patients with abnormal coronary arteries and in 70 patients the clinical diagnosis was proven angiographically by abnormal wall motion despite normal coronary angiogram. Therefore, at least in a few patients, combination of both normal findings can be accepted.

The fact that, in young patients, abnormally high physical workload can trigger MI, as described in the literature (see pp. 108, 115) cannot be documented from the data of our patients.

In conclusion, the majority of these young patients had one-vessel disease; more than those who had two- and three-vessel disease combined. The left anterior descending coronary artery is affected in more than half of the patients. In an important percentage (14%) the coronary arteries showed no important stenosis, and in 13 patients they were completely normal. Despite the fact that, in the majority, ventricular function could be preserved in 13%, the function was reduced severely to an ejection fraction of less than 40%. It therefore seems that in these young patients adaptation of the coronary vascular bed with the development of anastomoses is less common than in older age. That may be one explanation for the incidence of wall motion abnormalities in a patient group where one-vessel disease is present in more than 50%.

References

Burkart F, Meier C, Gutzwiller F, Moret P, Baumann PC, Rati R, Salzmann C, Rivier JL, Sigward U (1980) Die koronare Herzkrankheit beim jungen Patienten unter 35 Jahren in der Schweiz. Schweiz Med Wochenschr 110:1631–1643

Junod B, Alexander J, Wittlisbach V (1980) Evolution par cohorte et autres facteurs associés à la mortalité par maladie ischémique du cœur en Suisse. Schweiz Med Wochenschr 110:1701–1703

Maseri A, Mimmo R, Chierchia S, Marchesi C, Pesola A, d'Abbate A (1975) Coronary artery spasm as a cause of acute myocardial ischemia in man. Chest 68:625

Widmer L, Stähelin HB, Nissen C, da Silva A (1981) Venen-Arterien- und Herzkrankheiten bei Berufstätigen. Huber, Bern (Basler Studien I–III)

Coronary Angiographic Findings and Risk Factors in Postinfarction Patients Under the Age of 40

H. Gohlke, P. Stürzenhofecker, A. Thilo, C. Droste, L. Görnandt, and H. Roskamm [1]

Introduction

Myocardial infarction (MI) is – together with sudden cardiac death and angina pectoris – one of the three major manifestations of coronary artery disease.

MI is usually considered a disease of middle age, but epidemiological [1–3], clinical [4–7] and pathological [8] data indicate that 3%–6% of MIs occur under the age of 40. This percentage appears remarkably similar in different countries, irrespective of the overall incidence of MI [1].

Although this percentage may appear small, MI at young age is an important cause of longterm disability and has a great impact on the future job activity of the individual patient [9]. Therefore it appears necessary to evaluate the underlying risk factors in young patients who have suffered an MI to determine whether MI at young age represents an accelerated form of the same disease seen in older patients or whether there are features to suggest that different disease mechanisms may be operative in young patients.

The present study was undertaken to determine the angiographic findings and the constellation of risk factors in patients who survived a transmural MI under the age of 40.

Patient Material

Between 1973 and 1980, 844 patients with a documented transmural MI under the age of 40 were referred to our Rehabilitationszentrum in Bad Krozingen, Germany, for evaluation. The diagnosis of transmural MI was based on the WHO ECG criteria. In addition most of the patients had a clinical event with pain followed by a characteristic rise and fall of serum enzymes. A detailed history was taken from all patients with regard to the presence or absence of risk factors.

Coronary angiography and left ventriculography were performed using Sones or Judkins technique. Multiple projections including caudocranial views were performed to ensure adequate visualization of all vessels. A more than 50% narrowing of the luminal diameters of one of the three main vessels as measured with a caliper was considered a significant lesion.

Left ventricular angiography was performed in the 30° right anterior oblique (RAO) position and the left ventricle was divided into 5 segments (anterobasal, anterolateral, apical, diaphragmal, and posterobasal); except in a few patients examined in the initial study period, LV-angiography was also performed in the left

---

1 Rehabilitationszentrum, Südring 15, 7812 Bad Krozingen, FRG

anterior oblique (LAO) position where the LV circumference was divided into two segments (septal and posterolateral).

Left ventricular (LV) dysfunction was graded on a scale of 1 to 4 depending on the number of hypo- or akinetic segments. LV function was considered as normal, with one mildly hypokinetic segment, as mildly impaired with two or less hypo- or akinetic segments, as moderately impaired with three or more hypo- or akinetic, segments and as severely impaired when nearly all segments of the left ventricle showed severe hypo- or akinesis.

Results

Coronary Angiography

Of the patients referred 80%, gave informed consent and underwent angiography. There were 649 male patients and 30 female patients. The mean age at the time of MI was 35.9 years. The median time interval between the acute event and angiography was three months.

Patients were divided into three groups according to age: those less than 30 years old at the time of myocardial infarction, those 30–34 years old, and those 35–39 years old (Table 1).

Only 8% of patients were in the age-group below 30; 25% were in the age-group 30–34, and 67% were in the age-group 35–39 years.

Whereas the number of male patients increases more than ninefold from the younger group to the older group, there is only a two-and-a-half-fold increase in the number of female patients in the corresponding groups, indicating that in females

Table 1. Age distribution of 679 patients with transmural MI under the age of 40, who underwent coronary angiography

	Male	Female	Total	%
< 30 years	46	6	52	8
30 – 34 years	166	8	174	25
35 – 39 years	437	16	453	67
Total	649	30	679	100

Table 2. Coronary angiographic findings in 679 patients with the distribution of zero-, single-, double-, and triple-vessel disease

Disease	%
Zero-vessel disease	8.4 (3.7 normal coronary arteries, 4.7 less than 50% narrowing)
1-vessel disease	57.3
2-vessel disease	19.1
3-vessel disease	15.2

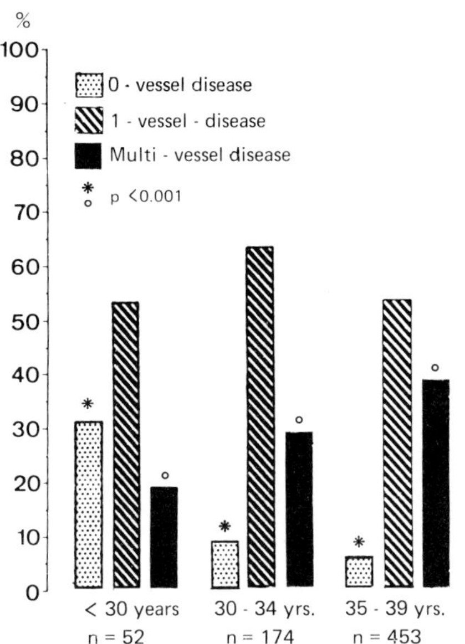

Fig. 1. Distribution of zero, single-, and multi-vessel disease in patients below 30, age 30–34, and age 35–39 at the time of MI

the mechanisms leading to myocardial infarction are predominantly age-independent.

The angiographic findings of the 679 patients are listed in Table 2. In 3.7% of patients we found entirely normal coronary arteries and an additional 4.7% had less than 50% luminal diameter narrowing, i.e., 8.4% of the patients were classified als "zero-vessel disease".

Single-vessel disease was present in 57.3%: thus two thirds of patients had zero- or single-vessel disease. This is in marked contrast to older patients after MI where multi-vessel disease predominates [10, 11].

In our young patients where the only selection criterion for coronary angiography was the presence of a documented transmural MI, the prevalence of zero-vessel disease decreased with increasing age. 31% of patients under the age of 30 had zero-vessel disease, 9% in the age group 30–34 and 6% in the age-group 35–39. Multi-vessel disease showed a corresponding increase with increasing age and the percentage in the three age-groups was 13%, 29% and 39% respectively (Fig. 1).

Both these differences in the prevalence of zero-vessel disease and multi-vessel disease with increasing age are statistically highly significant ($P < 0.001$).

In 19.4% of patients there was only a single stenosis in the entire coronary tree; this stenosis correlated with the site of MI. Approximately 50% of these patients had this single lesion in the proximal portion of the left anterior descending artery (LAD), prior to the first septal perforator.

Left Ventricular Angiography

The percentage of patients with normal or mildly and moderately or severely impaired left ventricular function in the three different age-groups is listed in Figure 2.

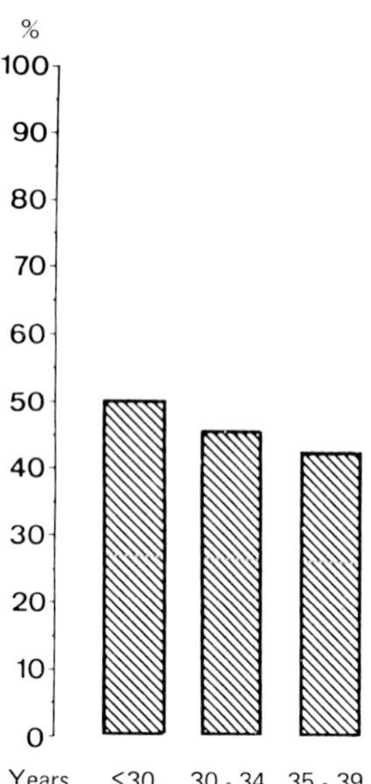

Fig. 2. Percent of patients with moderately or severely impaired left ventricular function in three different age groups

Although the incidence of multi-vessel disease is significantly higher in the older age-groups, the percentage of patients with moderately or severely impaired LV function tended to be higher in the group under age 30.

This can be explained by the significantly higher percentage of anterior wall infarctions in patients with zero- and single-vessel disease. This percentage of anterior wall infarction is 67% in patients with zero-vessel disease as compared to only 36% in patients with triple-vessel disease (Fig. 3).

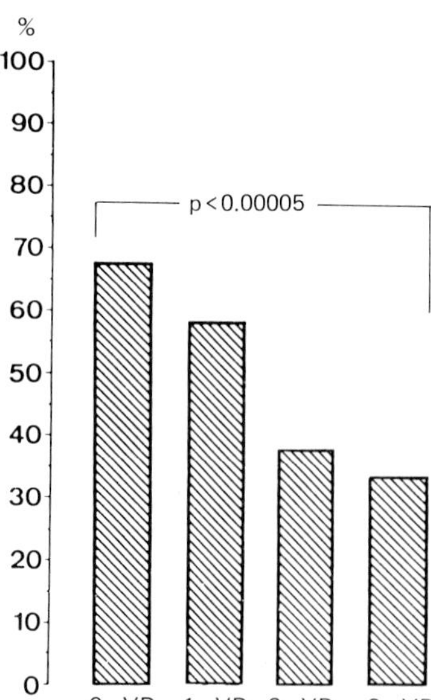

Fig. 3. Prevalence of anterior wall infarction in patients with "zero-vessel disease", single-, double-, and triple-vessel disease

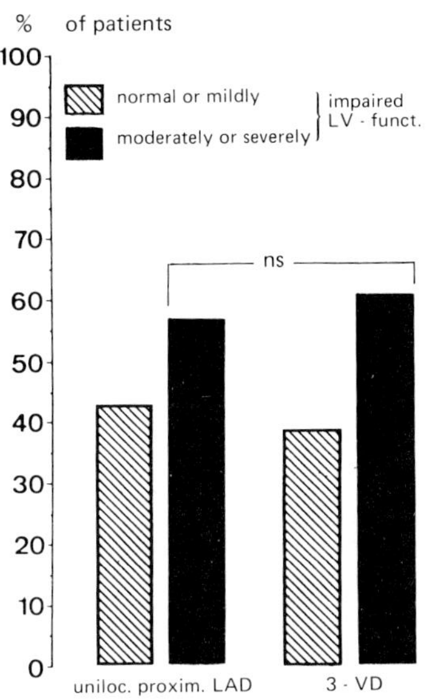

Fig. 4. Extent of left ventricular dysfunction in patients with unilocular proximal LAD disease and in patients with triple-vessel disease

The extent of coronary artery disease correlated only roughly with the degree of LV dysfunction after MI; it was the location of the lesion that determined the size of MI. Figure 4 compares two groups of patients with respect to LV dysfunction: one group with unilocular coronary artery disease but in a strategically important location in the proximal portion of the LAD prior to the origin of the first septal perforator; the second group of patients with triple-vessel disease. Despite the marked difference in the extent of coronary artery disease, the percentage of patients with moderately or severely impaired LV dysfunction is similiar.

Risk Factors

Eight risk factors were evaluated. The definition for the individual risk factors is given in Table 3. In addition the use of oral contraceptive drugs was registered. The

Table 3. Risk factor definition for the eight risk factors examined

Factor	Definition
Nicotine	> 10 cigarettes/day
Hypercholesterolemia	> 260 mg%
Hypertriglyceridemia	> 150 mg%
Hyperurecemia	7 mg% in males/6.5 mg% in females
Obesity	Broca Index > 10%
Arterial Hypertension	syst. $\geq$ 160 mmHg/diast. $\geq$ 90 mmHg
Family history	for AP, MI, stroke, HTN in first degree relatives
Diabetes mellitus	clinically manifest DM

Table 4. Prevalence of risk factors in 649 male and 30 female patients

649 ♂ patients		30 ♀ patients	
Nicotine	86.0%	Orale contraceptives	86%
Hypertriglycerid.	80.0%	Nicotine	67%
Family Hx	56.0%	Family Hx	67%
Hypercholest.	47.0%	Hypertriglycerid.	47%
Obesity	46.0%	Obesity	40%
Hyperuricemia	28.0%	Hypercholest.	33%
Art. HTN	27.0%	Art. HTN	20%
Diabetes	0.3%	Hyperuricemia	7%
		Diabetes	0%

prevalence of the individual risk factors in the male and female patients is given in Table 4.

The prevalence of risk factors in a normal population of similiar age in the south-western part of Germany has been examined by Nüssel et al. [12]. Their definitions were similiar to ours, except smokers were not divided into those with more than 10 cigarettes and those with less than 10 cigarettes per day; also a family history was not obtained. The incidence of risk factors in this normal male population is compared to the incidence of risk factors in our male patients (Fig. 5).

The most frequent risk factor is nicotine abuse with 63% (including ex-smokers) in the normal population and 93% in our male patients, including those patients who smoked less than 10 cigarettes per day. Hypertriglyceridemia (79%) and hyper-

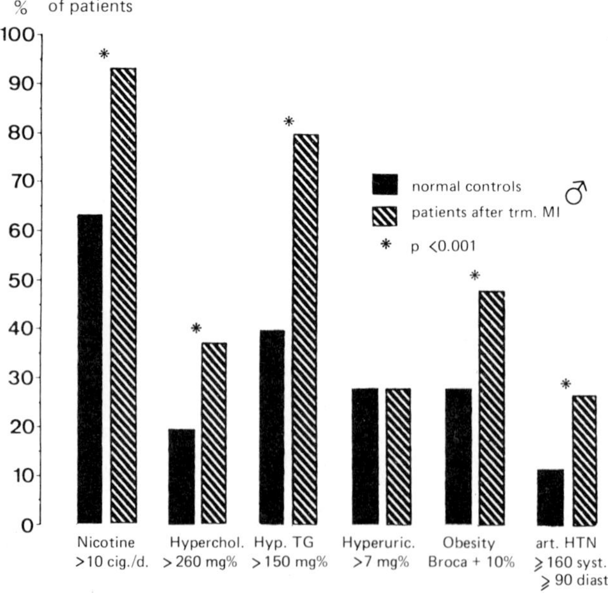

Fig. 5. Comparison of the prevalence of risk factors in our 649 male patients with transmural MI under the age of 40, and 1465 male controls age 30 to 39 [12]

cholesterolemia (47%) are approximately twice as frequent in postinfarction patients as in controls ($P < 0.001$). The same is true for arterial hypertension and obesity. There was no difference in the prevalence of hyperuricemia or diabetes as compared to controls.

In the female patients the most frequent risk factor was the use of oral contraceptives in 86% of patients (19 out of 22 patients where this information was available). Although the percentage of normal controls taking oral contraceptive drugs in Germany is not known, it is estimated at 25%–30% (Professor Breckwoldt, University of Freiburg). 90% of patients taking oral contraceptive drugs are also smokers. The combination of oral contraceptive use and smoking appears to be the typical risk factor constellation for female patients under the age of 40.

The correlation of the individual risk factors with the extent of coronary artery disease is shown in Figure 6.

Patients with zero-vessel disease are compared to patients with single-, double-, and triple-vessel disease. Three risk factors show a statistically significant correlation with the extent of coronary artery disease: Hypercholesterolemia, hypertriglyceridemia, and arterial hypertension ($P < 0.05$).

Figure 7 shows the mean serum cholesterol levels in subgroups with different degrees of coronary atherosclerosis: patients with normal coronary arteries, patients with unilocular disease, zero-, single-, double-, and triple-vessel disease, and triple-vessel disease with more than 75% stenosis in all three vessels. Cigarette consumption was uniformly high in all groups. The correlation of hyperuricemia, obesity, and a positive family history with increasing number of vessels diseased, does not reach statistical significance. Patients with zero-vessel disease had a mean number

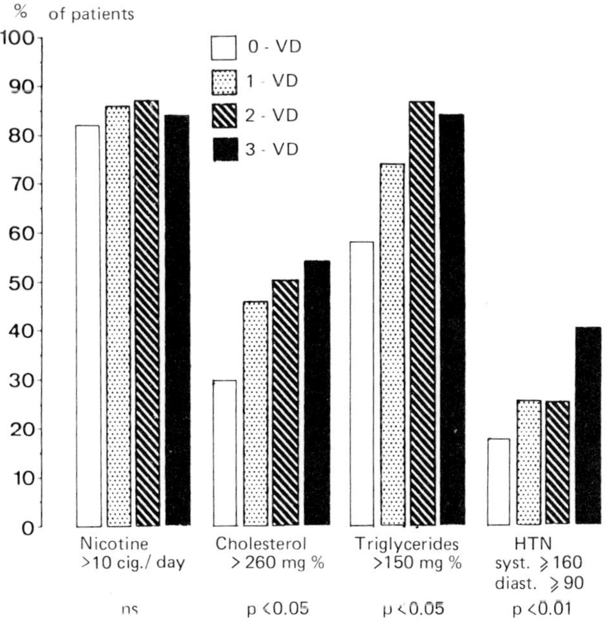

Fig. 6. Comparison of risk factors with extent of coronary artery disease: prevalence of risk factors in subgroups of patients with zero-, single-, double-, and triple-vessel disease

of 2.5 risk factors per patient, and patients with triple-vessel disease a mean number of 3.5 risk factors per patient compared to only 1.9 risk factors for the normal population.

Approximately 25% of patients after MI have a risk factor constellation that is not markedly different from controls. These patients are younger and have less extensive vessel disease than patients with more risk factors.

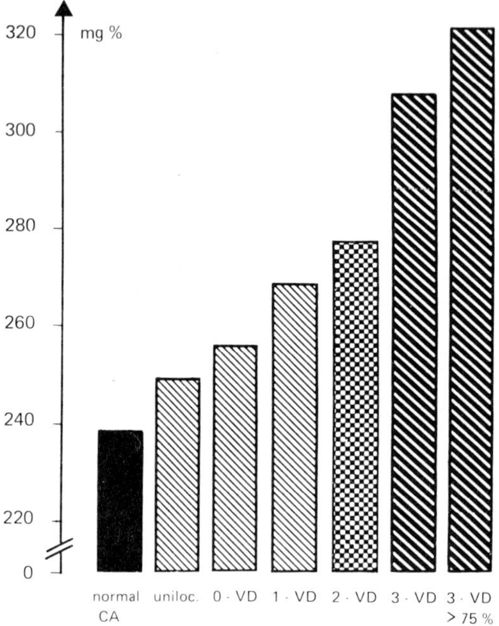

Fig. 7. Mean serum cholesterol levels in subgroups of patients with different extent of coronary artery disease: mean serum cholesterol levels increase with more advanced coronary disease

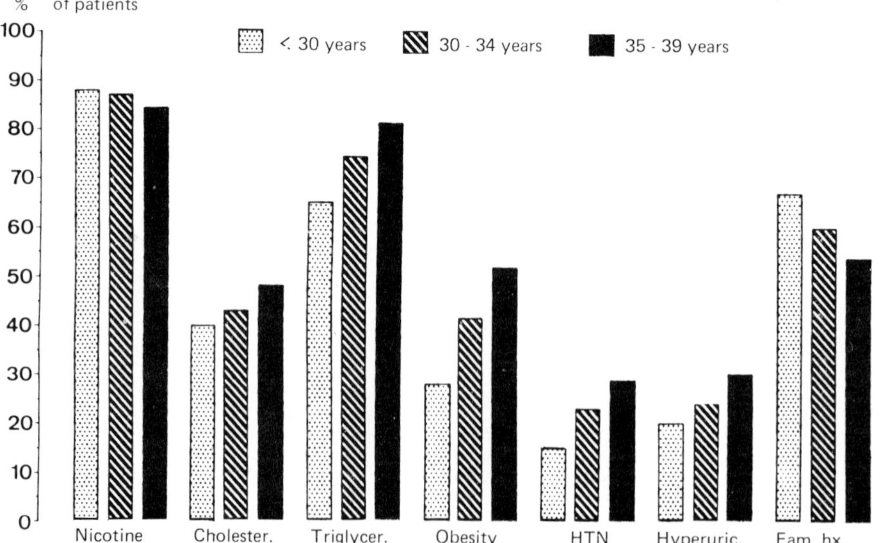

Fig. 8. Prevalence of the risk factors in patients in the three age groups

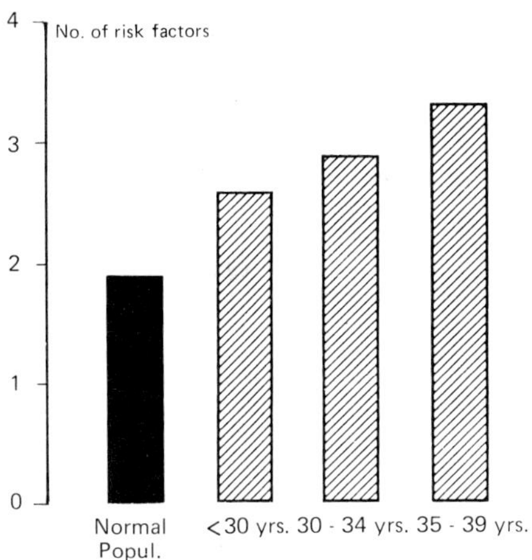

Fig. 9. Mean number of risk factors in patients with transmural MI in the three different age groups, compared to normal controls [12]

The prevalence of the individual risk factors in the three different age-groups is shown in Figure 8. The prevalence of five risk factors increased with age; the prevalence of cigarette smoking declined slightly with age and there was a moderate decrease of the frequency of a positive family history as the age at MI increased. Overall the mean number of risk factors increased with age (Fig. 9).

Discussion

Patient Material

Our series of patients with transmural MI under the age of 40 who underwent coronary angiography is the largest single series of such patients reported in the literature. A part of this series has been reported on previously [13–17].

Our series differs from most others in that the inclusion criterion was uniform throughout the entire study period: the only requirement was a documented transmural MI under the age of 40.

Other series of patients after MI at young age include patients with subendocardial (nontransmural) MI, or patients who show both normal coronary arteries and normal LV function after infarction [18, 19], leaving some doubt about the validity of the diagnosis. None of these patients are included in our series. In the initial study period a few patients were included in whom a transmural MI was documented by history, serial ECG and enzyme changes, but whose LV angiogram, performed only in the RAO projection, showed no abnormality. Alle these patients had significant coronary stenoses corresponding with the site of MI as determined by ECG.

Patients with normal LV angiogram in the RAO and LAO projection were not included in our series. Also excluded were patients with congenital anomalies presenting with an infarction pattern patients with associated valvular disease, and patients after chest trauma.

Virtually all patients seen in our institution are referred from community hospitals, largely from the state of Baden-Württemberg. We think that our patients are representative of young patients in Germany who survive the acute phase of transmural MI for the following reasons: (a) the referring community hospitals had been asked to send all their patients with MI under age 40, irrespective of their symptomatology, and (b) coronary angiography was recommended to all patients, irrespective of their clinical status or symptoms. This gives us the opportunity to compare the younger to the older patients within this group with respect to risk factors and angiographic findings.

Patients in other countries with different diet habits may have different risk factor constellations or may present with different findings [20].

Angiographic Findings

A remarkable finding in this group of young patients is the relatively high percentage of patients who have no significant obstruction at the time of angiography, in contrast to older postinfarction patients where this is rare. This finding is not explained by different selection criteria for coronary angiography in older patients; within our series where the indication for angiography was applied uniformly, the prevalence of zero-vessel disease decreases with increasing age, from 31% of patients under 30 to 6% of patients between 35 and 39.

This is in agreement with reports in the literature where it has been emphasized that patients with normal coronary arteries after MI tend to be younger than patients with atherosclerotic changes [18, 19, 21–25].

The true prevalence of MI and normal coronary arteries has not been established. Bruschke et al. [26] reported a 4.2% prevalence in patients undergoing coronary angiography after documented MI. Khan and Haywood [27] reported a prevalence of 11% (9 out of 78 patients). Despite this relatively high prevalence, Erlenbacher [24], in a review of the literature, compiled less than 100 cases and of these only 56 had truly normal coronary arteries. Our study is the first series of a defined population after transmural MI to show a clearly age related prevalence of normal coronary arteries. The prevalence in the small number of patients under 30 is high, but it declines rapidly as the age at MI increases.

It has to be assumed that in these patients a high grade stenosis or obstruction at the time of MI has regressed to a non-significant stenosis at the time of coronary angiography [28]. Coronary embolism, platelet aggregation with later fragmentation, and thrombosis with later recanalization, as well as the interaction of platelet aggregates with coronary spasm and atherosclerotic lesions or endothelial damage, have all been suggested as possible mechanisms for this phenomenon [22, 24, 28–33].

It appears less likely that a stenosis due to an atherosclerotic lesion would undergo regression within the short time interval between MI and angiography. James [34] has questioned the entity of normal coronary arteries after MI and claimed that lesions have been overlooked by the angiographer or that the quality of the film may not be sufficient to pick up lesions that may be very localized. It is the general impression that the degree of coronary atherosclerosis is usually underestimated by coronary angiography [28, 34–39].

This is particularly the case in vessels with a more than 50% narrowing of the luminal diameter, because the diffuseness of the disease may not allow estimation of the true diameter of the original lumen [36]. Although this may be a valid argument and may indeed apply to single cases, this is not true for the majority of patients in our series. If normal coronary arteries are found after MI, particular care is taken by the angiographer to visualize the portion of the coronary artery responsible for the MI.

The argument that a small side branch of a coronary artery may be occluded at the origin, and may not visualize, is not valid for the majority of our patients because the size of MI is substantial and cannot be explained by the occlusion of a side branch. Also autopsy findings in patients with normal coronary arteries after MI have been reported [21, 40–42]. The prevalence of infarction without morphologic evidence of an acute occlusion and without pre-existent severe coronary artery disease was 7% in a consecutive series of 100 autopsied cases [40].

If coronary spasm plays a role in the development of MI it must be an entity that is distinctly different from the *Prinzmetal-angina syndrome,* because of our 169 patients with zero-vessel disease or unilocular disease there is not a single patient who had a history of repeated episodes of angina suggestive of coronary spasm prior to MI.

The prevalence of single-vessel disease is more than 50% in all three of our age groups which is in contrast to older patients after MI, where multi-vessel disease predominates [10, 11].

Our findings are in agreement with other series of young postinfarction patients reported in the literature [43–45].

In our younger age-group, the patients had a higher incidence of zero- and single-vessel disease, and in turn patients with zero- and single-vessel disease had a significantly higher incidence of anterior wall infarction than patients with multi-vessel disease (Fig. 3). This is in agreement with other reports in the literature on young patients after MI [42]. Also several autopsy series on young patients after sudden death or MI report a high incidence of involvement of the left anterior descending artery with associated anterior wall infarction [46–49]. This may explain why the extent of LV dysfunction is at least as great in the younger patients as in older patients, despite the lesser degree of coronary artery disease.

In patients with multi-vessel disease the growth of stenoses is slower and leaves time for the development of collaterals in a significant number of patients.

An interesting subgroup of patients is those who have only unilocular diseae, i.e., a single stenosis in the entire coronary tree. Depending on the location of the stenosis, the size of the MI may be very large, e.g., in patients with unilocular disease in the proximal portion of the LAD. This subgroup of patients is unique in so far as repeat angiograms after more than three years have shown that a regression of stenosis occurs in a significant percentage of cases [17]. We do not know the histology in these patients, but the rather rapid development of a single stenosis and its subsequent regression make a thrombotic origin more likely than an atherosclerotic origin.

Risk Factors

The risk factor profile in these patients was obtained prospectively in a standardized manner to avoid bias of the interviewer. The likelihood that abnormal values will be found increases in a population that is examined repeatedly, like our patients; this makes a comparison to normal controls difficult because the controls are usually examined at a single point in time. Nevertheless, the comparison is useful in estimating the prevalence of different risk factors in a normal population because risk factors may vary from country to country [20], and from age-group to age-group [50].

Nicotine. Cigarette smoking has been mentioned as one of the most important risk factors in virtually all studies of MI in the young age-group [4, 20, 25, 43, 44, 50, 51–55]. Elmfeldt et al. (50) showed that cigarette comsumption was a stronger risk factor for MI in young age groups. In one autopsy series of young patients with MI or sudden cardiac death, excessive cigarette consumption preceeded death in a significant number of cases [46]. A particularly noteworthy finding in this series was the high incidence of intimal edema, which contributed to the luminal narrowing.

In our study the percentage of patients smoking ten or more cigarettes per day is above 80% in all age-groups. It is similarly high in patients with zero-, single-, double-, and triple-vessel disease. Nicotine abuse probably plays a role as a trigger mechanism [56, 57] for the initiation of MI; in several studies it is not associated with a higher incidence of angina pectoris [58, 59]. In our study the extent of vessel involvement in smokers and non-smokers was not different.

Nicotine abuse as a risk factor has been particularly stressed in series of patients with normal coronary arteries [24, 25, 55] and has been related to reinfarction in such patients [25]. However, comparable data on patients of similar age with MI and coronary disease are not available in those studies. Our data indicate that smoking is a very important risk factor in young patients, regardless of the number of vessels involved.

Hypercholesterolemia is one of the most important risk factors for the development of coronary atherosclerosis in young individuals [60, 61]. Our study showed a clear relationship between the extent of coronary atherosclerosis and the mean serum cholesterol level. Patients with zero- oder single-vessel disease had significantly lower serum cholesterol levels than patients with multi-vessel disease. However, 27% of our male patients and 40% of our female patients had serum cholesterol levels of less than 220 mg%, which can be considered normal in this age group.

The prevalence of *hypertriglyceridemia* is similarly related to the extent of coronary artery disease, although the relationship is not quite as close. Smokers with comparable levels of serum cholesterol had significantly higher serum triglycerides as compared to nonsmokers. This is in agreement with reports in the literature on other patient populations [62].

Arterial hypertension is a well established risk factor for the development of coronary heart disease [57]. The prevalence of arterial hypertension in our patients is twice that of the general population, but lower compared to older patients after MI [63]. However, the correlation with the extent of coronary artery disease was highly significant ($P < 0.01$). Within our age groups the prevalence of hypertension increases with age. Our findings are in agreement with other reports on young patients after MI where the hypertension risk factor was of less importance than in older patients [7, 20, 44, 50, 52, 64].

Family History. The familial occurrence of coronary heart disease has been the subject of several studies [65–70]. Rissanen [70] has investigated the incidence of cardiac deaths and the prevalence of coronary risk factors in first degree relatives of patients who had suffered a coronary event. Both risk factors and coronary deaths were more frequent in first degree relatives of patients who had suffered their coronary event before age 45, as compared to those who had suffered their coronary event at a later age.

In our study, a similiar tendency is shown; the results do not reach statistical significance, probably because our age range is too narrow and the number of patients in the age-group under 30 years is small. The tendency is, however, opposite to the other risk factors which show an increase with age. Does the positive family history reflect a genetic trait, or merely the influence of environmental factors like diet and smoking habits?

While our study was not designed to answer this question, the lower number of risk factors in the younger patients, together with a higher prevalence of a positive family history do suggest that for the very young patients heritable rather than environmental factors may play an important role in the early manifestation of coronary heart disease.

Obesity. The prevalence of obesity in our patients was almost twice as high as in the control population. Obesity as a risk factor varies in different populations, in a study in young patients after MI performed in 9 countries [20], obesity was especially common in Heidelberg, Cape Town, and Tel Aviv, whereas it was distinctly uncommon in Bombay, Melbourne, Singapore, and Edinburgh. Obesity has been questioned as a risk factor per se [17]; if hypertensive subjects are eliminated, obesity may add little to the risk of coronary artery disease. However, several series of young patients after MI describe a high prevalence of obesity [4, 53, 54, 72]. In the Framingham study, weight was a significant risk factor although of less importance than cholesterolemia, nicotine and blood pressure [60].

Hyperuricemia was no more prevalent in our patients than in our controls; like obesity, the prevalence in different populations differs [20].

Diabetes mellitus was rare in our patients which is in agreement with other series of MI at young age [44, 52].

Oral Contraceptives. The use of oral contraceptives has been shown to increase the incidence of myocardial infarction and cardiac deaths in young women [73–76]. The increased risk is particularly evident in patients with other risk factors. The annual risk of MI for female patients aged 38–40 has been estimated to increase by a ratio of 50 if both cigarette smoking and oral contraceptive use are present, compared to patients where only one of these is present [76].

Our data are in agreement with these reports. None of our female patients was free of the conventional risk factors; in addition 86% of female patients – where this information was available (19/22) – were using oral contraceptives prior to MI. Of the women using oral contraceptives, 90% were also smokers. Thus the combination of oral contraceptive medication and cigarette smoking appears to be the typical risk factor constellation for MI in young women.

Ot has been suspected that the effects of oral contraceptive drugs on the clotting system, and of nicotine on the platelet aggregability, may potentiate and lead to thrombosis in the coronary artery. The high number of anterior wall infarctions with subsequent normal coronary arteries in our patients seems to support this hypothesis. Engel and Lichtlen [33] have observed angiographic regression in a female patient and also speculated that this probably represented recanalization or lysis of a thrombus.

Summary

The angiographic findings of patients with a transmural MI under the age of 40 are characterized by a high prevalence of zero- and single-vessel disease with an associated high prevalence of anterior wall infarction.

In spite of the lesser extent of coronary artery disease in patients under 30, the extent of LV dysfunction equals that of patients with more extensive coronary artery disease over 30.

These findings suggest that the development of coronary artery stenosis in these young patients occurs rather rapidly, leaving no time for adequate collateralization. The result is an extensive MI.

Smoking is the most important risk factor for MI in young male patients, the combination of smoking and oral contraceptive use the most important risk factor constellation in young females.

The lower prevalence of risk factors in younger patients suggests that other mechanisms than atherosclerosis may play an important role in the development of coronary stenosis. These mechanisms may be thrombosis, coronary spasm, or a combination of the two.

Acknowledgment. This work was supported by grants of the BMA and BMFT (Bundesministerium für Arbeit und Sozialordnung and Bundesministerium für Forschung und Technologie).

References

1. Lamm G (1981) The epidemiology of acute myocardial infarction in young age groups. This vol pp 5–12
2. Nüssel E, Buchholz L, Scheidt R (1981) Juvenile myocardial infarction in the Heidelberg register area. This vol pp 13–16
3. Bergstrand R, Vedin A, Wilhelmsson C et al. (1978) Myocardial infarction among men below age 40. Br Heart J 40:783–788
4. Tiso B, Herrlein A (1973) Zur Ätiologie des jugendlichen Herzinfarktes. MMW 115:2129–2136
5. Gurevich MA (1970) Myocardial infarction in young age. Kardiologiia 10:152, cited in (7)
6. Romanov YD (1963) Certain clinical features of myocardial infarction in young people. Klin Med Mosk 44:32, cited in (7)

7. Simonson E, Berman R (1972) Myocardial infarction in young people: Experience in USSR. Am Heart J 84:814–821
8. Silver MD, Baroldi G, Mariani F (1980) The relationship between acute occlusive coronary thrombi and myocardial infarction studied in 100 consecutive patients. Circulation 61:219–227
9. Samek L, Spinder M, Müller F et al. (1981) Occupational situation in postinfarction patients under age 40. This vol pp 174–186
10. Proudfit WL, Shirey EL, Sones MF (1966) Selective cinecoronary arteriography: Correlation with clinical findings in 1000 patients. Circulation 33:901–910
11. Samek L, Roskamm H, Rentrop P et al. (1975) Belastungsprüfungen und Koronarangiogramm im chronischen Infarktstadium. Z Kardiol 64:809–814
12. Nüssel E, Buchholz L, Ebschner KJ et al. (1980) Die Gemeinde als Ansatzstelle für eine Prävention. Internist (Berlin) 21:437–445
13. Kovacsics H, Weisswange A, Rentrop P, Roskamm H (1976) Der jugendliche Herzinfarkt. Therapiewoche 26:1768–1770
14. Kovacsics H, Roskamm H, Stürzenhofecker P, Petersen J (1977) Risikofaktoren und Koronarmorphologie bei 218 männlichen Infarktpatienten unter 40 Jahren. Z Kardiol 66:685–689
15. Kovacsics H, Kovacsics A, Petersen J et al. (1978) Langzeitschicksal nach Myokardinfarkt bei Männern unter 40 Jahren. Dtsch Z Sportmed 1:1–5
16. Gohlke H, Gohlke-Bärwolf C, Stürzenhofecker P et al. (1980) Myocardial infarction at young age – correlation of angiographic findings with factors and history in 619 patients (Abstr). Circulation (Suppl III) 62:39
17. Gohlke H, Stürzenhofecker P, Görnandt L et al. (1980) Progression und Regression im chronischen Infarktstadium bei Patienten unter 40 Jahren. Schweiz Med Wochenschr 110:1663–1665
18. Thompson SI, Vieweg WVR, Alpret JS, Hagan AD (1977) Incidence and age distribution of patients with myocardial infarction and normal coronary arteriograms. Cathet Cardiovasc Diagn 3:1–9
19. Warren E, Thompson I, Vieweg WVR (1979) Historic and angiographic features of young adults surviving myocardial infarction. Chest 75:667–670
20. Dolder MA, Oliver MF (1975) Myocardial infarction in young men – study of risk factors in nine countries. Br Heart J 37:493–503
21. Brest AN, Wiener L, Kasparian H et al. (1974) Myocardial infarction without obstructive coronary artery disease. Am Heart J 88:219–224
22. Rosenblatt A, Selzer A (1977) The nature and clinical features of myocardial infarction with normal coronary angiogram. Circulation 55:578–580
23. Russel RO, Eslami B, Rackley CH (1977) Acute myocardial infarction without coronary arteriographic abnormalities. Chest 72:133–134
24. Erlebacher JA (1979) Transmural myocardial infarction with "normal" coronary arteries. Am Heart J 98:421–430
25. McKenna WJ, Chew CYC, Oakley CM (1980) Myocardial infarction with normal coronary angiogram. Possible mechanism of smoking risk in coronary artery disease. Br Heart J 43:493–498
26. Bruschke AVG, Bruyneel KJJ, Bloch A, van Herpen G (1971) Acute myocardial infarction without obstructive coronary artery disease demonstrated by selective cineangiography. Br Heart J 33:585–594
27. Khan AH, Haywood LJ (1974) Myocardial infarction in nine patients with radiographically patent coronary arteries. New Engl J Med 291:427–431
28. Arnett EN, Roberts WC (1976) Acute myocardial infarction and angiographically normal coronary arteries: An unproven combination. Circulation 53:395–400
29. Oliva PB, Breckenridge JC (1977) Acute myocardial infarction with normal or near normal coronary arteries. Am J Cardiol 40:1000–1007
30. Henderson RR, Hansing CE, Razavi M, Rowe GG (1973) Resolution of an obstructive coronary lesion as demonstrated by selective angiography in a patient with transmural myocardial infarction. Am J Cardiol 31:785–788

31. Kimbiris D, Segal BL, Munir M et al. (1972) Myocardial infarction in patients with normal patent coronary arteries as visualized by cinearteriography. Am J Cardiol 29:724–728
32. Glancy DL, Marcus ML, Epstein SE (1971) Myocardial infarction in young women with normal coronary arteriograms. Circulation 544:495–502
33. Engel HJ, Lichtlen P (1978) Evidence of spontaneous thrombolysis in the human coronary system. In: Kaltenbach M, Lichtlen P, Balcon R, Bussmann WD (eds) Coronary heart disease. 3rd International Symposium Frankfurt. Thieme, Stuttgart, p 127
34. James TN (1970) Angina without coronary disease (Sic). Cirulation 42:189–191
35. Vlodaver Z, Frech R, van Tassel RA, Edwards JE (1973) Correlation of the antemortem coronary angiogram and postmortem specimen. Circulation 47:162–169
36. Arnett EN, Isner JM, Redwood DR et al. (1979) Coronary artery narrowing in coronary heart disease: Comparison of cineangiographic and necropsy findings. Ann Intern Med 91:350–356
37. Grondin CH, Dyrda J, Pasternac A et al. (1974) Discrepancies between cineangiographic and post mortem findings in patients with coronary artery disease and recent myocardial revascularization. Circulation 49:703–708
38. Schwarz JN, Kong Y, Hackel DB, Bartel AG (1975) Comparison of angiographic and post mortem findings in patients with coronary artery disease. Am J Cardiol 36:174–178
39. Hutchins GM, Bulkley BH, Ridolfi RL (1977) Correlation of coronary arteriograms and left ventriculograms with post mortem studies. Circulation 57:32–37
40. Eliot RS, Baroldi G, Leone A (1974) Necropsy studies in myocardial infarction with minimal or no coronary luminal reduction due to atherosclerosis. Circulation 49:1127–1131
41. Regan TJ, Wu CF, Weisse AB et al. (1975) Acute myocardial infarction in toxic cardiomyopathy without coronary obstruction. Circulation 51:453–461
42. Kordasz B, Oczkowicz-Palatyńska A, Rafalska K et al. (1979) Myocardial infarction in young men. In: Florence International Meeting on Myocardial Infarction. Mason DT, Neri Serneri GG, Oliver MF (eds) vol I. Excerpta Medica, Amsterdam Oxford Princeton, p 450–452
43. Savran SV, Bryson AL, Welch TG et al. (1976) Clinical correlates of coronary angiography in young males with myocardial infarction. Am Heart J 91:551–555
44. Recusani F, de Servi S, Fatica N et al. (1977) L' infarto miocardico in eta giovanile. G Ital Cardiol 7:441–447
45. Davia JE, Hallal FJ, Cheitlin MD et al. (1974) Coronary artery disease in young patients: Arteriographic and clinical review of 40 cases aged 35 and under. Am Heart J 87:689–696
46. Müller E (1949) Die tödliche Koronarsklerose bei jüngeren Männern. Beitr Pathol Anat 110:103–157
47. Meessen H (1944) Über den plötzlichen Herztod bei Frühsklerose und Frühthrombose der Koronararterien bei Männern unter 35 Jahren. Z Kardiol 7/8:185–201
48. Yater WM, Traum AH, Brown WG et al. (1948) Coronary artery disease in men eighteen to thirtynine years of age. Am Heart J 36:334–372, 481–526, 683–722
49. Virmani R, McAllister HA (1981) Myocardial infarction in patients under age 40 (autopsy findings). This vol pp 92–103
50. Elmfeldt D, Wilhelmsson C, Vedin JA et al. (1976) Characteristics of representative male survivors of myocardial infarction compared with representative population samples. Acta Med Scand 199:387–398
51. White PD (1935) Coronary disease and coronary thrombosis in youth. J Med Soc NJ 32:596
52. Moll A, Hamacher F (1962) Der Herzinfarkt im jüngeren Lebensalter. Enke, Stuttgart
53. Roth O, Berki A, Wolff GD (1967) Long range observations in fiftythree young patients with myocardial infarction. Am J Cardiol 19:331–338
54. Walker WJ, Gregoratos G (1967) Myocardial infarction in young men. Am J Cardiol 19:339–343
55. Oliver MF (1974) Ischemic heart disease in young women. A re-apparaisal of the sex factor. Acta Cardiol (Brux) 20:59–68
56. Gordon T, Kannel WB, McGee D, Dawber TR (1974) Death and coronary attacks in men after giving up cigarette smoking: A report from the Framingham study. Lancet II: 1345–1348

57. Wilhelmsen L, Wedel H, Tibblin G (1973) Multivariate analysis of risk factors for coronary heart disease. Circulation 48:950–958
58. Simborg DW (1970) The status of risk factors and coronary heart disease. J Chronic Dis 22:515
59. Jenkins CD, Rosenman RH, Zyzanski SJ (1968) Cigarette smoking: Its relationship to coronary heart disease and related risk factors in the western collaborative group study. Circulation 38:1140–1155
60. Truett J, Cornfield J, Kannel W (1967) A multivariate analysis of the risk of coronary heart disease in Framingham. J Chronic Dis 20:511–524
61. Kannel WB, Castelli WP, Gordon T, McNamara P (1971) Serum cholesterol, lipoproteins and the risk of coronary disease. Ann Intern Med 74:1–12
62. Erikssen J, Enger SC (1978) The effect of smoking on selected heart disease risk factors in middle aged men. Acta Med Scand 203:27–30
63. Schimmler W, Neef C, Schimert G (1968) Risikofaktoren und Herzinfarkt. MMW 110:1585–1593
64. Burkart F, Meier C, Gutzwiller F et al. (1980) Die koronare Herzkrankheit beim jungen Patienten unter 35 Jahren in der Schweiz. Schweiz Med Wochenschr 110:1631–1643
65. Rose G (1954) Familial patterns in ischemic heart disease. Br J Prev Soc Med 18:75–80
66. Thomas BC, Cohen BH (1955) The familial occurrence of hypertension and coronary artery disease, with observations concerning diabetes and obesity. Ann Intern Med 42:90–127
67. Shanoff HM, Little A, Murphy EA, Rykert HE (1961) Studies of the male survivors of myocardial infarction due to "essential" atherosclerosis. I. Characteristics of the patients. Can Med Assoc J 84:519–530
68. Deutscher S, Ostrander LD, Epstein FH (1970) Familial factors in premature coronary heart disease – a preliminary report from the Tecumseh community health study. Am J Epidemiol 91:233–237
69. Rissanen AM, Nikkilä EA (1977) Coronary disease and its risk factors in families of young men with angina pectoris and in controls. Br Heart J 39:875–883
70. Rissanen AM (1979) Familial occurrence of coronary heart disease: Effect of age at diagnosis. Am J Cardiol 44:60–66
71. Keys A, Blackburn H (1964) Background of the patient with coronary heart disease. Prog Cardiovasc Dis 6:14
72. Gertler MM, White PD (1954) Coronary heart disease in young adults: A multidisciplinary study. Cambridge, Harvard University Press
73. Mann JI, Vessey MP, Thorogodd M, Doll R (1975) Myocardial infarction in young women with special reference to oral contraceptive practice. Br Med J II:241–245
74. Mann JI, Inman WHW (1975) Oral contraceptives and death from myocardial infarction. Br Med J II:245–248
75. Shapiro S (1975) Oral contraceptives and myocardial infarction (editorial). N Engl J Med 293:195–196
76. Jick H, Dinan B, Rothman KJ (1978) Oral contraceptives and nonfatal myocardial infarction. JAMA 239:1403–1407

Evolution of Ventricular Function in Young Patients with Myocardial Infarction and Normal Coronary Arteries: Advantage of Isotopic Methods

M. Amor, J. L. Bourdon, M. Fischer, N. Danchin, A. Bertrand, G. Karcher, and F. Cherrier [1]

Myocardial infarction (MI) with normal coronary arteries is uncommon and only recently described [1, 2]. Few Studies have been devoted to its long term prognosis [3]

A first assessment, published 2 years ago [5], where patients were studied regardless of their ages, showed a good midterm prognosis. The present paper studies long-term prognosis in young patients (under age 40).

Patients and Methods

The following criteria were considered necessary for inclusion: age under 40 years; typical chest pain at acute stage; increase of serum enzymes creatine phosphokinase (CPK) and SGOT; ECG typical of MI; and normal coronary angiograms.

A total of 1600 coronary angiograms were performed in patients with previous MI in our department between 1969 and 1979. Thirty-nine patients had normal coronary arteries and 22 were age 40 years or less at the time of MI. Mean age of the group was 35.5 years (23–40 years) and four patients were under 30 years old.

ECG abnormalities were located in the anterior leads in 12 patients, in the posterior or inferior leads in eight patients, and in the lateral leads in two patients.

All patients had first undergone a selective coronary angiogram, with at least four different views, for each coronary artery (left coronary artery was frontal, RAO 30°, LAO 60°, lateral; right coronary artery was frontal, RAO 30°, LAO 45°, lateral) and left ventriculogram in the RAO 30° view. All angiograms were reviewed by at least three independent observers. Global ejection fraction (GEF) was determined according to Simpson's method [5], and wall motion abnormalities (WMA) were studied by our quantitative method [6]. Mean time interval between the acute episode and hemodynamic investigations was 4 months (2–12 months).

A second survey was carried out after a mean follow-up period of 5.2 years (18–120 months) and included a clinical examination as well as the following:

1. Standard exercise test on bicycle at heart rate higher or equal to 85% of maximal heart rate.
2. Thallium imaging (TI) after injection of 2 mCi of thallium 201 at maximal exercise at four different views (frontal, LAO 30°, LAO 60°, lateral) coupled with redistribution study (RS) after 4 h at the LAO 30° view or the view best showing a

1 Centre Hospitalier Regional Nancy, Clinique des Maladies Cardio-Vasculaires, Hopital des Brabois, Route de Neufchateau, F-545000 Vandœvre – Les Nancy, France

cold spot. The results were studied by three independent observers who had no knowledge of the site of ECG abnormalities.

3. Radionuclide angiography (RNA) by multiple-gated equilibrium scintigraphy, after injection of red blood cells marked by 20 mCi technetium Tc 99 m, was performed at LAO and frontal views. The GEF was determined at the LAO view. For the regional study the left ventricle was divided into 16 angular sectors around the center of gravity at final diastolic time [7].

Results

At follow-up, all patients were alive and no further episode of MI was noted. No patient complained of chest pain, but two patients described exertional dyspnea and received medical treatment. Among the 22 patients, 20 were smokers before MI (15 cigarettes/day or less), and all had stopped smoking. Among the three females, two had been taking oral contraceptives and subsequently stopped and one female had experienced MI 2 months after her pregnancy.

Standard exercise testing was normal in 18 patients, and four patients had ST segment elevation at the site of MI.

With TI (Table 1), cold spots were noted in 13 cases. All were concordant with the ECG location and stable on RS, confirming myocardial injury [8].

Table 1. Thallium imaging at maximal exercise and redistribution in the patients with anterior, postinferior, and lateral MI

	Cold spot	
	Maximum exercise	Redistribution
Anterior	10	10
Postinferior	3	3
Lateral	0	0

Table 2. The second column gives mean global ejection fraction (GEF) at the first study by angiography and at the second study by radionuclide angiography (RNA). The three last columns show the number of cases according to the value of GEF

		No. patients		
GEF	Mean $\pm$ SEM	EF$\leq$0.40	0.40<EF<0.50	EF$\geq$0.50
First angiography	54.0$\pm$4.1	4	2	16
Second RNA	53.9$\pm$5.3	4 [a]	2 [a]	16
Wall motion abnormalities		4	2	3
Location of wall motion abnormalities		4 ant.	2 ant.	3 ant.

[a] Two patients showed significantly deteriorated GEF values

Table 3. Comparison of the results of thallium scanning and quantitative analysis (REF) of wall motion abnormalities (WMA) according to the value of global ejection fraction (GEF). All patients with WMA had a cold spot, but four patients without WMA also had a cold spot

		WMA (REF)		Cold spot	
	Location	With	Without	With WMA	Without WMA
GEF $\geq$ 0.50	Anterior	3	3	3	1
	Postinf.	0	8		3
	Lateral	0	2		0
GEF < 0.50	Anterior	6		6	

By multiple-gated equilibrium scintigraphy (RNA) (Tables 2, 3), GEF remained stable (54.0±4.1 versus 53.9±5.3) and all patients ($N = 16$) with an initial GEF higher than 50% remained stable. But GEF decreased in four patients with anterior MI (42.4±4.8 versus 30.5±7.4) whose initial GEF was lower than 45%. Two of these patients consented to a second coronary angiography and left ventriculography. These examinations confirmed the decreased GEF and normal coronary angiogram. The regional ejection fraction (REF), a quantitative regional study, showed WMA in nine patients, all of whom had anterior MI. All patients with WMA showed a cold spot at the same location on TI, but four patients without WMA showed a cold spot.

Discussion

The recent development of nuclear cardiology explains why our patients did not undergo TI and RNA at the time of MI. Still, in a previous study [9], GEF and REF determined by contrast angiography at the RAO 30° view and by RNA at the LAO view were found to be closely correlated (GEF $r=0.90$, REF $r=0.84$), and we think that ejection fractions determined by RNA during follow-up could be safely compared to the initial ejection fractions obtained by contrast angiography.

The condition of the coronary arteries was not studied systematically during the follow-up survey, but TI showed no cold spot outside the infarcted area, during exercise as well as RS and allows one to think that coronary anatomy is not markedly altered [10]. Indeed, two of the four patients with a decrease in GEF were assessed by a second coronary angiography that confirmed the integrity of the coronary arteries.

Furthermore, TI seems useful chiefly in patients showing no WMA, since four cold spots were detected in 13 patients with no WMA. This confirms the ability of thallium scanning to detect myocardial extraction abnormalities even in the absence of injured large coronary arteries.

Conclusion

A favorable 5-year prognosis in young patients with MI and normal coronary angiograms appears plausible. In fact, all our patients are alive and none complain of any residual typical chest pain. Furthermore, most have a stable ejection fraction.

Nevertheless, we observed a significant deterioration of GEF in four patients who had a low initial GEF (under 0.45), which confirms the prognostic significance of left ventricular function.

Nuclear cardiology appears particularly helpful, as it allows a noninvasive follow-up of young patients with MI.

References

1. Campeau L, Lesperance J, Bourassa MG, Ashekian PB (1968) Myocardial infarction without obstructive disease at coronary ateriography. Can Med Assoc J 99:837
2. Bruschke AVG, Bruyneel KJ, Bloch A, van Herpen G (1971) Acute myocardial infarction without obstructive coronary artery disease demonstrated by selective cinearteriography. Br Heart J 33:585
3. Ravazi M, Lynch J, Singh K et al. (1980) Long-term follow-up of patients with myocardial infarction and normal coronary arteries. Circulation Suppl III 62:39
4. Cherrier F, Breton C, Bourdon JL et al. (1979) Profil épidémiologique des sujets porteurs d'un infarctus avec coronarographie normale. Arch Mal Cœr 72:26
5. Cherrier F, Ethevenot G, Beissel J, Neimann JL (1977) Etude comparative des différentes méthodes d'évaluation du volume ventriculaire gauche par angiocardiographie monoplane. Arch Mal Cœur 7:699
6. Ethevenot G, Beissel J, Neimann JL, Cherrier F (1977) Tentative d'appréciation de la valeur contractile du myocarde dans les anévrismes ventriculaires gauches. Arch Mal Cœur 70:819
7. Amor M, Bertrand A, Karcher G et al. (to be published) Une nouvelle méthode radioisotopique d'étude des fractions d'éjection locales. Arch Mal Cœur
8. Pohost GM, Alpert NM, Ingwall JS, Strauss HW (1980) Thallium redistribution: Mechanisms and clinical utility. Semin Nucl Med 10:70
9. Ethevenot G, Amor M, Betrand A et al. (to be published) Comparaison de la contractilité locale du ventricule gauche par les méthodes volumétriques isotopiques et angiographiques. Arch Mal Cœur
10. Pitt B, Strauss HW (1979) Clinical application of myocardial imaging with thallium 201. In: Willerson JT (ed) Nuclear cardiology. Davis, Philadelphia, p 125

Prognosis of Coronary Heart Disease
and Progression of Coronary Arteriosclerosis in
Postinfarction Patients Under the Age of 40

P. Stürzenhofecker, L. Samek, C. Droste, H. Gohlke, J. Petersen, and H. Roskamm [1]

The course of coronary heart disease may be evaluated by two different approaches:

I. By determination of the annual mortality in relation to different clinical and angiographic parameters.
II. By evaluation of changes in coronary morphology by means of follow-up coronary angiographies.

Regarding the first approach, studies in the literature mainly deal with older coronary heart disease patients, mostly with angina pectoris, who are not exclusively postinfarction patients [1–4]. Some of these studies include small numbers of young patients. Regarding the second approach, our knowledge derives (a) from follow-up angiographies in operated patients [5–8], and (b) from follow-up angiographies in nonoperated patients with clinical deterioration [6, 9].

There is no systematic study in young patients with repeated angiographies performed independent of the development of the patients' symptoms and signs.

Annual Mortality in Relation to Clinical
and Angiographic Parameters

Patients and Methods

From January 1973 to December 1979, 774 postinfarction patients under 40 years of age were admitted to our clinic. Coronary angiography was recommended to all of them, and 620 accepted. After excluding women and those who had to undergo aortocoronary bypass surgery, 537 were left; of these 465 had a coronary angiography within 12 months after the acute event. They were followed up for 1–7 years, on average 3.5 years. The following parameters were determined on average 6 months after myocardial infarction (MI) and tested for their prognostic value: (a) multi-vessel disease (MVD), > 50% reduction of luminal diameter; (b) moderate and severe left ventricular dysfunction (SVD), 2 or more out of 9 segments in the left ventriculogram being severely hypo-, a-, or dyskinetic; (c) significant ventricular arrhythmias (SVA), ≥ 1 ventricular premature contraction (VPC) in ECG at rest, > 10 VPCs in 1 h of Holter monitoring or per examination (exercise test or physiotherapy) multiform or paired VPCs, ventricular tachycardias, or R/T phenomenon.

Statistics: Differences in the frequency of parameters were analyzed by the chi-square test.

1 Rehabilitationszentrum, Südring 15, 7812 Bad Krozingen, FRG

Results

Annual mortality for the whole group of patients from cardiac causes was 2.7%. The prognostic significance of the following parameters was evaluated (risk predictors of cardiac death):

Vessel Involvement. Annual mortality from cardiac causes increased with the number of vessels involved: In patients with zero- and one-vessel disease annual mortality was 1.8%, in those with two-vessel disease it was 2.1%, and in patients with three-vessel disease it was 6.2%.

Left Ventricular Dysfunction. Annual mortality also increased with deterioration of left ventricular function: In the patient group with only mild left ventricular dysfunction it was 1.5%, in patients with moderate left ventricular dysfunction 2.5%, and in patients with severe left ventricular dysfunction 8.9%.

Arrhythmias. The annual mortality was related to the presence of significant arrhythmias. In the patient group without significant arrhythmias it was 1.6%, in the presence of significant arrhythmias 3.6%.

Combination of Risk Predictors for Cardiac Death

Furthermore, we examined the relationship between annual mortality and the combination of one or more of the above mentioned risk predictors for cardiac death.

Table 1. Mortality of 465 postinfarction patients in relation to the number of positive risk predictors for cardiac death

Risk predictors present	Patients	All deaths	Annual mortality
	n	n	(%)
None	160	5	0.9
One	170	12	2.0
Two	106	14	3.8
Three	29	6	5.9

$P < 0.005$

Table 2. Mortality of 465 postinfarction patients in relation to different combination of positive risk predictors for cardiac death (SVA = significant ventricular arrhythmias, MVD = multi vessel disease, SVD = severe ventricular dysfunction)

	Patients	All deaths	Annual mortality (%)
	n	n	
No SVA/MVD/SVD	160	5	0.9
SVA alone	51	4	2.2
SVA with SVD/MVD	149	19	3.6

$P < 0.005$

If none of these factors was present, annual mortality was 0.9%; in the presence of one of these factors it was 2%, and if all three factors were present, annual mortality increased significantly ($P < 0.005$) to 5.9% (Table 1).

The presence of significant arrhythmias alone (in the absence of moderate or severe left ventricular dysfunction and of multi-vessel disease) seems to have only little prognostic relevance (Table 2). The annual mortality in this subgroup was 2.2% versus 0.9% in the group without any of the three risk predictors positive. In arrhythmia patients – including those with moderate or severe left ventricular dysfunction and multi-vessel disease – the annual mortality increased significantly ($P < 0.005$), to 3.6%.

Changes in Coronary Morphology

To evaluate changes of coronary morphology and left ventricular function, 293 patients whose first angiography was done more than 3 years previously were asked to have a second angiography done. 54 did not respond, 47 refused, 21 had died, and 7 were excluded for medical reasons (colon-carcinoma, hepatitis). The remaining 164 patients underwent a second coronary angiography an average of 3.8 years after the first, irrespective of the clinical course during this time interval. Progression or regression of coronary arteriosclerosis was assumed, if there was a difference of at least two grades, based on the AHA classification of stenoses [10].

Results

The majority of patients (58%) showed no change of coronary morphology, 28.6% progression, and 13.4% regression (Fig. 1).

Progression was present in 24% of one-vessel disease patients; in two- and three-vessel disease patients it was more frequent with 37.7%. Regression was found in 16% of the patients with one-vessel disease and it was less frequent (7%) in patients with multi-vessel disease but none of this differences are statistically significant ($P < 0.1$).

The group was divided into those patients who showed an unilocular disease in the first angiogram, i.e., with only one stenosis or occlusion in one vessel and the other vessels totally normal, and into those who had a multilocular disease. For example, a patient with a $> 50\%$ stenosis in one vessel only, and one or more $< 50\%$ stenoses in the same or other vessels is a *one-vessel disease* patient but with a *multilocular disease*.

In the unilocular group, progression was very rare with 3.6% and regression was rather frequent with (28.6%) (Figure 2). In the multilocular group, progression was frequent with 34.3% and regression rather rare with 10.4% ($P < 0.001$). These differences are significant.

Progression was equally frequent in each of the three vessels; the left anterior descending (LAD) with 18%, the circumflex artery with 17% and the arteria coronara dextra (ACD) with 17%. Regression occurred predominantly in the proximal portion of the LAD: of the 21 regressions, 17 were found in the proximal LAD, only 4 in the ACD, and none in the circumflex artery.

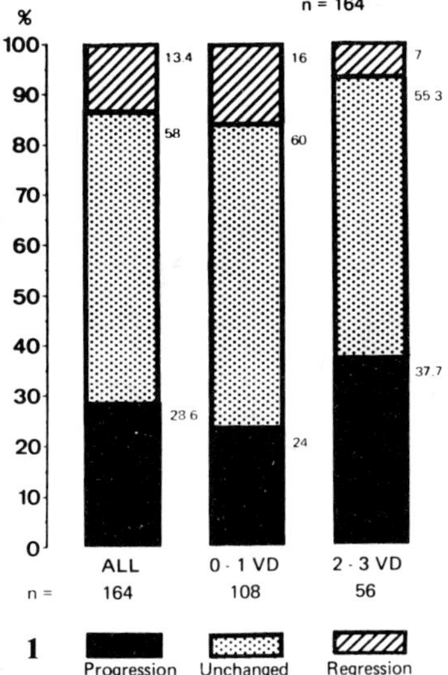

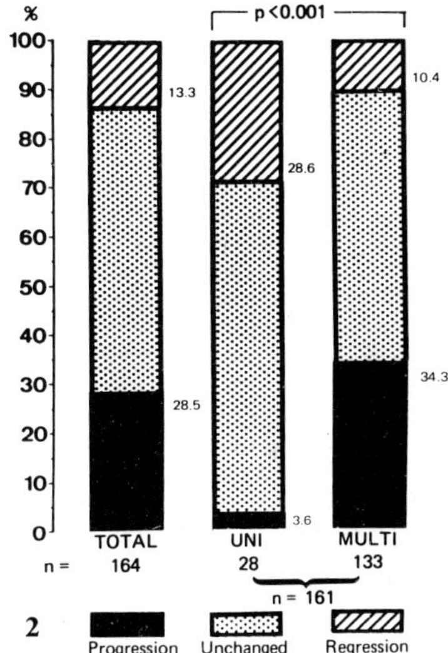

Fig. 1. Frequency of patients with unchanged morphology, progression and regression of angiographic findings after 3.8 years on average. Figures are given for the whole group of patients ($n = 164$), as well as those with zero- and one-vessel disease, and those with two- and three-vessel-disease

Fig. 2. Frequency of patients with unchanged morphology, progression and regression of angiographic findings after 3.8 years on the average. Figures are given for the whole group of patients ($n = 164$), and for those with uni- and multilocular disease

The degree of progression (47 patients with 56 stenoses) is shown in Figure 3. By definition, the difference between the two coronary angiographies had to be at least two grades, based on the AHA classification of stenoses. This figure does not include 9 patients whose 90%–99% stenosis progressed to total occlusion. 7 patients developed a more than 50% stenosis in previously normal vessels.

The degree of regression (22 patients) is shown in Figure 4. Excluded are 15 patients with total occlusion at the first angiography who showed an opening of the vessel to 90–99% stenosis at the second angiography. A typical example of regression is shown in Fig. 5 on p. 3 in this book.

Regression was found to be age-dependent. It is more frequent at a very young age, i.e., under 35; the frequency decreases already in the age-group 35–39 years. In older patients as far as we know it is very rare.

Relationship Between Control of the Risk Factor Smoking and Progression of Coronary Artery Disease

The group was divided into one subgroup with progression and one with no change or regression. Before the infarction the frequency of cigarette smoking was comparably high in both groups, 89% and 79% respectively. In the progression group at the time of the second angiogram 38% were still smoking; in the group without progression there were only 14% smokers. This difference is significant (Table 3).

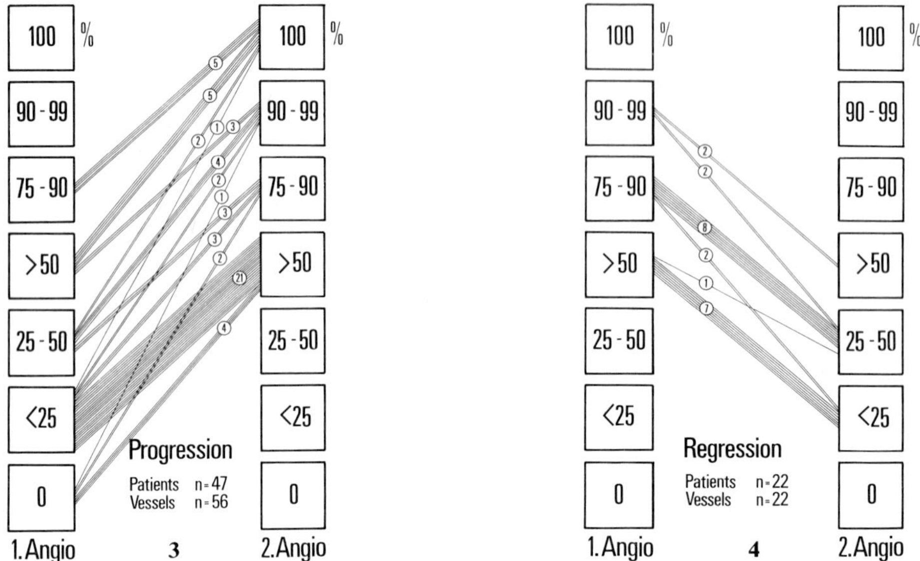

Fig. 3. Degree of stenosis at the first and second coronary arteriography in 47 patients who showed a progression of stenosis of at least two grades, based on the AHA classification of stenoses

Fig. 4. Degree of stenosis at the first and second coronary arteriography in 22 patients who showed a regression of stenosis of at least two grades, based on the AHA classification of stenosis

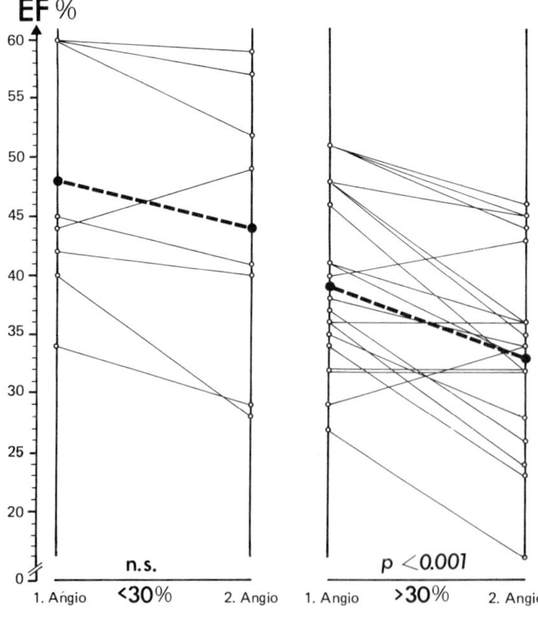

Fig. 5. Ejection fraction (EF%) at the first and second angiography (time interval $\bar{x}$ 3.8 years) in 28 patients with anterior wall infarction who did not show progression of coronary arteriosclerosis

Table 3. Frequency of smokers before MI (I), and at the time of the second angiography (II), in 47 patients with and 117 patients without progression of coronary arteriosclerosis during a mean follow-up of 3.8 years

		Progression	No. progression
		$n = 47$	$n = 117$
Cigarette smoking	I.	89.4%	78.6%
		└─── ns ───┘	
	II.	38.4%	14.5%
		└─── $P < 0.01$ ───┘	

Changes in Left Ventricular Function

We were mainly interested to see if left ventricular function deteriorated in patients with large infarctions who did not show progression of coronary arteriosclerosis. 28 patients with anterior wall infarctions and one-vessel disease who had no change in coronary morphology were divided into those with a scar of above or below 30% of the total circumference in the RAO ventriculogram. At the first angiography the first group had an ejection fraction of 48, the second of 40%. In the first group, the ejection fraction did not change during the follow-up of 3.5 years, in the second group there was a slight but significant deterioration (Fig. 5).

Discussion

Annual Mortality

It has been stated that annual mortality of young postinfarction patients is lower than in older age-groups [11–14]. In our study, annual mortality was 2.7%; in relation to older age groups this is indeed a rather low figure. But it is about ten times higher than in an age-matched normal population, where it is 0.29% [15].

Risk Predictors of Cardiac Death

In our young postinfarction patients as in older coronary heart disease patients, multi-vessel disease [1, 3, 16–18], myocardial dysfunction [2, 19, 20], and ventricular arrhythmias [21–25] have been found to be important risk predictors of cardiac death in the years following the infarction. The occurrence of arrhythmias is related to left ventricular dysfunction or heart volume enlargement [26–29]. In some studies, arrhythmias per se have been shown to be of prognostic relevance [25, 30, 31], in others only if they are combined with left ventricular dysfunction [32–36]. In our study, for postinfarction patients with arrhythmias, but without moderate or severe left ventricular dysfunction or multi-vessel disease, prognosis is somewhat worse than in those without any of the mentioned risk predictors positive (annual mortality 2.2 versus 0.9%). However, prognosis is significantly better than in arrhythmia patients with moderate or severe left ventricular dysfunction or multi-vessel disease (annual mortality 2.2 versus 3.6%).

Progression of Coronary Arteriosclerosis

In young patients with coronary arteriosclerosis, progression of the disease was found to be more frequent and more pronounced than in older age groups [37, 38, 39]. According to the experience of this study, subgroups with different frequency of progression exist. Postinfarction patients with unilocular disease, show only little progression of coronary arteriosclerosis in the following three years. On the other hand, in patients who in their first coronary angiography already show multi-vessel or multilocular disease, a high frequency of progression could be demonstrated. In 3.8 years, on average, 37.7% and 34.3% respectively show significant progression of one or more stenoses. The frequency of progression can apparently be reduced by risk factor correction [37–40]; in this study, this could be confirmed with the risk factor smoking.

Regression of Coronary Angiographic Findings

Regression of coronary angiographic findings has been repeatedly described in single case reports in the literature [9, 41–43]. In our patients, 21 stenosed vessels showed regression in the second angiogram; 17 of these regressions were found in the LAD. What is the mechanism behind regression of coronary angiographic findings? Two explanations may be discussed:

1. There was a spasm during the first catheterization.
2. There was recanalization and organization of the thrombus since the time of the first angiogram.

We think spasm during the first angiogram is unlikely, at least in the majority of patients, for the following reasons:

– In most patients with regression nitroglycerine was also given during the first angiogram;
– the site of regression was always in the infarction-related vessel, i.e. in the proximal anterior descending artery, and never in the proximal right coronary artery where spasm is common.

Occurrence of regression is age-dependent (as it was with zero-vessel disease (see p. 65). It is rather frequent at a very young age, i.e., under 35 years. The frequency already decreases in the age-group 35–39 years. In older patients, as far as we know, it is very rare. In our opinion most cases of regression have to be explained by recanalization and organization of a thrombus. Thus, it should be called regression of a coronary angiographic finding rather than regression of coronary arteriosclerosis. Actual regression of arteriosclerosis has only been reported in the early stages of femoral arteriosclerosis in patients treated for hyperlipoproteinemia [44].

Two Types of Coronary Heart Disease in Young Patients

In our opinion, MI at young age can be caused by two different types of disease. The first is a one-vessel disease, with the non-infarction-related vessels being normal or showing only minimal narrowing. Coronary thrombosis may primarily play an important role, intima oedema and spasm as a trigger mechanism cannot be excluded. If there is a spontaneous lysis of the thrombus, we may find normal coronary arteries or zero-vessel disease; these are more often seen in young patients. If the lysis is ineffective, one-vessel disease will be the result. However, in some of these patients recanalization and organization of the thrombus may occur later, even after months or years. In these cases we find regression in the second angiogram.

In this type of disease there is a rare incidence of progression and the prognosis is good if the risk factors, especially smoking, are controlled. There is only little tendency for deterioration of left ventricular function, but the patients will have to be observed over a longer period of time.

The second type of disease is what is better known in older patients; multi-vessel disease. It is premature in the age-group below 40 years. In this type of disease, progression is very common even after a 3- or 4-year period of time. Of course we have to expect combinations of these two types of coronary artery disease in young patients.

Acknowledgment. This work was supported by grants of the BMA and BMFT (Bundesministerium für Arbeit und Sozialordnung and Bundesministerium für Forschung und Technologie).

References

1. Bruschke AVG, Proudfit WL, Sones FM Jr (1973) Progress study of 590 consecutive non-surgical cases of coronary disease followed 5–9 years. I. Arteriographic correlations. Circulation 47:1147–1153
2. Bruschke AVG, Proudfit WL, Sones FM Jr (1973) Progress study of 590 consecutive non-surgical cases of coronary disease followed 5–9 years. II. Ventriculographic and other correlations. Circulation 47:1154–1163
3. Burggraf G, Parker J (1975) Prognosis in coronary artery disease. Angiographic, hemodynamic and clinical factors. Circulation 51:146
4. Steinbrunn W, Lichtlen P (1976) Spontanverlauf der koronaren Herzkrankheit. Schweiz Med Wochenschr 106:1538–1540
5. Benchimol A, Harris CL, Flemming H, Desser KB (1974) Progression of obstructive coronary artery disease after implantation of aorto-coronary saphenous vein bypass grafts. J Thorac Cardiovasc Surg 68:257–262
6. Ben-Zvi J, Hildner FJ, Javier RP et al. (1974) Progression of coronary artery disease. Am J Cardiol 34:295–301
7. Maurer BJ, Oberman A, Holt JH Jr et al. (1974) Changes in grafted and nongrafted coronary arteries following saphenous vein bypass grafting. Circulation 50:293–300
8. Bourassa MG, Corbara F, L'Esperance I, Campeau L (1978) Progression of coronary disease five to seven years after aortocoronary bypass surgery. In: Kaltenbach M, Lichtlen P, Balcon R, Bussmann WD (eds) Coronary heart disease. Third International Symposium. Thieme, Stuttgart, p 139
9. Gensini GG, Kelly AE (1972) Incidence and progression of coronary artery disease. Arch Intern Med 129:814–827
10. Austen WG, Edwards JE, Frye RL et al. (1975) A reporting system on patients evaluated for coronary artery disease. AHA Committee Report. Circulation [Suppl] 51:7–40

11. Helmers C (1973) Short and long-term prognostic indices in acute myocardial infarction. A study of 606 patients initially treated in a coronary care unit. Acta Med Scand [Suppl] 555
12. World Health Organization Regional Office for Europe (1976) Myocardial infarction community registers. Public Health in Europe 5. Copenhagen, p 123
13. Nüssel E, Buchholz L, Bergdolt H et al. (1977) Daten des Heidelberger Herzinfarkt-Registers im internationalen Vergleich. Med Tech 97:118–122
14. Bergstrand R, Vedin A, Wilhelmsson C, Wilhelmsen L (1981) Myocardial infarction among men below age 40 in Göteborg. This vol pp 23–28
15. Statistisches Bundesamt Wiesbaden (ed) (1978) Gesundheitswesen: Fachserie 12, Reihe 4, Todesursachen. Kohlhammer, Stuttgart Mainz
16. Webster JS, Moberg C, Rincon G (1974) Natural history of severe proximal coronary artery disease as documented by coronary cineangiography. Am J Cardiol 33:195
17. Lichtlen PR (1978) Natural history of coronary artery disease based on coronary angiography. Cleve Clin Q 45:153–155
18. Read RC, Murphy ML, Hultgren HN (1978) Survival of men treated for chronic stable angina pectoris: A cooperative randomized study. J Thorac Cardiovasc Surg 75:1
19. Parker JO (1978) Prognosis in coronary artery disease. Cleve Clin Q 45:145–146
20. Proudfit WL (1978) Minor prognostic associations. Cleve Clin Q 45:141–142
21. Kotler MN, Tabatznik B, Mower MM, Tominaga S (1973) Prognostic significance of ventricular ectopic beats with respect to sudden death in the late postinfarction period. Circulation 47:959–966
22. Moss AJ, DeCamilla J, Mietlowski W et al. (1975) Prognostic grading and significance of ventricular premature beats after recovery from myocardial infarction. Circulation [Suppl III] 51/52:III 204–210
23. Ruberman W, Weinblatt E, Frank CW et al. (1976) Prognostic value of one hour of ECG monitoring of men with coronary heart disease. J Chronic Dis 29:497–512
24. Tabatznik B (1976) Ambulatory monitoring in the late postmyocardial infarction period. Postgrad Med J [Suppl 7] 52:56–59
25. Hammermeister KE, DeRouen TA, Dodge HT (1979) Variables predictive of survival in patients with coronary disease. Circulation 59:421–430
26. Lown B, Calvert AF, Armington R, Ryan M (1975) Monitoring for serious arrhythmias and high risk of sudden death. Circulation [Suppl III] 51/52:III 189–198
27. Bethge K-P, Bethge H-C, Graf A et al. (1977) Kammer-Arrhythmien bei chronisch koronarer Herzkrankheit. Z Kardiol 66:1–9
28. Calvert A, Lown B, Gorlin R (1977) Ventricular premature beats and anatomically defined coronary heart disease. Am J Cardiol 39:627–634
29. Samek L, Kirste D, Roskamm H et al. (1977) Herzrhythmusstörungen nach Herzinfarkt. Herz Kreislauf 9:641–649
30. Coronary Drug Project Research Group (1973) Prognostic importance of premature beats following myocardial infarction. JAMA 223:1116–1121
31. Moss AJ, DeCamilla J, Davis H et al. (1976) Use and limitations of ventricular premature beats as prognostic indicators of the posthospital course of myocardial infarction. Am J Cardiol 37:158
32. Schulze RA Jr, Strauss HW, Pitt B (1977) Sudden death in the year following myocardial infarction. Relation to ventricular premature contractions in the late hospital phase and left ventricular jection fraction. Am J Med 62:192–199
33. DeBusk RF, Davidson DM, Houston N, Fitzgerald J (1980) Serial ambulatory electrocardiography and treadmill exercise testing after uncomplicated myocardial infarction. Am J Cardiol 45:547–554
34. Lichtlen PR, Bethge K-P, Platiel H (1980) Inzidenz des plötzlichen Herztodes bei Koronarpatienten in Abhängigkeit von Anatomie und Rhythmusprofil. Z Kardiol 69:639–648
35. Samek L, Stürzenhofecker P, Görnandt L, Roskamm H (1980) Prognosis of 343 post-infarction patients under age 40. Abstr. VIII. European Congress of Cardiology, Paris, p 227
36. Califf RM, Wagner GS, Rosati RA (1981) Prognostic value of ventricular arrhythmias (Abstr). Am J Cardiol 47:397

37. Sanmarco ME, Selvester RH, Brooks SH, Blankenhorn DH (1976) Risk factors reduction and changes in coronary arteriography (Abstr). Circulation [Suppl II] 56:140
38. Selvester RH, Camp J, Sanmarco ME (1977) Effects of exercise training on progression of documented coronary arteriosclerosis in men. In: Milvy P (ed) The marathon: Physiological, medical, epidemiological, and psychological studies. New York Academy of Sciences, New York, pp 495–508
39. Selvester RH, Blessey RL, Sanmarco ME (1981) Risk reduction and coronary progression/regression in man. This vol pp 196–200
40. Nash DT, Gensini G, Simon H et al. (1977) The erysichthon syndrome. Circulation 56:363–365
41. Henderson RR, Hansing CE, Razavi M, Rowe GG (1973) Resolution of an obstructive coronary lesion as demonstrated by selective angiography in a patient with transmural myocardial infarction. J Cardiol 31:785–788
42. Spring DA, Thomsen JH (1973) Recanalization in a coronary artery thrombus. JAMA 224:1152–1155
43. Kavanagh-Gray D (1974) Angiographic evidence of coronary occlusion and resolution. Can Med Assac J 110: 945–946
44. Brandt R Jr, Blankenhorn DH, Crawford DW, Brooks SH (1977) Regression and progression of early femoral atherosclerosis in treated hyperlipoproteinemic patients. Ann Intern Med 86:139–146

Myocardial Infarction in Patients Under the Age of 40 Autopsy Findings [1]

R. VIRMANI and H. A. MCALLISTER, JR. [2]

During the last 20 years most of the autopsy reports on patients with coronary heart disease have concentrated on patients in decades 5–7 [1–15]. Although the greatest incidence of coronary heart disease is found in this age group [16–18], selective studies on patients under the age of 40 years are lacking. The present report attempts to fill this void by describing cardiovascular observations at autopsy in 112 patients under the age of 40 who died with myocardial infarction (MI).

Materials and Methods

The files of the Armed Forces Institute of Pathology, which includes case material from military, Veterans Administration, and civilian sources, were searched for patients 40 years and younger with fatal coronary heart disease recorded consecutively during 1954–1979. In all, there were 201 patients who had died from coronary heart disease, and 186 of these had adequate descriptions of the heart and circumstances of death. Of the 186 who died of coronary heart disease, 112 had MI and they form the basis for this study. Of the 112 patients, 110 had adequate descriptions of the maximal amount of coronary artery narrowing in each of the three major epicardial coronary arteries, i.e., right, left anterior descending, and left circumflex coronary arteries: Only 60 had adequate descriptions of the left main coronary artery. The coronary arteries had been previously cut at 5-mm intervals, and the area of maximal narrowing selected by gross examiniation was submitted for histologic examination. The paraffin blocks were available for further sectioning and staining with hematoxylin and eosin, and Movat's pentachrome stain. The gross descriptions of the myocardium documented the presence or absence of macroscopic myocardial fibrosis and/or necrosis, and at least three sections of the left ventricular myocardium were submitted for histologic examination. Microscopic examination confirmed the presence of acute and/or healed MI and documented the infarcts as subendocardial (infarcts that did not extend from endocardium to the epicardium) or transmural (infarcts extending from the endocardium to epicardium). Among the patients with both healed and acute infarcts, infarcts were classified as subendocardial if both types of infarcts did not extend to the epicardium, and as transmural if one and/ or both types of infarcts extended to the epicardium.

---

1 The opinions or assertions contained herein are the private views of the authors, and are not to be construed as official or as reflecting the views of the Department of the Army or the Department of Defense
2 Department of Cardiovascular Pathology, Armed Forces Institute of Pathology, Washington, D.C., 20306, USA

Results

The sample of 112 patients with MI at autopsy were 18–40 years old (mean 33 years; 103 men and 9 women) (Table 1), and 91 (81%) were active-duty military personnel. Thirty patients were under 30 years, and 82 were 31–40 years of age.

The mode of presentation was sudden death in 66 patients (59%) (defined as death occurring instantaneously or within 1 h of the onset of symptoms), 40 patients (36%) had symptoms of chest pain for more than 1 h, two patients (2%) had a history of chronic congestive heart failure, and four (3%) died within 1 day after aortocoronary bypass surgery. Thirty-two (29%) of the patients developed symptoms during or soon after exercise.

A history of predisposing conditions known to accelerate coronary atherosclerosis was available in 73 (Table 2): Of these, 41 (56%) had known risk factors, including systemic hypertension, diabetes mellitus, hyperlipoproteinemia, family history of coronary heart disease, mediastinal irradiation, and prolonged corticosteroid therapy. A history of smoking was not uniformly available, and when available most of the details specifying number of cigarettes consumed per day and duration in years was not mentioned. A history as to the presence or absence of prior cardiac disease was available in 85 of the 112 patients and, of these, 47 (55%) had been symptomatic (Table 2).

At autopsy the heart weights were increased in 61 (54%), with "normal" for men as less than 400 g and for women less than 350 g (Table 3). Of 112 patients, the infarcts were subendocardial in 30 (27%) and transmural in 82 (73%).

The amount and extent of coronary artery narrowing is summarized in Tables 4–7. Of the four major epicardial coronary arteries examined, for severe atherosclerosis (greater than 75% cross-sectional area luminal narrowing by atherosclerotic plaque), only one artery was involved in 24 patients (21%), two coronary arte-

Table 1. MI in patients under age 40 (autopsy findings). Clinical observations in 112 autopsy patients

	No. pts. < 30 yrs	No. pts. 31 – 40 yrs	Total
	30	82	112
Age in years, range (Avg)	18 – 30 (25)	31 – 40 (37)	18 – 40 (33)
Sex: M:F	28:2	75:7	103:9
Mode of presentation			
Sudden death (< 1 h)	16 (54%)	50 (61%)	66 (59%)
Chest pain (> 1 h)	13 (43%)	27 (33%)	40 (36%)
Chronic CHF	1 (3%)	1 (1%)	2 (2%)
Post-op SVBG (< 1 day)	0	4 (5%)	4 (3%)
Circumstance of death			
During exercise	15 (50%)	7 (8%)	22 (22%)
Soon after exercise	6 (20%)	4 (5%)	10 (9%)
At rest	9 (30%)	71 (86%)	80 (71%)

ries in 49 (44%), three coronary arteries in 34 (30%), and four arteries were infrequently involved in three patients (3%) (Table 4, Fig. 1).

Of the 390 coronary arteries examined in 110 patients, 234 (60%) were greater than 75% narrowed in the cross-sectional area by atherosclerotic plaque, for an average of 2.14 coronary arteries/patient. The most frequent artery of involvement was the left anterior descending, in 99 patients (90%). Thrombus was present in 51 (13%) of the coronary arteries (Table 6).

Table 2. MI in 112 Autopsy patients under age 40: History of risk factors

	No. pts. < 30 yrs	No pts. 31 – 40 yrs	Total
	22	51	73
History of risk factors (RF) available			
Risk factors			
Systemic hypertension	3	15	18
Diabetes mellitus	1	7	8
Hyperlipoproteinemia (cholesterol > 250 mg %)	1	15	16
Family history of CHD	3	10	13
Mediastinal irradiation	2	0	2
Prolonged corticosteroid therapy	1	0	1
No. pts. with 1 or more RF present	8 (36%)	33 (65%)	41 (56%)
Obesity	3 (10%)	26 (32%)	29 (26%)
History of prior cardiac disease available	22	63	85
Angina pectoris (AP)	1	18 (29%)	19 (22%)
Acute myocardial infarction (AMI)	0	5 (8%)	5 (6%)
AP + AMI	0	15 (24%)	15 (18%)
Chronic congestive heart failure (CCHF) after AMI + AP	0	6 (9%)	6 (7%)
CCHF	1	1 (1%)	2 (2%)
Total no. pts. with prior cardiac disease	2 (9%)	45 (71%)	47 (55%)

Table 3. Morphologic observations in 112 autopsy patients under age 40 with MI

	Pts < 30 yrs 30	Pts 31 – 40 yrs 82	Total 112
Heart weight (gs)			
Range (avg)	275 – 525 (381)	260 – 860 (435)	260 – 860 (421)
Increased	12 (40%)	49 (60%)	61 (54%)
Type of infarct			
Acute myocardial infarct (AMI)	16 (53%)	24 (29%)	40 (36%)
Healed myocardial infarct (HMI)	6 (20%)	40 (49%)	46 (41%)
AMI + HMI	8 (27%)	18 (22%)	26 (23%)
Total	30	82	112
Complications			
Aneurysms	0	5 (6%)	5 (4%)
Rupture	0	2 (2%)	2 (2%)

Table 4. Comparison of the amount of severe coronary artery (CA) atherosclerosis in patients with (112) and without (74) MI at autopsy

No. of four Major CA'S narrowed > 75% in cross-sectional area	Patients with MI at autopsy				Patients with coronary heart disease without infarct MI at autopsy				P value of totals
	Pts < 30 yrs	Pts 31 – 40 yrs	P value	Total	Pts < 30 yrs	Pts 31 – 40 yrs	P value	Total	
1	10 (33%)	14 (17%)	0.07	24 (21%)	11 (61%)	24 (43%)	NS	34 (46%)	0.02
2	15 (50%)	34 (41%)	NS	49 (44%)	4 (22%)	15 (27%)	NS	19 (26%)	0.02
3	4 (13%)	30 (37%)	0.05	34 (30%)	2 (11%)	12 (21%)	NS	15 (20%)	NS
4	1 (3%)	2 (2%)	NS	3 (3%)	1 (6%)	2 (4%)	NS	3 (4%)	NS
Severe	0	2	NS	2 (2%)	0	3 (5%)	NS	3 (4%)	NS
Total	30	82		112	18	56		74	

NS = not significant

Table 5. Comparison of the amount of severe coronary atherosclerosis in patient with and without prior cardiac disease

No. of four major coronary arteries narrowed > 75% in cross-sectional area	Patients with prior cardiac disease	Patients without prior cardiac disease	P value	Total
	47	38		85
1	4 (8%)	13 (34%)	0.01	17 (20%)
2	20 (43%)	16 (42%)	NS	36 (43%)
3	22 (47%)	7 (18%)	0.01	29 (34%)
4	1 (2%)	1 (3%)	NS	2 (2%)
Severe	0	1 (3%)	NS	1 (1%)

The artery most commonly involved in single-vessel disease was the left anterior descending (Table 7). When two arteries were involved, the most frequent combination was left anterior descending and right, and in three vessel disease the arteries most commonly involved were the left anterior descending, left circumflex, and right.

The number and percentage of severely narrowed coronary arteries were evaluated according to the type of infarction, as follows: acute MI, 39 patients; healed MI, 45 patients; acute and healed MI, 26 patients. There was no significant differ-

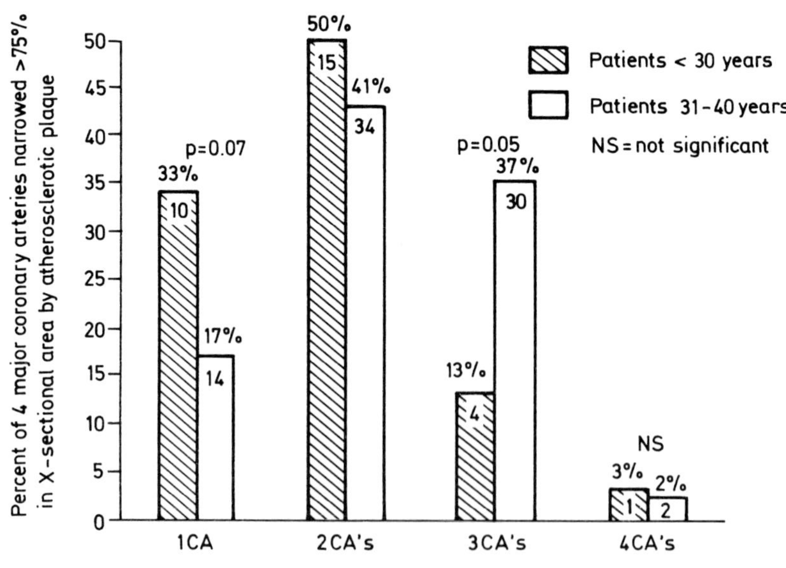

Fig. 1. Comparison of the percent and number of four major coronary arteries narrowed more than 75% in a cross-sectional area by atherosclerotic plaque in 30 patients less than 30 years and 80 patients 31–40 years of age with MI at autopsy

Table 6. Comparison of the amount of severe coronary artery (CA) atherosclerosis (Ath) in the four major coronary arteries in patients with (110) and without (71) MI at autopsy

Coronary artery	Patients under 40 years with MI at autopsy			Patients under 40 years with coronary heart disease without MI			P value	
	No. CA's examined	No. CA's narrowed > 75% in cross-sectional area by Ath. plaque (%)	No. CA's containing thrombi (%)	No. CA's examined	No. CA's narrowed > 75% in cross-sectional area by Ath. plaque (%)	No. CA's containing thrombi	CA narrowing	CA thrombi
Right	110	73 (66)	12 (11)	71	40 (56)	5 (7)	NS	NS
Left main	60	13 (22)	3 (5)	40	8 (20)	1 (2)	NS	NS
Left anterior descending	110	99 (90)	29 (26)	71	60 (84)	15 (21)	NS	NS
Left circumflex	110	49 (44)	7 (6)	71	24 (34)	2 (3)	NS	NS
Total	390	234 (60)	51 (13)	253	132 (52)	23 (9)	0.05	NS

NS = not significant

Table 7. Type and combination four major epicardial coronary arteries narrowed $>75\%$ in cross-sectional area by atherosclerotic plaque in 110 patients with MI and 71 patients without MI at autopsy. Abbreviations: LAD = left anterior descending; LC = left circumflex; LM = left main; NS = not significant; R = right

Coronary arteries	Patients with MI				Patients without MI				Total P value
	< 30 yrs	$31 - 40$ yrs	P value	Total	< 30 yrs	$< 31 - 41$ yrs	P value	Total	
LAD	8 (27%)	12 (15%)	NS	20 (18%)	9 (50%)	14 (26%)	0.07	23 (32%)	0.05
R	0	1		1	0	8 (15%)		8 (11%)	
LM	2	0		2	0	2		2	
LC	0	1		1	2	0		2	
LAD + R	10 (33%)	23 (29%)	NS	33 (30%)	2	10 (19%)	NS	12 (17%)	0.05
LAD + LC	2	6		8	1	4		5	
LAD + LM	3	2		5	1	0		1	
R + LC	0	4		4	0	1		1	
LAD + LC + R	3 (10%)	28 (35%)	NS	31 (28%)	1	11 (21%)	NS	12 (17%)	0.09
LM + LAD + R	1	1		2	1	0		1	
LM + LAD + LC	0	0		0	0	1		1	
LM + LAD + LC + R	1	2		3	1	2		3	
Total	30	80		110	18	53		71	

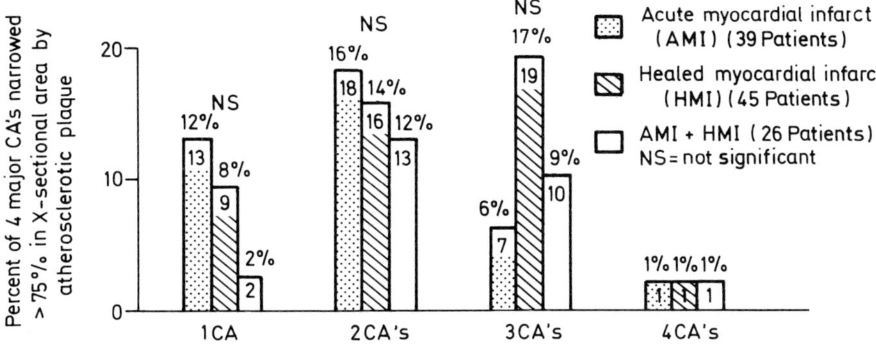

Fig. 2. Comparison of number and percent of four major coronary arteries narrowed greater than 75% in a cross-sectional area by atherosclerotic plaque in 110 autopsy patients according to the type of MI

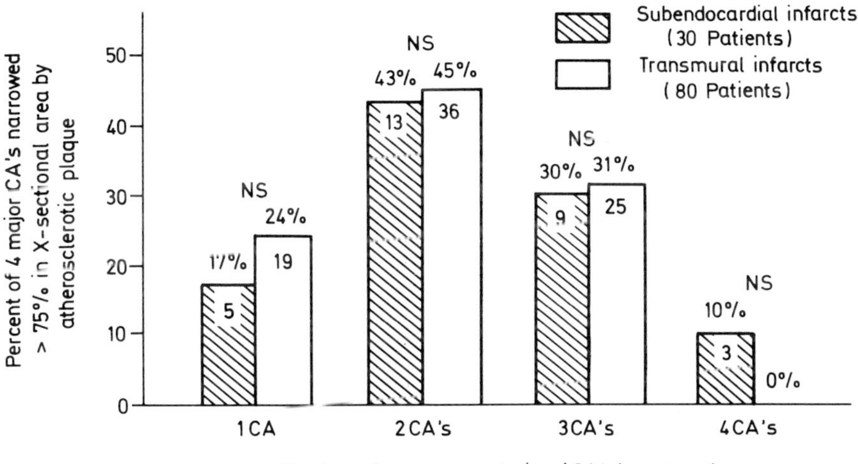

Fig. 3. Comparison of number and percent of four major coronary arteries narrowed greater than 75% in a cross-sectional area by atherosclerotic plaque in 30 patients with subendocardial infarct and 80 patients with transmural infarct

ence (Fig. 2). Likewise, patients with subendocardial infarcts had similar degrees of coronary artery involvement when compared to patients with transmural MI (Fig. 3).

Discussion

Few autopsy studies in the last 2 decades have concentrated specifically on coronary heart disease in the young. Most of the knowledge of this young population based

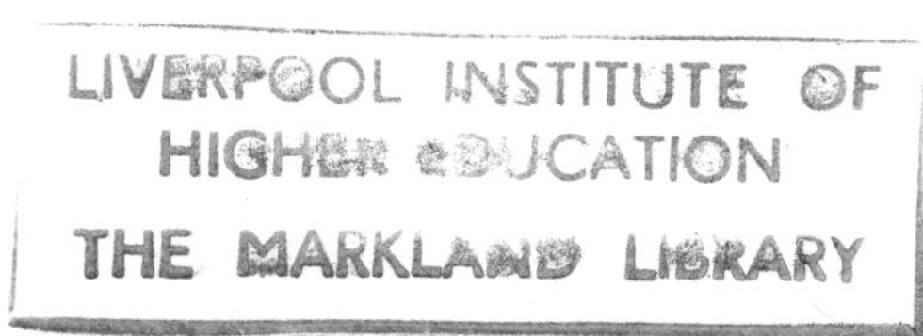

on autopsies comes from studies performed in the second quarter of this century [19–26].

Most recent data on coronary atherosclerosis in young patients is clinical. Since the advent of coronary angiography [27], some clinical studies have concentrated not only on the amount of coronary atherosclerosis seen in symptomatic young adults, but have also shown progression and regression of coronary artery disease in patients less than 40 years of age [28]. The present study describes clinical and autopsy findings in 112 patients under 40 years of age with MI at autopsy. The mode of presentation in the majority of our patients was sudden death, and in approximately one-third of the patients chest pain was the presenting symptom. Of the patients less than 30 years of age, 70% died during or soon after exercise, whereas in the majority of patients 31–40 years of age, the terminal event occurred at rest. Of the 73 patients in whom a history of risk factors could be elicited, 56% had one or more. The incidence of the presence of risk factors was significantly greater in patients 31–40 years (65%) than in patients less than 30 years (36%). The reason for these differences is unclear.

A history of prior cardiac disease was more frequent in patients 31–40 years of age (71%) than in patients under 30 years (9%). This difference may have been accentuated because symptoms of chest pain in patients under 30 years of age conceivably could have been interpreted as noncardiac in origin. Indeed, 47% of patients less than 30 years with healed MI at autopsy had either silent infarcts or the symptoms of chest pain had been ignored.

At autopsy, isolated healed MI was the most frequent finding (41%) and acute and healed MI was present in 23%. Thus, 64% of our patients at autopsy had prior MI. This incidence is similar to the 59% reported by Roberts and Buja [10] in 107 autopsy patients, average age 59, who died of acute MI.

Of the four major coronary arteries examined at autopsy in the 112 patients with MI, one or two coronary arteries were severely narrowed in two-thirds of the patients, and only one-third had three-vessel disease. This finding is different from the previous reports on patients with fatal acute infarction [14], sudden death [12], angina pectoris [13], and healed MI [15], in which the average involvement was narrowing of at least two or three of the four major coronary arteries. However, in these previously reported studies the average age of the patients was 53 years. Comparison of the degree of luminal compromise and extent of coronary artery atherosclerosis in patients with and without a prior history of cardiac disease showed significantly greater atherosclerosis in patients with prior cardiac disease.

Comparison of the severity of coronary artery disease in patients with MI at autopsy to patients with coronary heart disease without MI at autopsy showed significantly greater disease in patients with MI. This finding is similar to that reported in 27 patients (average age 59) who died of acute transmural MI [14]. The degree of luminal compromise and extent of coronary atherosclerosis was greater in patients with healed left ventricular scars as compared to those without [14].

Our patients 31–40 years of age had significantly greater disease than patients under 30 years. This finding is contrary to that reported by Roberts et al. [14] in patients with acute transmural MI, sudden death [12], angina pectoris [13], and healed MI [15]. Of our 110 patients with MI at autopsy, 30 had subendocardial infarcts, and 80 had transmural infarcts: The degree of luminal compromise and extent of severe atherosclerosis was similar in the two groups, which is similar to previous reports [10].

Of the total 390 coronary arteries examined in 110 patients, 234 (60%) were greater than 75% narrowed in the cross-sectional area by atherosclerotic plaque for an average of 2.14 coronary arteries per study patient. This ratio is less than previous reports of patients with various types of coronary heart disease [12–15]. Our patients under 30 had, on an average, less disease (1.8/patient) than patients 31–40 years (2.3/patient).

Coronary artery thrombi were present in 38% of our patients, and were more frequent in patients less than 30 years than in patients 31–40 years. The reasons for this difference are unclear. The reported incidence of thrombi has varied from 7% to 91% [2–12, 19–21, 26]. Our overall incidence of coronary thrombi is similar (39%) to that reported by Roberts and Buja in their 107 patients with fatal myocardial infarction [10].

The artery most commonly involved with atherosclerosis was the left anterior descending (90%), followed by the right (60%), left circumflex (44%), and left main (22%). Vlodaver and Edwards [29] have studied the maximum distribution of atheromatous lesions in 50 unselected adult subjects and found the middle third of the right coronary artery to be the artery most commonly involved: The second most common site was the proximal half of the left anterior descending coronary artery. Roberts et al. report almost similar amounts of severe narrowing in the right, left anterior descending, and left circumflex coronary arteries in patients with coronary heart disease [12–15]. These differences are possibly because of patient selection and methods of study, though the ages of the patients may also be a determining factor.

Summary

Clinical and morphologic observations in 112 patients (103 men, 9 woman) with MI under the age of 40 are described. Sixty-six (59%) died suddenly, 40 (36%) had a history of chest pain greater than 1 h in duration, two died in chronic congestive heart failure, and four died shortly after aortocoronary bypass operations. Of the 73 patients in whom a history of risk factors could be elicited, 41 (56%) had predisposition to coronary atherosclerosis. The presence of risk factors was significantly higher in patients 31–40 years of age compared to patients less than 30 years. A history as to the presence or absence of prior cardiac disease was available in 85 of the 112 patients and of these, 47 (55%) had been symptomatic. Heart weight was increased in 61 (54%).

At autopsy, acute MI was present in 40 patients (36%); healed MI in 46 (41%); and both acute and healed MI in 26 (23%). One of the four major coronary arteries was severely compromised in 24 patients (21%) two in 49 (44%), three in 34 (30%), and all four coronary arteries in only three patients (3%). Patients with prior cardiac disease had significantly greater severity of coronary atherosclerosis than patients without. Patients 31–40 years of age had significantly greater coronary atherosclerosis than patients under 30 years. There was no significant difference in the severity of coronary artery disease in patients with subendocardial infarct compared to those with transmural infarcts. The severity of coronary atherosclerosis in the 112 patients was compared to that in 74 age-matched patients who died of coronary heart disease without evidence of MI at autopsy. The patients with MI had a greater severity of coronary artery disease. The coronary artery most commonly involved was the left anterior descending in 90% of our patients and, in 18%, it was the only artery of involvement. The most frequent type and combination of the four major coronary arteries involved were left anterior descending and right (30%), and left anterior descending, left circumflex, and right (28%). Coronary artery thrombi were present in 42 of the patients (38%), and were more frequent in patients less than 30 years (67%) than in patients 31–40 years of age (27%).

References

1. Allison RB, Rodriguez FL, Higgins EA Jr et al. (1963) Clinicopathologic correlations in coronary atherosclerosis: Four hundred-thirty patients with postmortem coronary angiography. Circulation 27:170–184
2. Baroldi G (1965) Acute coronary occlusion as a cause of myocardial infarct and sudden coronary heart death. Am J Cardiol 16:859–880
3. Harland WA, Holburn AM (1966) Coronary thrombosis and myocardial infarction. Lancet II:1158–1159
4. Chapman I (1968) Relationships of recent coronary artery occlusion and acute myocardial infarction. J M Sinai Hosp 35:149–154
5. Jorgensen L, Holrem JW, Chandler AB, Borchgrevink CF (1968) The pathology of acute coronary death. Acta Anaesthesiol Scand [Suppl] 29:193
6. Edwards JE (1969) What is myocardial infarction? Circulation [Suppl IV] 40:IV-5-IV-11
7. Spain CM, Bradess VA (1970) Sudden death from coronary heart disease: Survival time, frequency of thrombi, and cigarette smoking. Dis Chest 58:107–110
8. Bouch DC, Montgomery GL (1970) Cardiac lesions in fatal cases of recent myocardial ischemia from a coronary care unit. Br Heart J 32:795–803
9. Edwards JE (1971) The value and limitations of necropsy studies in coronary arterial disease. Prog Cardiovasc Dis 13:309–323
10. Roberts WC, Buja IM (1972) The frequency and significance of coronary arterial thrombi and other observations in fatal acute myocardial infarction. A study of 107 necropsy patients. Am J Cardiol 52:425–443
11. Roberts WC, Ferrans VJ, Levy RI, Fredrickson DS (1973) Cardiovascular pathology in hyperlipoproteinemia: Anatomic observations in 42 necropsy patients with normal or abnormal serum lipoprotein pattern. Am J Cardiol 31:557–570
12. Roberts WC, Jones AA (1979) Quantitation of coronary arterial narrowing at necropsy in sudden coronary death: Analysis of 31 patients and comparison with 25 control subjects. Am J Cardiol 44:39–45
13. Roberts WC, Virmani R (1979) Quantification of coronary arterial narrowing in clinically isolated unstable angina pectoris. An analysis of 22 necropsy patients. Am J Med 67:792–799
14. Roberts WC, Jones AA (1980) Quantification of coronary arterial narrowing at necropsy in acute transmural myocardial infarction. Analysis and comparison of findings in 27 patients and 22 controls. Circulation 61:786–790
15. Virmani R, Roberts WC (1980) Quantification of coronary arterial narrowing and of left ventricular myocardial scarring in healed myocardial infarction with chronic, eventually fatal, congestive cardiac failure. Am J Med 68:831–838
16. Keyes A, Aravanis C, Blackburn H et al. (1972) Probability of middle-aged men developing coronary heart disease in five years. Circulation 45:815–828
17. Kannel WB (1976) Some lessons in cardiovascular epidemiology from Framingham. Am J Cardiol 37:269–282

18. Monthly Vital Statistics Report (1971) National Center for Health Statistics, Washington, D.C., 26, No 12
19. Glendy RE, Levine SA, White PD (1937) Coronary disease in youth. Comparison of 100 patients under 40 with 300 persons past 80. JAMA 109/22:1775–1781
20. Master AM, Dack S, Jaffe HL (1939) Age, sex and hypertension in myocardial infarction due to coronary occlusion. Arch Intern Med 64:767–786
21. Blumgart HL, Schlesinger MJ, David D (1940) Studies on the relation of the clinical manifestations of angina pectoris, coronary thrombosis, and myocardial infarction to the pathologic findings with particular reference to the significance of the collateral circulation. Am Heart J 19:1–91
22. French AJ, Dock W (1944) Fatal coronary arteriosclerosis in young soldiers. JAMA 124:1233–1237
23. Poe WE (1947) Fatal coronary artery disease in young men. Am Heart J 33:76–83
24. Yater WM, Trau AH, Brown WG et al. (1948) Coronary artery disease in men 18 to 39 years of age. Am Heart J 36:334–372
25. Dry TJ (1950) The relationship of the degree of coronary atherosclerosis with age in men. Circulation 1:645–654
26. Spain DM, Brades VA (1960) The relationship of coronary thrombosis to coronary atherosclerosis and ischemic heart disease. A necropsy study covering a period of 25 years. Am J Med Sci 240:701–721
27. Baltaxe HA, Amplatz K, Levin DC (1973) Coronary angiography. Thomas, Springfield
28. Roskamm H, Sturzenhofecker P, Gornandt L et al. (1980) Progression and regression of coronary artery disease in postinfarction patients less than 40 years of age. Cleve Clin Q 47:192–194
29. Vlodaver Z, Edwards JE (1971) Pathology of coronary atherosclerosis. Prog Cardiovasc Dis 14/3:256–274

Comparison of Luminal Narrowing by Atherosclerotic Plaques in Young and Very Old Necropsy Patients with Fatal Coronary Events

B. F. WALLER and W. C. ROBERTS [1]

This study compares the amounts of luminal narrowing by atherosclerotic plaques in necropsy patients with fatal coronary events at 40 years of age and younger to those 90 years and older.

Materials and Methods

Certain clinical observations in 69 study patients, 59 patients aged 40 years or less and ten patients 90 years or more, are summarized in Table 1. The type and frequency of fatal coronary events in the study patients are summarized in Table 2.

Table 1. Certain clinical observations in 69 necropsy patients with fatal coronary events: 59 patients age $\leq$ 40 years and 10 patients $\geq$ 90 years

Item	$\leq$40	$\geq$90
1. Age (years)	22 – 40 (34)	90 – 99 (93)
2. No. (%) men	41 (69)	3
3. Angina pectoris	33 (56%)	5
4. History of hypertension	28/48 (58%)	8
5. Cigarette smoking	22/30 (73%)	5
6. Diabetes mellitus	9 (15%)	1
7. Estrogen therapy	2 (3%)	0
8. Total cholesterol (mg/dl)	210 – 700 (341)* (30 patients)	236 – 283 (259)* (4 patients)

* $P < 0.05$

The epicardial coronary arteries in all 69 patients were studied at necropsy in a similar fashion. The entire lengths of the right, left main, left anterior descending, and left circumflex coronary arteries were removed from the heart, fixed in formalin, radiographed, decalcified, cut transversely into 5-mm long segments, processed in alcohols and xylene for histologic study, and a histologic section was prepared from each segment and stained by the Movat method. The degree of luminal narrowing in all segments was determined by examination of the histologic sections magnified 25–50 times. The percent of cross-sectional area luminal narrowing by atherosclerotic plaques was divided into the following five categories: 0–25, 26–50, 51–75, 79–95 and 96–100.

1 Pathology Branch, National Heart, Lung and Blood Institute, National Institutes of Health, Bethesda, Maryland, USA

Table 2. Types of fatal coronary events in 69 necropsy patients: 59 patients, age ≤ 40 years and 10 patients age ≥ 90 years

Event	No. (%) Pts	
	≤ 40 ($n = 59$)	≥ 90 ($n = 10$)
1. Sudden coronary death	35 (59)	1
2. Acute MI	7 (12)	5
3. Healed MI with chronic congestive heart failure	7 (12)	4
4. Pure angina pectoris[a]	10 (17)	0
Totals	59 (100)	10

[a] Death during cardiac catheterization or at time of aortocoronary bypass operation. Never clinical evidence or acute myocardial infarction or congestive heart failure.

Results

The results of quantitative analysis of 3178 5-mm coronary segments (2673 in patients 40 years or less and 415 in patients 90 years or more) are summarized in Table 3 and Figure 1. Both groups of study patients had a similar percent of coronary segments narrowed 76%–100% in the cross-sectional area by atherosclerotic plaques: 775 of 2763 (28%) and 92 of 415 (22%) (Table 3). The patients 40 years or less had significantly more coronary segments narrowed 96%–100% in the cross-sectional area

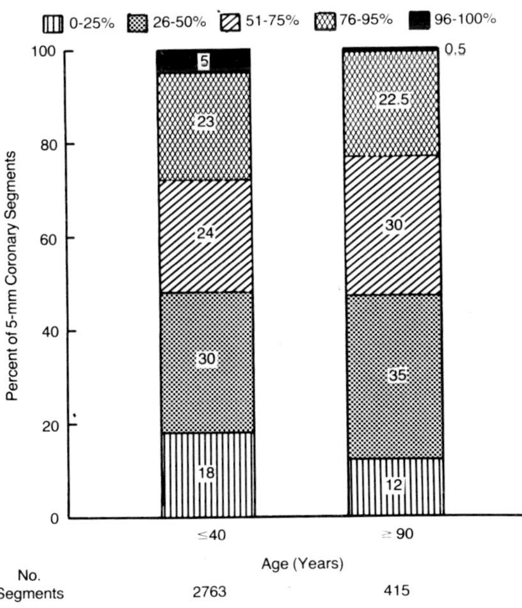

Fig. 1. Percent of 5-mm long coronary arterial segments narrowed to various degrees in the cross-sectional area by atherosclerotic plaques in 69 necropsy patients (59 patients 40 years or more and ten patients 90 years or more) with fatal coronary events

Table 3. Number and percent of 5-mm segments of 271 major coronary arteries (right, left main, left anterior descending, left circumflex) and the grade of cross-sectional area luminal narrowing by atherosclerotic plaques in 69 necropsy patients with fatal coronary events: 59 patients (231 arteries) age $\leq$ 40 years (Y) and 10 patients (40 arteries) age $\geq$ 90 years (0)

Coronary artery	0 – 25 No. (%)		26 – 50 No. (%)		51 – 75 No. (%)		76 – 95 No. (%)		96 – 100 No. (%)		Totals No. (%)	
	Y	O	Y	O	Y	O	Y	O	Y	O	Y	O
R	207 (21)	21 (15)	230 (23)	46 (33)	260 (26)	43 (30)	244 (24)	29 (21.5)	60 (6)	2 (0.5)	1001 (36)	141 (34)
LM	9 (17)	3	13 (24)	6	13 (24)	1	18 (33)	0	1 (2)	0	54 (2)	10 (2)
LAD	166 (16)	16 (11)	283 (28)	51 (36)	273 (27)	44 (30)	238 (24)	34 (23)	52 (5)	0 (0)	1012 (37)	145 (35)
LC	119 (17)	12 (10)	174 (25)	41 (35)	241 (35)	39 (32)	126 (18)	27 (23)	36 (5)	0 (0)	696 (25)	119 (29)
Total	501 (18)	52 (12)	700 (30)	144 (35)	787 (24)	127 (30)	626 (23)	90 (22.5)	149 (5)	2 (0.5)	2765 (100)	415 (100)

Table 4. Amount of calcific deposits in coronary atherosclerotic plaques in 69 necropsy patients with fatal coronary events: 59 patients age ≤ 40 years and 10 patients age ≥ 90 years

Calcific deposits in atherosclerotic plaques ($0 - 4^+$)	No. (%) patients	
	≤ 40	≥ 90
0	39 (66)	0
$1^+ - 2^+$	20 (34)	8
$3^+ - 4^+$	0	2
Totals	59 (100)	10

by atherosclerotic plaques (i.e., virtually total lumen occlusion). Furthermore, the frequency of left main coronary arteries narrowed 76%–100% in the cross-sectional area was much higher in the younger patients than in the older patients [19 of 54 (35%) versus 0 of 10]. The amounts of calcific deposits in coronary atherosclerotic plaques in each age group are summarized in Table 4. In 20 (34%) of 59 patients 40 years or less and in all ten patients over age 90 years, calcific deposits were found.

Discussion

This is the first study to compare quantitatively at necropsy the degree and extent of coronary arterial luminal narrowing by atherosclerotic plaques in patients with fatal coronary events 40 years or less to those 90 years or more.

Both groups had a similar percent of 5-mm coronary segments narrowed 76%–100% in the cross-sectional area by plaques: 28% in patients 40 years or less and 22% in patients 90 years or more. Both young and old patients also had *diffuse* coronary narrowing with only 18% and 12% of the coronary segments, respectively, narrowed 0%–25% in the cross-sectional area.

Three major differences between the two groups were noted. The patients 40 years or less had a higher frequency of severely narrowed (96%–100%) coronary arterial segments [149 of 2763 (5%) versus 2 of 415 (0.5%)], a higher frequency of severe (76%–100%) left main coronary narrowing [19 of 35 (35%) versus of 0 of 10], and a lower frequency of coronary arterial calcific deposits [20 of 59 (34%) versus 10 of 10].

Coexistence of Vigorous Exercise and Heavy Smoking in Triggering Acute Myocardial Infarction in Men Under 35 Years – Fact or Fiction?

A. PIC, J. P. BROUSTET, B. SALIOU, P. GOSSE, and P. GUERN [1]

We would like to put forward the following questions:
- What is the rate of myocardial infarction (MI) occurring during or immediately after severe physical exercise (these may also be called exercise MIs or ex. MIs).
- Do these ex. MIs show particular characteristics?
- Would these MIs have been predictable and if so could they have been avoided?

Patients

During the past four years patients who had MIs before the age of 35 were studied. There were 26 of them with a mean age of 29.2 years. Nine of them (35%), mean age 30, had MIs during or immediately following severe physical exercise. In three cases this was a football match, in three others a rugby match and in the remaining three cycling in mountainous regions. The other 17 cases had not undertaken severe physical exercise during or before their MIs.

In 1953 Morris et al. [4] reported that in a large series of 1653 MIs at all ages, only 1.9% could be related to inhabitual physical exercise.

Even when considering that a study group of 26 is rather small and that more young people do sports than older ones, the proportion of 35% of MIs due to severe physical exercise cannot in our opinion be accidental.

Risk Factors

Of all the risk factors smoking is by far the most frequent: 81% of all patients were smokers and 42% smoked more than 30 cigarettes per day. This frequency does not vary between the ex. MI group and the entire group of patients under 35.

Hyperlipidemia was found in 31% of patients and was of Type II and IV according to Frederickson's classification. Here, too, the frequency did not vary from one group to the other. High blood pressure appears to be rare. 31% of the patients had a parent with a history of coronary heart disease before the age of 60. Only 2 patients appeared to be free of the known risk factors for coronary heart disease.

Results of Coronary Angiography (Table 2)

Coronary angiography was performed approximately three months after the infarction and analysed independently by two investigators. As one patient died on the

1 Hopital Cardiologique du Haut Lévêque, Avenue de Magellan, F-33604 Pessac, France

Table 1. Risk factors

Tobacco: smokers 81% (more than 30 cigarettes a day 42%)

cig/day	0	≤ 10	$10 - 30$	≥ 30
Ex. MI (9 pts)	2	1	2	4
Others (17 pts)	3	1	6	7

Hyperlipidemia: 31%
    Ex. MI 3 pts   others 5 pts

High blood pressure: 8%

Family: 31%
    Ex. MI 2 pts   others 6 pts

No risk factors: 2 pts (Ex. MI)

Table 2. Coronary angiography

	All (25 pts)	Ex. MI (9 pts)	Others (16 pts)
Normal C. A.	9 (36%)	3	6
slender coronary artery	3 (12%)	2	1
One-V. D.	8 (32%)	3	5
Two- or three-V. D.	5 (20%)	1	4

first day after admission we can consider only 25 patients here. In 9 patients (36%) the coronary arteriogram was normal. Three patients showed no stenoses but one or more coronary arteries appeared narrowed. Eight patients had one-vessel disease: (five with stenoses and three with occlusions). Five patients had two-vessel disease.

The main results were as follows:
- The frequency of normal coronary arteries is rather high; of course, the presence of very small lesions cannot be ruled out.
- The frequency of normal coronary arteries is not significantly higher in the ex. MI group.
- All patients with normal coronary arteries smoked more than 20 cigarettes per day.

Follow-up of Patients (Table 3)

The follow-up period was 7–40 months.

In 67% of the patients there were no clinical events during the follow-up period. Maximal exercise tests were normal and exercise capacity was excellent. In the ex. MI group prognosis was even better than in the entire group. "All or nothing"

Table 3. Evolution

	Ex.-MI (9 pts)	Others (17 pts)
Without sequelae (67%)	7	11
Death (first day)		1
Angina		3
Heart failure		1
Aneurysm op.	2	1

seems to be the law. Two of nine ex. MI patients had ventricular aneurysms which were operated on. Surgery was very beneficial in one case but the other patient died 6 months later after a period of heart failure.

To illustrate this law of all or nothing, we give the example of a famous French cyclist who was second in the "Tour de France" in 1948 (Fig. 1). While struggling up a mountain pass in the 1952 Tour de France he had an MI. 38 years later we can only detect a slight abnormality in the ECG in V1 and V2. The maximal exercise test is normal and his exercise capacity is excellent at 62 years of age.

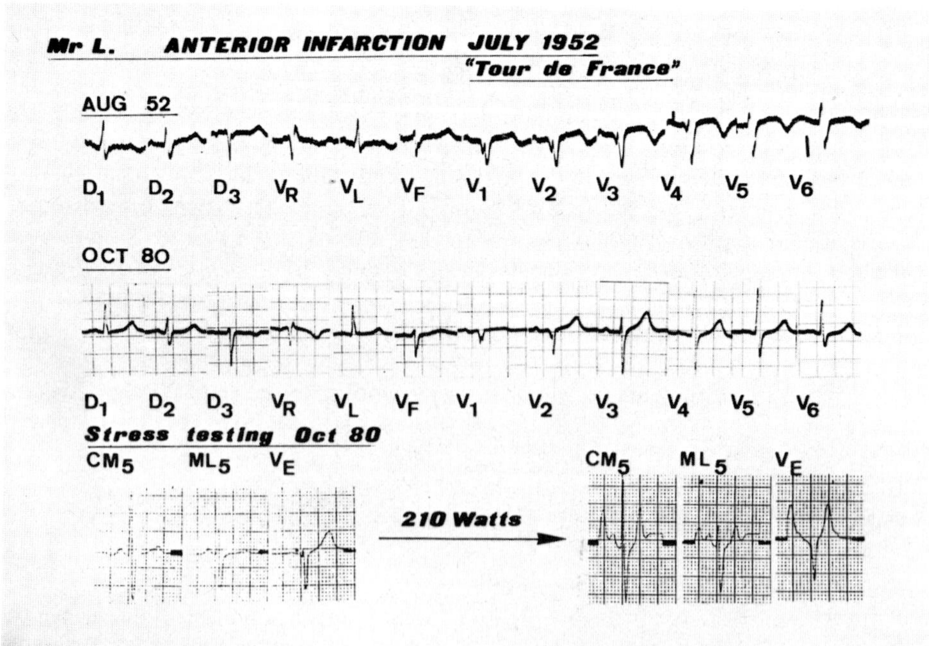

Fig. 1. MI in young sportsmen: evolution without sequelae

Identification of Infarction-prone Patients

Sometimes MI patients at a young age had had chest pain in the preceding weeks or months, but this was often not a typical angina pectoris.

Eleven patients (42%) suffered from chest pain before their MI and this induced three of them to have a heart check-up. Two had a normal ECG at rest and a normal maximal exercise test. The third, an active sportsman, had an abnormal ECG at rest with a negative T wave and up-sloping ST segment in the anterior region. The correction of these abnormalities under exercise wrongly reassured both the physician and the patient. 2½ years later he suffered an MI at the end of a rugby match. The coronary angiography taken one month later was normal and the ergonovine tests were negative.

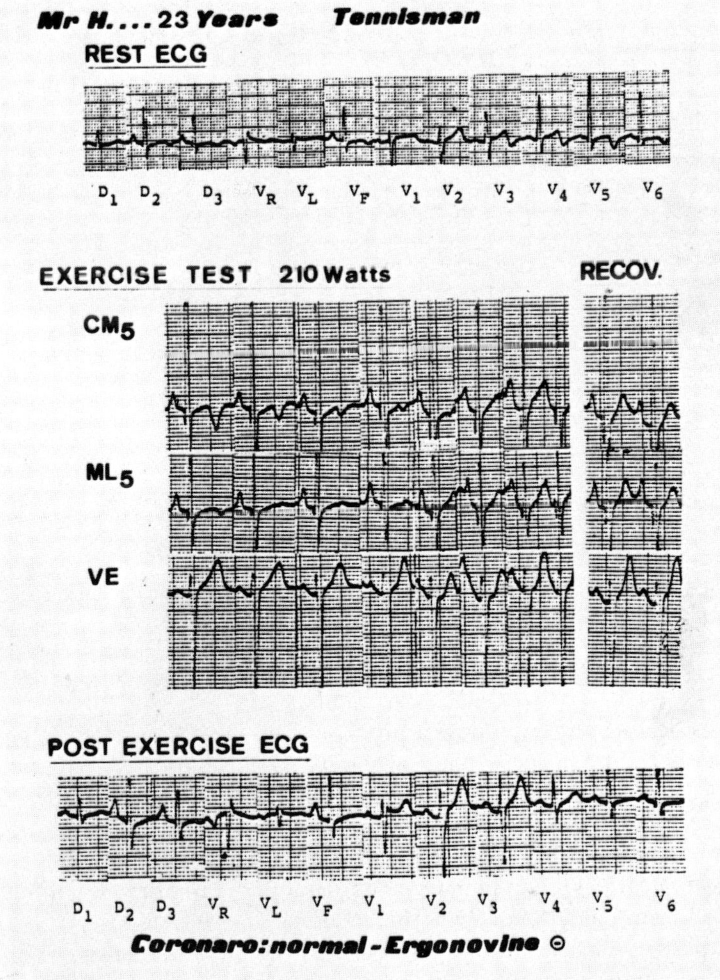

Fig. 2. Benign rest ECG abnormalities disappearing during stress testing

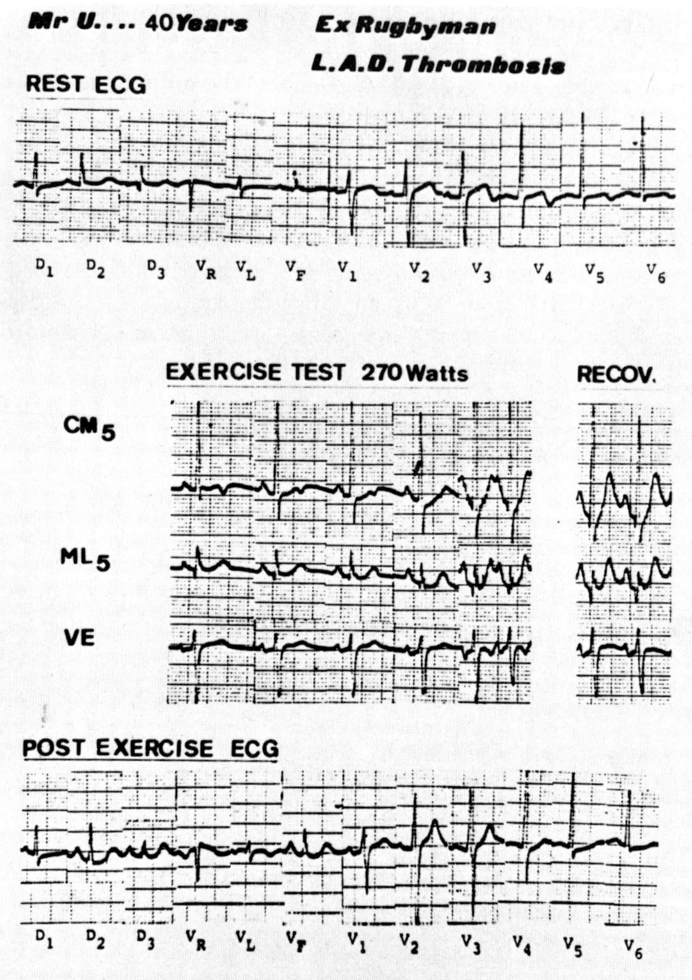

Fig. 3. Rest ECG abnormalities, sequelae of recent anterior MI, disappearing during stress testing. *LAD*, left anterior descending

ECG abnormalities in sportsmen pose a problem. The fact that they disappear during exercise is considered a sign of their benignity. For example, a young male tennis player (Fig. 2) came to see us about ECG abnormalities and regardless of their disappearance during exercise we carried out a coronary angiography. Normalisation of ST/T alterations during exercise is also possible in patients after a recent anteroseptal infarction with akinesia in the left ventriculogram. In our case coronary arteriogram and left ventriculogram were normal (Fig. 3).

Sportsmen displaying such abnormalities in the resting ECG should in our opinion undergo further studies, as should those who suffered chest pain. In addition to an exercise test at least thallium scintigraphy should be performed.

Coronary Spasm Triggered by Physical Exercise – Role of Smoking

This paper cannot forego mentioning coronary spasm triggered by physical exercise. Fig. 4 shows a 33-year old athlete who smoked and who complained of chest pain after exercise. Resting ECG and ECG during maximal exercise were normal, but

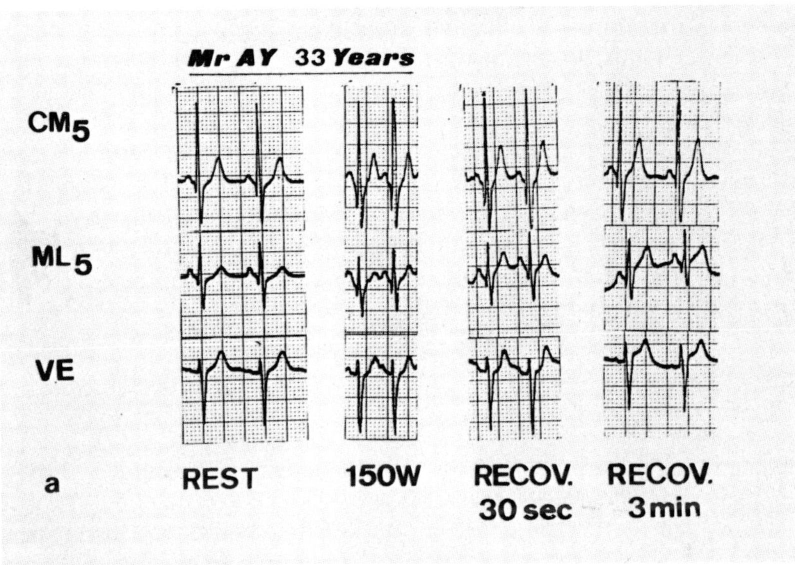

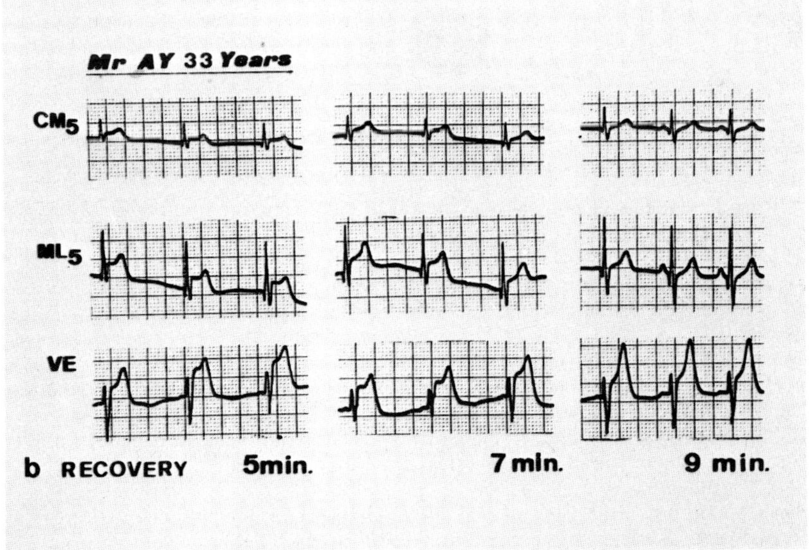

Fig. 4a, b. Variant angina occurring after exercise: normal coronary arteriography. During and immediately after exercise ECG is normal (a), 5 minutes after exercise there is a significant ST segment elevation (b)

five minutes after finishing the exercise we can see an ST segment elevation typical of the variant form of angina pectoris which disappeared a few minutes later. We have observed this phenomenon in five patients whose coronary arteriograms were normal [3]. Under treatment with a calcium antagonist, we have never been able to reproduce this phenomenon.

We cannot help thinking that those patients were destined to suffer an MI one day, perhaps even while using a calcium antagonist (Fig. 4b).

It is well-known that during severe physical activity there is an increase of coagulability. Fortunately this is associated with an activation of fibrinolytic activity [1]. These modifications are less important after physical training or after beta-adrenergic antagonist [2, 6]. Platelet aggregation is also encouraged by smoking, leading to aggregation of platelets on the pathologic arterial intima. Thromboxane A_2 released by activated platelets may trigger a spasm favoring thrombosis [5]. This mechanism may be exaggerated in smokers and result in MI during or after exercise. As thrombus would be a major key in the pathogenesis of myocardial infarction of this type, there may be spontaneous thrombolysis resulting in normal coronary arteries, at least in a coronary arteriogram taken some time afterward.

Conclusion

We can conclude that intense physical activity is able to trigger an acute MI. Generally this event occurs in patients who are heavy smokers.

Atypical chest pain or ECG abnormalities are a frequent reason for medical consultation. The physician has to be very careful; it would be dramatic to interrupt the career of a sportsman but sometimes this is necessary in order to save a life.

Perhaps myocardial thallium scintigraphy and ergonovine tests are useful in the detection of MI in such cases.

References

1. Astrup T (1979) The effects of physical activity on blood coagulation and fibrinolysis. In: Naughton JP, Hellerstein HK (eds) Exercise testing and exercise training in coronary heart disease, vol 1. Academic Press, New York, p 169
2. Broustet JP, Boisseau M, Bouloumie J et al. (1976) L'influence de l'effort aigu et de l'entraînement physique sur la fonction plaquettaire du coronarien. Arch Mal Coeur 3:305
3. Broustet JP, Griffo R, Series E et al. (1979) Angor de Prinzmetal déclenché par l'arrêt de l'effort. Cinq cas à coronarographie normale. Arch Mal Coeur Vaiss 72:385
4. Morris JN, Heady JA, Raffle PAG et al. (1953) Coronary heart disease and physical activity of work. Lancet II:1053
5. Scheele K, Muller KM (1980) Acute cardiac death caused by an increase of platelet aggregation during and after maximal physical stress In: Lubich T, Venerando A (eds) Sports cardilogy, vol 1. Aulogaggi, Bologne, p 449
6. Series E, Broustet JP, Boisseau M, Bricaud H (1978) Hémolyse et fonction plaquettaire chez les porteurs de prothèses valvulaires cardiaques. Modifications à l'effort et sous propranolol. Arch Mal Coeur Vaiss 71:1129

Myocardial Infarction at Young Age During High Physical Exercise

J. Delaye, J. Beaune, and J. P. Delahaye[1]

It is a widely held opinion that sport and physical exercise protect against coronary heart disease; hence the present fashion of physical exercise.

Many prospective studies on the effect of sports activities are under way and they may allow an objective evaluation of the roles attributed to tobacco supression and weight reduction in association with the direct effect of physical training [6].

Except for patients with known coronary disease, the occurrence of coronary events during physical exercise is extremely rare. Studies of the relationship between myocardial infarction (MI) and physical exercise are still few. There is a study, however, published in 1952, of 1347 cases which estimates the percentage of high effort infarctions at 1.9% [2, 3], while another study published in 1974 puts the figure of sudden death triggered by high effort between 2% and 5% [30]. (Sudden death defined as infarction with fatal evolution within 24 hours). None of these general studies specify the type of effort.

Other studies about MI in young and relatively young patients (less than 40 years) also do not regularly deal with the circumstances of the infarction [4, 16, 31, 32]. Moreover, very few of the studies mentioned in literature include coronary angiographic data [17, 21].

This paper presents a study of 12 cases of MI during sports activities in young men. All had a coronary angiography performed. The results of the clinical and angiographic findings as well as a practical conclusion will follow.

Material

Twelve patients from 1600 submitted for coronary angiography were selected. As shown in Table 1 they were all males between 17 and 39 years of age (mean 27 years) with regular physical exercise. Four patients (cases 4, 6, 9, and 10) had usually had two training sessions per week. Five patients (cases 1, 5, 7, 8, and 12) had done moderate regular training once a week. Cases 2, 3, and 11 had done little training once a week irregularly.

Types of sport were football (five), cycling (three), rugby (two) and one patient lifted heavy weights. In all cases angina pectoris began during exercise. In case 2 it started 30 minutes afterwards.

Seven patients had suffered an anterior and five patients an inferior wall infarction. Enzyme studies were found to be positive in all but case 9.

---

1 Hospices Civils de Lyon, Hopital Cardio-Vasculaires et Pneumologique Louis Pradel, Lyon-Montchat, F-69394 Lyon Cedex 3, France

Table 1. Patients included in this study

No.	Age	Year	Site of infarction	Type of sport and level of training	Result of coronary angiography (C) and ventrilography (V)
1	20	1975	A.S.I.	Football (moderate)	C: ulcerated atheromatous plaques V: aneurysm 2, 3, 4
2	38	1973	A.S.I.	Cycling (little)	C: R 40%; LAD 80 Cir 40% V: akinesia 2, 3
3	39	1974	A.L.I.	Rugby (little)	C: R 40%; LAD 90% V: akinesia 4, 5
4	33	1978	I.I.	Basketball (important)	C: R 70% V: akinesia 5, 6
5	32	1977	I.I.	Football (moderate)	C: circ 80%, RC 80% V: posterior akinesia
6	22	1977	I.I.	Rugby (important)	C: circ 30% V: normal
7	29	1977	A.L.I.	Cycling (moderate)	C: normal V: aneurysm 3, 4
8	25	1978	A.S.I.	Football (moderate)	C: normal V: aneurysm
9	17	1969	I.I.	Cycling (important)	C: normal V: normal
10	26	1976	A.S.I.	Football (important)	C: normal V: hypokinesia 2, 3
11	23	1969	I.I.	Static effort (little)	C: right coronary artery dissection V: normal
12	25	1973	A.L.I.	Football (moderate)	C: fistula between pulmonary artery and LAD V: akinesia 2, 3, 4

ASI: anteroseptal infarction; ALI: anterolateral infarction; II: inferior infarction; 1, 2, 3: anterior segments of left ventricular wall; 4, 5, 6: inferior segements of left ventricle; R, RC = right coronary artery (better: ACD); Cir, Circ. = circumflex artery (better: Rcx)

Smoking was the most prevalent risk factor, with more than 20 cigarettes per day in 10 cases; cases 7 and 11 did not smoke. There was no patient with hypertension.

Coronary angiographies were performed in all patients (Sones technique) with ventriculography in the 30°-right anterior oblique projection, and interpreted by several observers with the following findings:

- Significant coronary atherosclerotic lesions in six patients; presenting as one-vessel disease in three patients, two-vessel disease in two patients and three-vessel disease in one patient.
- Coronary fistulae between the left anterior descending and the pulmonary artery was found in case 12.
- Localized dissection of the first two segments of the right coronary artery was seen in case 11.

– Normal coronary arteries with no significant lesions could be verified in four patients.
– Ventriculography was abnormal in all eight patients with coronary lesions. Myocardial damage corresponded to the arterial lesions. Of the four patients with normal coronary arteries an apical aneurysm was seen in two, an apical hypokinesis in one patient. In one patient with the clinical course of an inferior wall infarction the ventriculogram was normal.

Comments

Frequency of Coronary Events During Physical Exercise

It is difficult to estimate the frequency of sudden death in subjects under 40. The information concerning sudden cardiac death supplied by Opie in 1975 [29] was one death for 50 000 hours of rugby in subjects practicing this sport. This incidence is low when compared to that of sudden deaths in referees of the same sport, namely one for 30 000 hours. It is important to note here that the mean age for active players is 26 years, for referees it is 50 years.

As far as we know there is no information concerning the frequency of MI under these circumstances. It seems logical though, to assume that it is more frequent than sudden cardiac death due to coronary heart disease. The frequency of sudden death with regard to type of sport is also not exactly known.

In the above mentioned study [29], many types of sports were represented: Seven deaths in rugby, two in football, one each in golf, alpinism, tennis, jogging and yachting. To complete this list, let us include findings of other countries; three deaths in cycling, and one each in basketball, baseball, weightlifting, parachuting, fencing [22] and ice hockey [21]. As outlined by several authors, the accidents were sometimes associated with special emotional stress. It is important to note the absence of such incidences in endurance sports like marathon running [2] and cross-country skiing [19], in spite of the high physical demands involved. At this level of high and sustained effort, which usually demands regular training, subjects are beyond what is called by Morris et al. [25] "the protector threshold of exercise".

It is noteworthy that short distance runners burn essential carbohydrates while long distance runners also burn lipids [5, 18].

A classic example for the possible role of sports in the prevention of coronary heart disease is Clarence de Mar, the well-known marathon runner of Boston who died at the age of 69 of a noncardiac cause and whose coronaries were found to be free of atherosclerotic lesions [10].

Observations led Bassler [3] and Noakes et al. [26] to claim that marathon runners never die from MI. The case of a fatal infarction in such a subject published by Green et al. [15] in 1976 was thus the cause of prolonged controversy connecting the death to a heat stroke [33]. However, a study of 6 cases of MI in marathon-runners was reported by Noakes et al. [26].

We can summarise that MIs occur rarely in trained athletes and very rarely in endurance trained athletes with intensive regular training.

Types of Exercise and Environmental Influences

It is not necessary to discuss the differences between static and dynamic exercise per se at this point.

The importance of environmental influences on the other hand can clearly be demonstrated with the example of the marathon runner: a well-trained runner can run 35–45 km (approx. 1.6 km every 5–6 minutes). According to Costill [9] this corresponds to 90% of maximal oxygen uptake, with a fluid loss generally exceeding 3% [34]. It becomes evident that a change in temperature, humidity, and fluid intake alone is of considerable importance, not taking into account other influences like altitude and emotional stress. All these factors may play a role, even more so when training is insufficient or irregular.

Exercise Myocardial Infarction – Causes and Mechanisms

The differences between exercise MI with pre-existing coronary pathology and MI with normal coronaries should be emphasised.

a) Exercise MI with pre-existing coronary pathology:

Common atherosclerotic coronary lesions were found most frequently in our study as well as in other series described in the literature. They are most often located in the proximal part of the three important vessels (one-vessel or multi-vessel disease). In one of our patients, however, the stenosis was, according to usual angiographic criteria, nonsignificant at 30%. We should consider that in conditions of maximal exercise where vascular adjustment is the single factor allowing an increase of coronary flow, a moderate stenosis suffices to create an ischemia and lead to MI if the ischemia lasts more than 30 minutes. Such moderate stenoses may eventually be aggravated by thrombosis or spasm [27].

Lesions of uncommon type, congenital or dystrophic, are less frequent.

Congenital lesions: Coronary pulmonary fistulas are the main congenital lesions. Rupture of the distal vessel and coronary steel mechanism are important factors [11].

Abnormalities of origin: the small number of patients included in our series is probably due to the fact that congenital malformative coronary pathology is usually revealed earlier in life.

Susceptibility of the coronary artery wall: Coronary dissections can occur in normal or ectasic arteries [14].

b) Exercise myocardial infarction with a normal coronary arteriogram:

Four patients in our study fall into this group. Similar cases were reported in other studies [17, 21, 26]. We will view them together with the more numerous cases of MI with normal coronary findings, which are not related to physical exercise. There is no adequate explanation for these cases.

Coronary thrombosis already lysed at the time of coronary angiography [21] is very often proposed. This etiology is possible since the majority of patients underwent their coronary angiography more than a week after the acute phase of MI.

Coronary spasm as a cause has been proposed as a hypothesis by several authors [8, 13, 20] but up to date there is no documented evidence to support it. On the other hand the existence of authentic spasms observed in Prinzmetal angina supports this hypothesis [12, 28]. If the spasm lasts longer than 20 minutes. It is believed to be responsible for MI. In all cases described in the literature, spasms observed in Prinzmetal angina were relieved by nitrate derivatives.

Spasm may be due to either an increased sensitivity of the arterial wall or a spontaneous increase of catecholamines, or they may be elicited by physical exercise, as in the patients discussed here.

Coronary emboli [8] or angiographically *unidentifiable coronary lesions* are other hypotheses. Total occlusion of the diagonal branch and/or enzymatic problems may be the reasons for the imbalance due to an inadequate adjustment of coronary vascularization and myocardial mass. Disturbances of oxyhemoglobin-dissociation, enzymatic anomalies, particularly in the rate of hydrolysis of the ATP [29] have not been documented to support their role in the cause of exercise-induced MI.

Different mechanisms are responsible for MI occurring during exercise and those immediately after:

MI occurring during exercise: Exercise creates a significant increase in myocardial oxygen demand, which may not be satisfied. If the deficit exceeds 30 min (depending on individual myocardial bloodfow, this varies from one subject to the next) ischemia becomes irreversible and tissue necrosis occurs.

Myocardial infarction occurring immediately after exercise: The period following intense exercise is regarded as one of particular vulnerability [1]. It is a time when perfusion of the myocardium is still unstable. Several factors may cause deterioration of myocardial perfusion:

Arrhythmias: The most serious ones are ventricular fibrillation, responsible for causing deaths observed in treadmill tests (four in 18 000 as reported by Bruce [6a]).

Biochemical alterations: increase of free fatty acids which, exceeding a certain rate, can elicit arrhythmias and arterial thrombosis. The increase can be caused by circulatory catecholamines and precipitate arrhythmias as well as myocardial ischemia.

General vasomotor phenomena: elicited by peripheral vasodilatation due to ambient temperature; bath or shower immediately after exercise or cigarette smoking could amplify the effects of arrhythmias and myocardial biochemical disorders.

In practice the following recommendations should be observed [21]:

1. A sportsman with suspicious chest pain during intense exercise must always be taken seriously and be taken to hospital.
2. He should not walk off, the field by himself, but be carried.
3. Strenous efforts of competitive sports should not be started after the age of 25, without previous medical check-up and scrutinous supervision (clinical exams, treadmill tests, etc.)
4. The risk of coronary event is significantly higher in cigarette-smoking sportsmen.

The occurrence of MI during exercise does not offer arguments against practicing sports. On the contrary, it calls for regular training; for the continuous efforts to eliminate risk factors, smoking in particular; and last but not least for a better understanding of the physiology of sports by the sportsman himself.

Summary

Twelve cases of MI during exercise in men under 40 have been studied. All had coronary arteriography and ventriculography performed:

- Six subjects presented moderate or severe coronary atherosclerotic lesions.
- Four had normal coronary arteries.
- One presented a finding compatible with dissection of the right coronary artery.
- The last presented a decreased lumen of the left descending coronary above a coronary artery fistula.

Several hypotheses have been offered to explain the occurrence of MI in the four patients with normal coronary arteries, including thrombosis with secondary lysis, or spasm. There is no documented support for either hypothesis. These patients as well as the eight with previous coronary pathology run a higher risk of the occurrence of sudden death during exercise. This calls for a program of prudent exercise, particularly in those subjects who had stopped exercising. Special attention must be paid to those factors which cause inevitable deterioration of myocardial perfusion in patients with an exercise MI, such as abrupt changes of ambience and cigarette smoking.

References

1. Adams CW (1972) Symposium on exercise and the heart Introduction. Am J Cardiol 30:713–715
2. Bassler TJ (1972) Previous health and longevity of males athletes (letter). Lancet II:711
3. Bassler TJ (1975) Marathon running and immunity to heart disease. Phys Sports Med 3:77–80
4. Benacerraf A, Castillo-Fenoy A, Goffinet D, Krantz D (1978) L'infarctus du myocarde avant 36 ans. A propos de 20 cas. Arch Mal Coeur 71:756–764
5. Bleich HL, Boro ES (1975) Fuel homeostasis in exercice. N Engl J Med 293:1078–1084
6. Brown KS, Milvy P (1977) A critique of several epidemiological studies of physical activity and its relationship to aging, health and mortality. Ann NY Acad Sci 301:703–719
6a. Bruce RA (1977) Controversy in exercise testing: Old and new aspects. In: Topics in cardiovascular disease. Proceedings of an International Symposium, Basle/Switzerland, May 1976. Horsham/England:CIBA 1977
7. Cheitlin JN, Chave SPW, Adam C et al. (1973) Vigourous exercice in leisure time and the incidence of coronary heart disease. Lancet I:333–339
8. Cheng TO, Bashour T, Singh T, Kelser GA (1972) Myocardial infarction in the absence of coronary arterio-sclerosis; result of coronary spasm. Am J Cardiol 30:180–225
9. Costill DL (1970) Metabolic responsa during distance runing. J Appl Physiol 28:251–225
10. Currens JH, White PD (1961) Half a century of running. Clinical, physiologic, und autopsy finding in the case of Clarence de Mar (Mr Marathon). N Engl J Med 265:988–993
11. Delaye J, Janin A, Dupont JC et al. (1973) Shunt gauche – droite par des branches des artères coronaires droite et gauche communiquant avec l'artère pulmonaire. Son intervention dans l'insuffisance coronaire. Coeur Med Interne 12:659–667

12. Delaye J, Amiel M, Delahaye JP et al. (1976) Coronary artery spasm associated with variant angina pectoris. 7th Congress of European Cardiology Society. Amsterdam. Abstr n°465
13. Engel HJ, Page HL, Campbel WB (1976) Coronary artery spasm as the cause of myocardial infarction during coronary arteriography. Am Heart J 91:501–506
14. Gay J, Benoit P, Tcheroakoff P et al. (1974) Anévrysmes des artères coronaires. Arch Mal Coeur 67:1327–1338
15. Green LH, Cohen SI, Kurland G (1976) Fatal myocardial infarction in marathon racing. Ann Intern Med 84:704–706
16. Grosgogeat Y, Bessede P (1965) Aspects anatomopathologiques de l'infarctus myocardique a évolution mortelle du sujet jeune. Vie Med 46:385–392, 1693–1725
17. Guermonprez JL, Ponsonnaille J, Ruiz, Maurice P (1975) Infarctus myocardique et troncs coronariens normaux à l'angiographie. Am Cardiol Angéiol 2:115–118
18. Hunter R, Swale J, Peymann MA, Barnett UWH (1975) Some immediate and long terme effects of exercise on the plasma lipids. Lancet II:671–675
19. Karvonen MJ, Klemloca H, Virkajarvi J, Kerkonen A (1974) Longevity of endurance skiers. Med Sci Sports 6:49–51
20. Khan AH, Haywoud J (1974) Myocardial infarction in 9 patients with radiologically patent coronary arteries. N Engl J Med 291:427–431
21. Kimbiris D, Segal BL, Munir M et al. (1972) Myocardial infarction in patients with normal patent coronary arteries as visualized by cinearteriography. Am J Cardiol 29:724–728
22. Klein R (1967) Quelques cas d'infarctus du myocarde chez le sportif. Med Educ Phys Sport 4:211–213
23. Maseri A, L'Abrate A, Marzilli M, Ballestra AM, Cherchia S, Parodi O, Severi S (1978) Coronary vasospasm as a cause of acute myocardial infarction. Trans Eur Soc Cardiol 1:62
24. Master AM, Dacks S, Jaffre HI (1937) Factors and events associated with onset of coronary thrombosis. JAMA 109:546
25. Morris JN, Chave SPW, Adam C, Sirey C, Epstein L (1973) Vigourous exercise in leisure time and incidence of coronary heart disease. Lancet, I:333–339
26. Noakes TD, Opie LH, McKechnie J, Benchimol A, Dogsser K (1977) Coronary heart disease in marathon runners. Ann NY Acad Sci 301:593–619
27. Oliva PB, Breckinridge JC (1977) Arteriopathic evidence of coronary arterial spasm in acute myocardial infarction. Circulation 56:366–374
28. Oliva PB, Potts DE, Pluss RG (1973) Coronary arterial spasm in prinzmetal angina. N Engl J Med 288:745–751
29. Opie LH (1975) Sudden death and sport. Lancet I:263–266
30. Paul O (1974) Myocardial infarction and sudden death. In: Braunwald E (ed) The myocardium; failure and infarction. HP publishing Co, New York pp 273–282
31. Pernot C (1966) Infarctus du myocarde par effort violent et prolongé. Journ Reanim, Nancy, Spei Ed. 73–90
32. Raynaud R, Boivin JM, Brochier M et al. (1973) L'infarctus du myocarde de l'adulte jeune. Sem Hop Paris 49–25, 1809–1814
33. Scaff JH (1976) Letter to the editor. Ann Intern Med 85:391
34. Wyndham CH (1977) Heart stroke and hyperthermia in marathon runners. Ann NY Acad Sci 301:128–138
35. Wyndham CH, Strydom NB (1969) The danger of an inadequate water intake during marathon running. S Afr Med J, 43:896

Acute Myocardial Infarction in Young Women: Evidence for Spontaneous Lysis of a Coronary Thrombus

H. J. Engel, E. Engel, and P. R. Lichtlen[1]

The problem of myocardial infarction (MI) with angiographically and autoptically normal coronary arteries has received much interest in recent literature [1–5, 10]. While subendocardial disseminated MI may occur with normal coronary arteries in situations of very low oxygen supply (e.g., severe anemia, CO intoxication, or severe hypotension) or with markedly increased oxygen demand (e.g., hypertrophic cardiomyopathy or aortic stenosis), transmural MI with subsequently normal coronary arteries are most frequently attributed to spontaneous lysis of thrombotic occlusions [1, 5] and to coronary vasospasm [9, 13, 14].

After having seen three patients who showed the sequence of thrombotic coronary occlusion with resultant MI and complete normalization of the coronary arteriograms (with residual segmental left ventricular [LV] dysfunction) after a few months [7], we were interested to observe a series of young women who had undergone transmural MI during oral contraceptive medication and who subsequently had normal or almost normal coronary arteriograms [5, 11]. Since the phenomenon of MI with normal coronary arteries appeared to occur particularly frequently in young women, possibly enhanced by oral contraceptive use and cigarette smoking, we investigated the clinical and angiographic data of all females age 50 years or less who had undergone cardiac catheterization and coronary arteriography in our cardiovascular laboratories during the past 6 years.

Patients

Between October, 1974, and October, 1980, 329 females 50 years old or less underwent cardiac catheterization, including coronary arteriography, in our institution. Of these 329 women, 76 had abnormal coronary arteriograms and/or segmental LV dysfunction. This report primarily concerns 34 of the 76 patients who had undergone acute transmural MI and who were found to have segmental akinesis or hypokinesis, yet absolutely normal or almost normal coronary arteriograms. These 34 patients will be called group A (Fig. 1).

In contrast, advanced coronary artery disease was found in 42 young females who will be referred to as group B (Fig. 1). The mean age of group A was 39 years and the mean age of group B, 43 years. The 34 patients of group A will be analyzed with regard to clinical history, the incidence of five commonly acknowledged atherogenic risk factors (cigarette smoking, hypertension, hypercholesterolemia, diabetes mellitus, positive family history), use of oral contraceptives, coronary anatomy,

1 Abteilung für Kardiologie, Zentrum für Innere Medizin, Medizinische Hochschule Hannover, Karl-Wiechert-Allee 9, 3000 Hannover 61, FRG

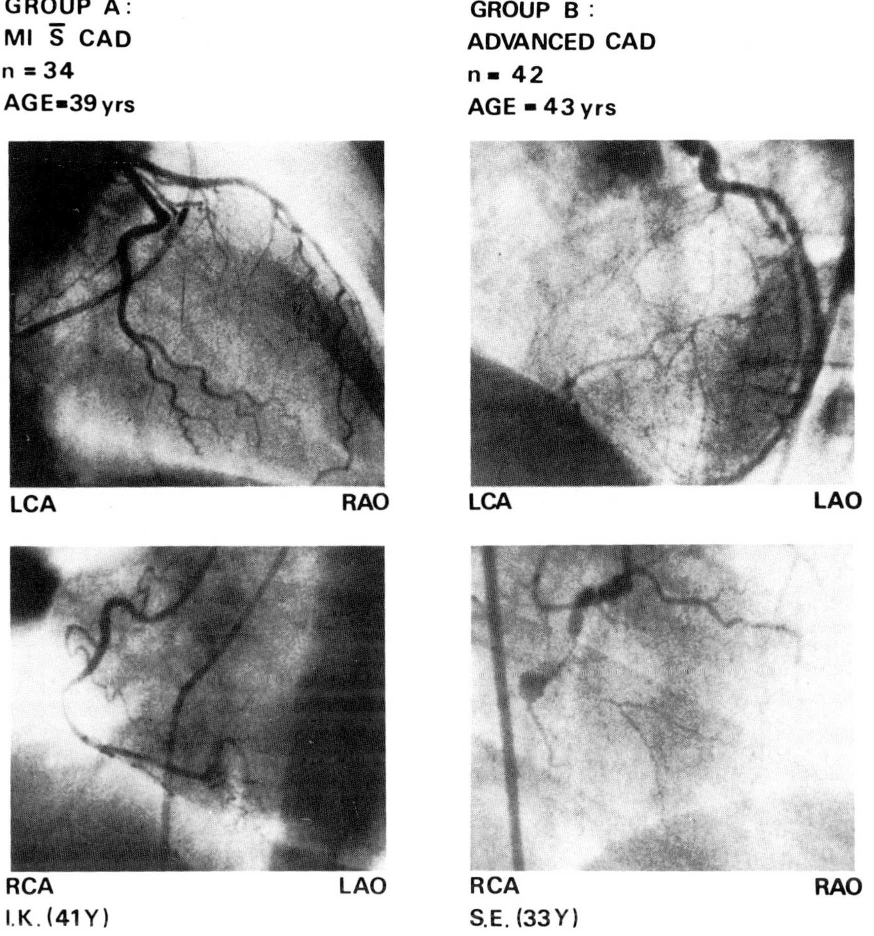

Fig. 1. Typical angiographic examples of group A (41-year-old woman with anterior MI and normal coronary arteries) and group B (33-year-old woman with occlusions of the LAD and RCA)

and LV function, and they will be compared to the other 42 females up to age 50 who had angiographically advanced coronary atherosclerosis (group B).

Results

A summary of the angiographic findings of the 34 MI patients without angiographic evidence of typical coronary atherosclerosis (group A) is contained in Table 1. Segmental akinesis was present in 21 and hypokinesis in 13 cases. The involved vessel was the left anterior descending (LAD) in 22 cases, i.e., almost two-thirds of the patients, the right coronary artery (RCA) in 11, and the left circumflex (LCx) in only two patients.

Table 1. Angiographic findings: group A (MI without coronary artery disease). All obstructions were isolated, focal, and smooth

Left ventricular:		
Akinesis	$n=21$	
Hypokinesis	$n=13$	
Vessels involved	LAD	$n=21$
	LCx	$n=2$
	RCA	$n=11$
Coronary obstructions (% luminal diameter)	100% $n=6$ 76% – 99% $n=5$ 50% – 75% $n=6$	47%
	20% – 40% $n=6$ Normal $n=12$	53%

In six patients there was total occlusion of a vessel, in five patients there was a severe obstruction (76%–99% luminal diameter), and in six patients there was a moderately severe (50%–75%) stenosis. On the other hand, 12 patients had absolutely normal vessels, and six patients had only mild focal narrowing or a localized luminal irregularity. Thus, more than half of the patients did not have a hemodynamically significant lesion at angiography, which was performed at an average interval of 9 (1–28) months following MI.

It is of interest to note that all lesions were unusually focal, isolated, and smooth, and that all other segments and branches were absolutely normal and free of even minimal luminal irregularities.

In contrast, the 42 group B patients (Table 2) had a total of 95 obstructions of at least 50% luminal diameter; among them 28 total obstructions. The location of the stenotic lesions was unremarkable; the main left coronary artery (MLCA) in three LAD in 35, LCx in 22, and RCA in 24 patients.

Concerning the clinical presentation, it is of interest that among the 34 patients without typical coronary atherosclerosis, only four (12%) had experienced chest pain prior to MI. This compares to 29 of 42 of group B patients (69%) who had complained of anginal pain prior to MI. Following MI, 70% of patients without typical

Table 2. Angiographic findings: group B (advanced CAD)

Left ventricular:		
Akinesis	$n=21$	
Hypokinesis	$n=21$	
Coronary obstructions (% luminal obstruction)	100% $n=28$ 76% – 99% $n=23$ 50% – 75% $n=44$	
Vessels involved	MLCA	$n=3$
	LAD	$n=35$
	LCx	$n=22$
	RCA	$n=24$

coronary atherosclerosis complained of angina pectoris, which was stress-induced in the majority of cases. Surprisingly, postinfarct angina was also observed in some patients without any residual hemodynamically significant coronary obstruction.

The analysis of atherogenic risk factors included:

hypertension (> 140/ > 90 mmHg);
hypercholesterolemia (> 250 mg%; > 6.5 mmol/liter);
diabetes mellitus;
cigarette smoking (more than 10 pack-years)
family history [MI and/or cerebrovascular accident (CVA) in parents or siblings prior to age 55].

Since oral contraceptives have been shown to increase the risk of MI [2, 12, 19], we also investigated this parameter in both groups of patients.

Figure 2 graphically demonstrates the incidence of atherogenic risk factors in group A and group B. It is obvious that patients who had sustained acute MI without coronary atherosclerosis (group A) had a low incidence of hypertension, hypercholesterolemia, diabetes, and positive family history, and that young females with advanced coronary atherosclerosis (group B) showed a high number of atherogenic risk factors. The majority of patients in both groups, however, were cigarette smokers. The average number of atherogenic risk factors in group A was 1.1 and, in group B, 2.7. An interesting finding is that, among patients with normal or almost normal coronary arteries, 79% (27 of 34) had been taking oral contraceptives at the time of MI. The average duration of oral contraceptive medication was 6.9 years. In group B, however, only 36% had ever used oral contraceptives.

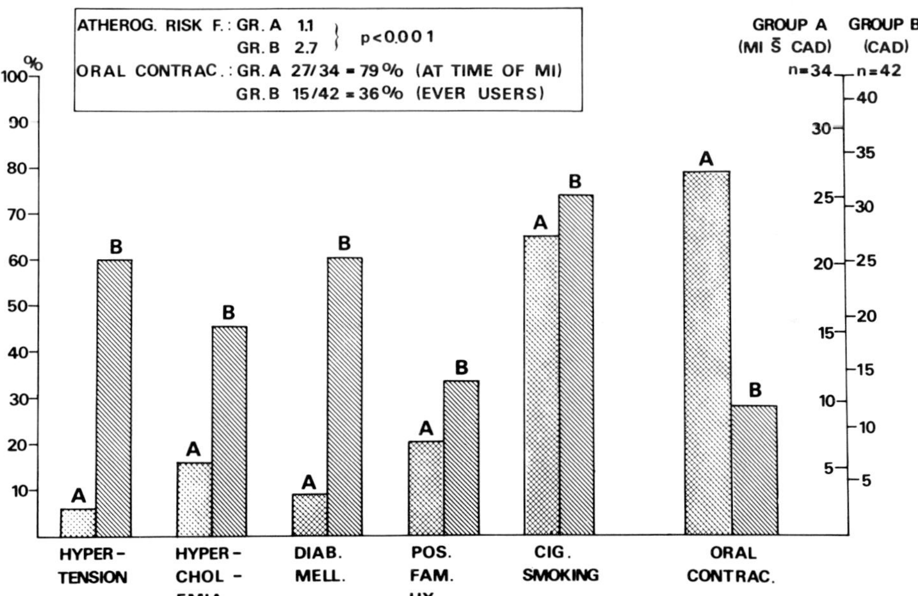

Fig. 2. Incidence of atherogenic risk factors and oral contraceptive use in patients of group A and B

Discussion

Young females with MI without typical coronary atherosclerosis differed from those with advanced coronary atherosclerosis, not only angiographically, but also with regard to the clinical presentation and the average number of atherogenic risk factors. In group A, MI mostly occurred without premonitory symptoms, and coronary arteriograms were either normal or showed one isolated smooth lesion with otherwise normal vessels. This is in clear contrast to patients with MI due to coronary atherosclerosis, where generalized and diffuse atherosclerosis of all vessels was generally present [17]. With the exception of cigarette smoking, atherogenic risk factors were rare in group A. Surprisingly, some patients developed typical angina pectoris following MI, although their arteriograms were free of stenotic lesions.

The mechanism responsible for acute transmural MI in the 34 group A patients remains speculative. The angiographic observation of spontaneous regression of a 75% proximal LAD stenosis at angiography performed 5 months after the first angiographic examination (Fig. in [6]) is of interest in this context: Since the stenosis had remained unchanged after nitroglycerin and nifedipine during the first angiogram, we conclude that spontaneous lysis of an occlusive thrombus is a possible mechanism for such events. The thrombus present at the time of acute MI may have been either primary or secondary. The data presented here contain no information to make inferences about the time course or cause-effect relationship.

Of our series of women 50 years old or less with MI, 45% did not show coronary atherosclerosis angiographically. Among this group, 79% had been taking oral contraceptives at the time of MI and the majority were habitual cigarette smokers.

The presented data confirm that use of oral contraceptives and cigarettes does represent a risk concerning acute MI, and suggest that this risk may be independent of the presence of atherogenic risk factors and coronary atherosclerosis. The latter statement is in contrast to findings of other authors [15, 16] who found the risk of MI during oral contraceptive medication particularly increased in women with atherogenic risk factors. Since MI during oral contraceptive medication may occur with and without coronary atherosclerosis, oral contraceptives do not appear to be an atherogenic risk factor. Although hypertension, diabetes mellitus, and hyperlipidemia are among the known side-effects of oral contraceptives [10], enhancement of these atherogenic risk factors by oral contraceptives did not contribute to the risk of MI in the present group of patients since the incidence of these risk factors was low (Fig. 2). The known effects of oral contraceptives on blood clotting factors and on the microstructure of the vessel wall [10] and synergistic effects of nicotine on platelet aggregation [18] suggest that thromboembolic mechanisms may be active in such cases, although coronary spasm and immunological phenomena have been considered as well.

Coronary atherosclerosis continues to be rare among young women. During a time interval of 6 years in which we performed 600–1000 coronary arteriograms annually, only 42 women 50 years old or less with advanced coronary atherosclerosis were observed. The high incidence of atherogenic risk factors in these patients supports our previous observation [4] that coronary atherosclerosis is practically nonexistent in premenopausal females in the absence of an unusually high number of risk factors.

In conclusion, MI in young women were not associated with typical coronary atherosclerosis in 45% of our series of 76 patients. Occlusion of macroscopically normal coronary arteries by formed elements of blood with subsequent spontaneous (partial or complete) lysis is among possible mechanisms for such events.

Summary

Among 76 women 50 years old or less with abnormal coronary and/or left ventricular angiograms studied in Hannover between 1974 and 1980, 34 had undergone myocardial infarction (MI) with subsequently normal or almost normal coronary angiograms (isolated smooth focal stenosis with otherwise absolutely normal coronary anatomy). These 34 females (group A) not only showed no coronary atherosclerosis angiographically, but also did not have atherogenic risk factors. The average number of five risk factors (cigarette smoking, hypertension, hypercholesterolemia, diabetes mellitus, and positive family history) was only 1.1 (cigarette smoking in the majority) whereas 42 females 50 years old or less with advanced coronary atherosclerosis had an average of 2.7 (group B). Of 34 group A patients, 27 (79%) had been taking oral contraceptives at the time of their MI, whereas only 15 of the 42 group B patients (36%) had ever used them. Among group A patients, sequential coronary arteriograms documented spontaneous regression of an isolated 75% LAD stenosis in a patient with transmural anterior MI under oral contraceptives. It, thus, appears that transmural MI may occur in the absence of coronary atherosclerosis, and the high incidence of oral contraceptive and nicotine users in this group (A) suggests that these factors are contributory in some cases. In conclusion, MI are infrequent in females of this age group, and in many instances they are not associated with typical coronary atherosclerosis angiographically. Occlusion of macroscopically normal coronary arteries by formed elements of blood with subsequent spontaneous (partial or complete) lysis is among possible mechanisms for such events.

References

1. Arnett EN, Roberts WC (1976) Acute myocardial infarction and angiographically normal coronary arteries – an unproven combination (editorial). Circulation 53:395–400
2. Dear HD, Jones WB (1971) Myocardial infarction associated with the use of oral contraceptives. Ann Intern Med 74:236
3. Eliot RS, Baroldi G, Leone A (1974) Necropsy studies in myocardial infarction with minimal or no coronary luminal reduction due to atherosclerosis. Circulation 49:1127–1131
4. Engel HJ, Lichtlen P (1976) Angina pectoris and myocardial infarction without coronary atherosclerosis (in German). Ther Umsch 33:75–86
5. Engel HJ, Lichtlen P (1978) Evidence of spontaneous thrombolysis in the human coronary system. In: Kaltenbach M, Lichtlen P, Balcon R, Bussmann WD (eds) Coronary heart disease. Thieme, Stuttgart, pp 127–132
6. Engel HJ, Lichtlen P (1980) Cardiovascular side-effects of oral contraceptives (in German). Ther Umsch 37:96–104
7. Engel HJ, Page HL Jr (1975) The problem of angiographically normal coronary arteries after myocardial infarction. Verh Dtsch Ges Kreislaufforsch 41:112–115
8. Engel HJ, Page HL Jr, Campbell WB (1974) Coronary artery disease in young women. JAMA 230:1531–1534

9. Engel HJ, Page HL Jr, Campbell WC (1976) Coronary artery spasm as the cause of myocardial infarction during coronary angiography. Am Heart J 91:501–506
10. Engel HJ, Hundeshagen H, Lichtlen P (1977) Transmural myocardial infarctions in young women taking oral contraceptives: Evidence of reduced flow in spite of normal coronary arteries. Br Heart J 39:477–484
11. Engel HJ, Page HL Jr, Lichtlen P (1978) Myocardial infarctions during oral contraceptive medication – a discrete disease entity unrelated to coronary atherosclerosis? (abstract). Am J Cardiol 41:408
12. Mann JI, Vessey MP, Thorogood M, Doll R (1975) Myocardial infarction in young women with special reference to oral contraceptive practice. Br Med J II:241
13. Maseri A, L'Abbate A, Baroldi G et al. (1978) Coronary vasospasm as a possible cause of myocardial infarction. N Engl J Med 299:1271–1277
14. Oliva PB, Breckinridge JC (1977) Arteriographic evidence of coronary arterial spasm in acute myocardial infarction. Circulation 56:366–374
15. Oliver MF (1970) Oral contraceptives and myocardial infarction. Br Med J II:210
16. Radford DJ, Oliver MF (1973) Oral contraceptives and myocardial infarction. Br Med J 3:428
17. Roberts WC, Buja LM (1972) The frequency and significance of coronary arterial thrombi and other observations in fatal acute myocardial infarction. Am J Med 52:425
18. US Public Health Service (1968) The health consequences of smoking: A Public Health Service review. Revised US Government Printing Office, Washington, D.C. (PHS Publication, No 1696)
19. Vessey MP, McPherson K, Johnson B (1977) Mortality among women participating in the Oxford Family Planning Association contraceptive study. Lancet 804 II:731

Major Role of Coronary Spasm in the Pathogenesis of Myocardial Infarction at Young Age

A. L'Abbate, A. Biagini, M. G. Mazzei, C. Brunelli, M. G. Trivella, S. Severi, M. Marzilli, and A. Maseri[1]

The role of coronary vasospasm in the genesis of angina, postulated many years ago, has been recently documented both in resting angina [6, 8] and in some cases of angina on effort [14]. Conversely, the role of coronary vasospasm in the genesis of myocardial infarction (MI), although postulated and even demonstrated in some cases, is still unclear [9]. Therefore, to discuss the role of spasm at young age is difficult.

It is well established, both from postinfarction angiographic studies and necroscopic examination, that approximately 10% of cases with MI show no significant coronary narrowings while approximately 20% of vascular occlusions are not accompanied by myocardial necrosis. In addition, no significant difference in severity or extension of coronary atherosclerosis has been found in patients with and without clinical manifestation of myocardial ischemia [1]. These data challenge the classic view of a direct cause-effect relationship between MI and coronary atherosclerosis, and should represent the background knowledge for the search of other factors that differ from the atherosclerotic plaque or are associated with it, but produce MI.

The role of thrombus and subintimal hemorrhage in the genesis of MI as factors which, superimposed on different degrees of atherosclerosis, can transform an non-CHD patient into a CHD patient has been challenged by morphological and nuclear studies respectively showing the lack of correlation between the presence of the thrombus and the presence and extension of MI, and on the other hand, the buildup of the thrombus during MI. Research on the pathogentic mechanism of MI is made difficult for a number of reasons mainly related to our retrospective approach to the phenomenon which, even in the animal model, may give information related to consequences rather than the cause of MI.

The ideal experimental basis for such research would be the study of the patient before the infarction and during its development. Unfortunately, this approach is complicated by the fact that patients come to medical attention only after the onset of MI. In the attempt to investigate this problem, a reasonable approach would be to identify a population of patients with high risk of MI, define their characteristics, and possibly study the transition from no-infarction to infarction. The achievement of this goal appears particularly hard in young people since, more than in older patients, MI frequently represents the first clinical manifestation for the CHD. However, as the indicence of MI is higher in patients with so-called unstable angina or angina at rest, this kind of population, irrespective of age, can represent the ideal subpopulation for a clinical pathogentic study of MI.

---

1 C.N.R. Institute of Clinical Physiology and Istituto di Patologia Medica I, University of Pisa, Pisa, Italy

In our institute we have studied cases of angina at rest since 1973 and we feel confident that coronary vasomotor changes play a dominant role in the genesis of transient ischemic attacks in these patients. Thus, it can be asserted that MI occurs more frequently in patients with vasospastic angina, as compared to other populations in which the role of vasospasm has not been defined or could not be relevant. This clinical evidence, however, is not sufficient to link coronary spasm to MI with a cause-effect relationship and additional information is required. We should first evaluate whether MI occurs in the myocardium perfused by the coronary vessel undergoing spasm. Once more this goal is a difficult one, as the angiographic documentation of a transient phenomenon like spasm can hardly be obtained in a large number of patients. For this reason, and on the basis of previous studies with hemodynamic monitoring, ECG monitoring, coronary sinus O_2 saturation monitoring, and myocardial scintigraphy [3, 6–8], the relationship between ECG-documented ischemia at rest and coronary vasospasm may be assumed. In these cases (absence of documented spasm, but presence of documented transient ischemia at rest) the ECG leads showing alterations can be compared during ischemia and infarction.

Documented Vasospastic Ischemia Before MI

In 44 patients, transient episodes of ischemia at rest were documented by ECG and/or scintigraphic studies before MI. In 11 of these patients we also obtained angiographic documentation of a coronary vasospasm during an ischemic attack.

All the patients developed MI in the same myocardial region showing ECG ST segment changes during transient ischemia.

Out of these 44, five were of or below age 40 (Table 1) and, of these, four showed ST segment elevation and one ST segment depression during angina at rest. Coronary angiography was performed before MI development in four patients: One had normal coronary vessels, the others 75%–90% stenosis of the vessel supplying the area subsequently infarcted. A complete coronary spasm of the LAD was documented in the patient with normal coronary arteries (a 24-year-old woman not taking oral contraceptives and without risk factors) (Fig. 1). In the fifth patient the coronary angiography, performed 1 month after an anteroseptal infarction, showed 90% and 75% stenosis of the LAD.

Therefore, it appears that the study of patients with recurrent anginal attacks allows the assessment of a topographic relation between transient ischemia and MI and between coronary vasospasm and MI. At the same time, this finding can reasonably rule out embolism as a precipitating event in MI, a pathogenic mechanism proposed by some authors especially in cases of MI and normal coronary arteries [2, 4, 5, 13]. In fact, it seems unlikely that embolus would consistently lodge in the previously ischemic territory.

Undocumented Ischemia Before MI

In 52 patients of or under the age of 40 it was not possible to document previous ischemic attacks because of the absence of symptoms in 40, or lack of ECG record-

Table 1. Patients of or under the age of 40 with documented transient ischemia before MI. Abbreviations are as follows: Old MI (OMI); left anterior descending (LAD); left circumflex (LC); first diagonal (1st D); branch to the obtuse margin (M); right coronary artery (RC)

Patient	Age (years), sex	ECG location of changes (leads)		Coronary angiography	
		Angina	MI	Time before MI	Time after MI
GN	24, F	↑ V_2–V_5	V_{1-3}	15 days	Normal LAD spasm 100%	
DA	40, M	↑ V_{1-2} ↓ V_{4-6}	V_{1-4} OMI (diaphragmatic)	2 days	LC occluded LAD 90% 1st D 75%	
LF	37, M	↓ V_{2-6}	V_{1-4}	2 days	LAD 90% LC 90% M 90%	
GO	40, M	↑ D_2, D_3, aVF ↓ V_{1-4}	D_2, D_3, aVF OMI (diaphragmatic) OMI (anterior)	4 years	LAD 90% + 50% LC 75% M 75% RC 75%	
AS	38, M	↑ D_1–aVl, V_{1-3}	V_{1-3}		1 month LAD 90% + 75%

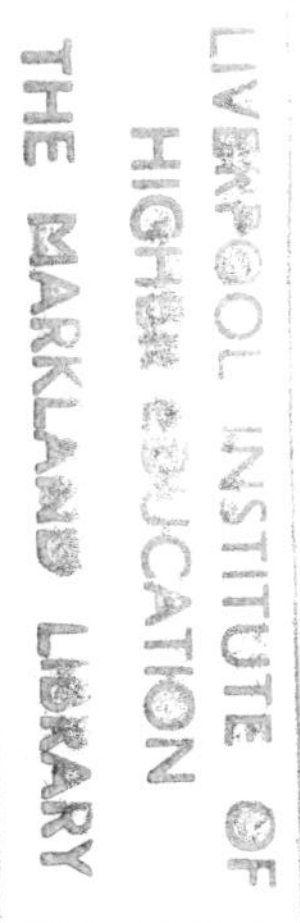

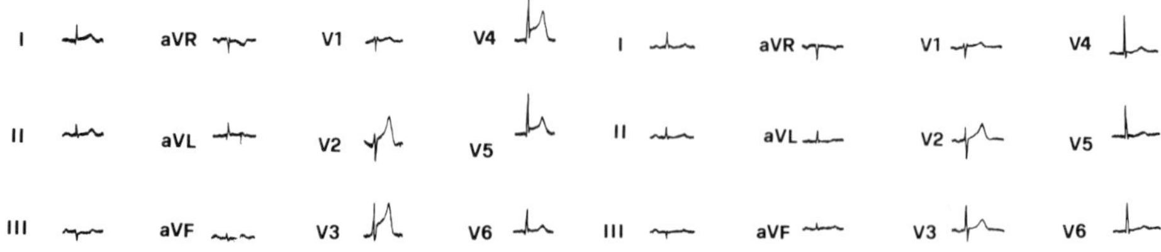

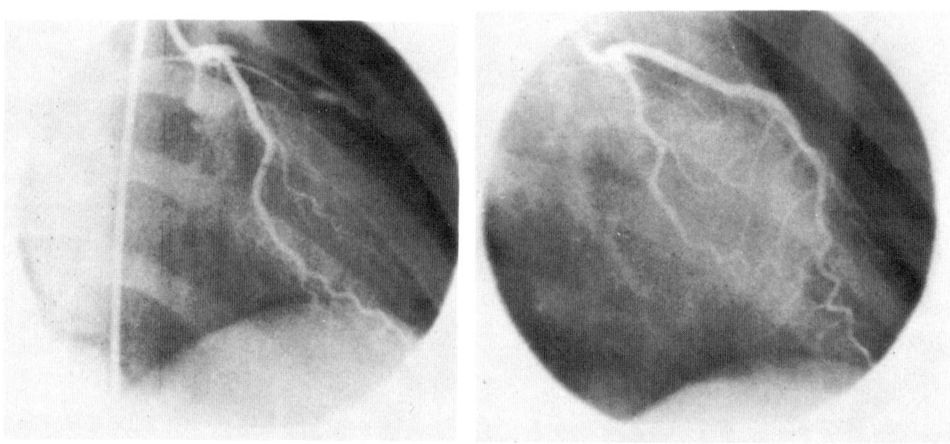

Fig. 1. Left coronary angiography showing a complete spasm of the LAD (*left*) during an ischemic episode with ST segment elevation on the precordial leads in a patient who sustained anterior MI 15 days later. Angiogram of control (*right*)

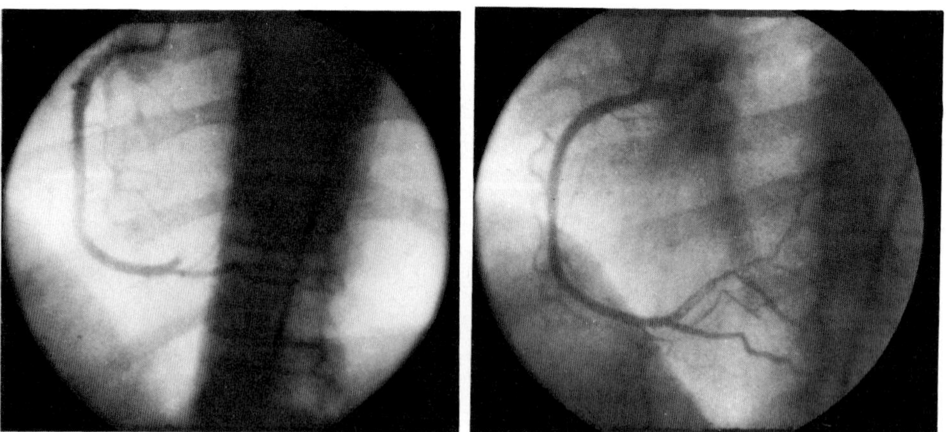

Fig. 2. Recanalization of the distal portion of the right coronary artery, previously occluded. Angiogram on the *left* was obtained a few hours after the onset of a diaphragmatic MI; a complete occlusion of the distal portion of the right coronary artery is present. Angiogram on the *right*, obtained 24 h later, shows the reperfusion of the vessel and an image of "minus" at the level of the previous occlusion, likely related to the presence of a thrombus

ing during symptoms in those remaining. None of these patients underwent coronary angiography before MI, while 51 were studied after MI (Table 2). Of these, 13 had normal vessels (less than 50% stenosis) 16 one-vessel disease, 14 two-vessel disease and 8 three-vessel disease. The main vessel supplying the infarcted region was normal in 13 instances, occluded in eight, and with variable stenosis in the remainder. Among the latter, in six instances the vessel showed the aspect of a recanalization (Fig. 2).

Table 2. Patients of or under the age of 40 without documented transient ischemia before MI. Results of coronary angiography after MI

Coronary disease		Anatomy of the vessel supplying the infarcted region	
0-vessel	13	normal	13
1-vessel	16	50% – 90%	30 (six recanalized)
2-vessel	14		
3-vessel	8	occluded	8
Total	51		51

Thus, in 51 postinfarction coronary angiographies performed in people under the age of 40, "normal" coronary arteries were present in 25% of the cases and in one case among five preinfarction angiographies.

The high frequency of normal coronary arteries found in patients at young age, before or after MI, makes the lack of correlation between atherosclerosis and MI even more striking than in the entire population of patients with MI.

Since a positive correlation exists between age and atherosclerosis, the lower degree of atherosclerosis in young people with MI does not imply that a mechanism differing from atherosclerosis can play a role in this subgroup as compared to the older group. On the contrary, it is reasonable to hypothesize that the same mechanism may also be operative in old age, where the presence of an high degree of atherosclerosis can confuse the picture of the pathogenic inter-relationships. This consideration, on the one hand, indicates that the young subgroup could be most suitable for pathogenic studies of MI, but does not justify an arbitrary subdivision of patients with MI according to the age on the assumption of different mechanisms operating at different ages.

Transition from Noninfarction to Infarction

As stated previously, more information on the genesis of MI could be obtained from studies performed with patients at high risk of MI during the time between the noninfarction and infarction state. The available information relating to this condition is scarce.

We had the opportunity to look at the beginning phase of MI in a few cases during hemodynamic and/or ECG monitoring or coronary angiography. Two of these cases have already been published [9], however, because of their interest it is worthwile to mention them here.

The first case, a 65-year-old male with previous MI and "crescendo" angina for 1 month, underwent ECG and hemodynamic monitoring for the study of his anginal episodes. During the 11 h before the onset of an anterior infarction, the patient showed 24 ischemic attacks. In the 3 h preceding the infarction (Fig. 3), nine attacks occurred. They became more prolonged, less sensible to nitroglycerin until the tenth episode, hemodynamically the same as the others, persisted with development of clear Q wave and typical serum enzyme elevation.

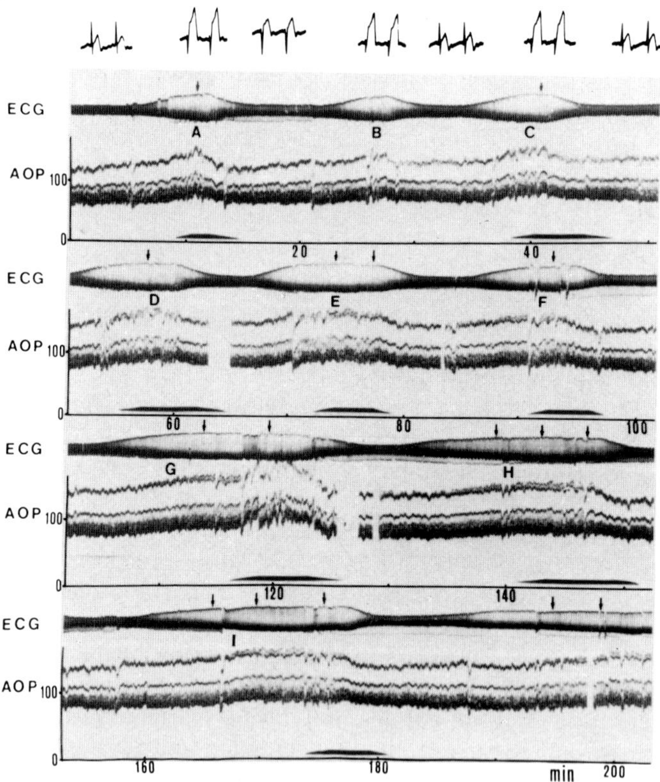

Fig. 3. Low-speed analog playback of *ECG* lead V_4 and aortic pressure (*AOP*) (mmHg) recorded for 200 min showing nine successive reversible ischemic episodes, characterized by ST segment elevation (*A–I*), up to the onset of acute MI. Pain (indicated by the black areas on the abscissa) always occurred late in relation to the onset of ECG changes, and the second episode (*B*) and the last irreversible episode were asymptomatic. The ECG pattern at rest and during attacks is shown at the top for episodes *A, B* and *C*. Both at rest and during attacks, the QRS complex shows sudden changes in the direction of activation. The duration of the attacks increases progressively until the last episode of ST segment elevation (*bottom right*), unresponsive to nitrates, persisted with development of Q waves. Arrows indicate nitroglycerin administration. Maseri et al. (1977) [9]

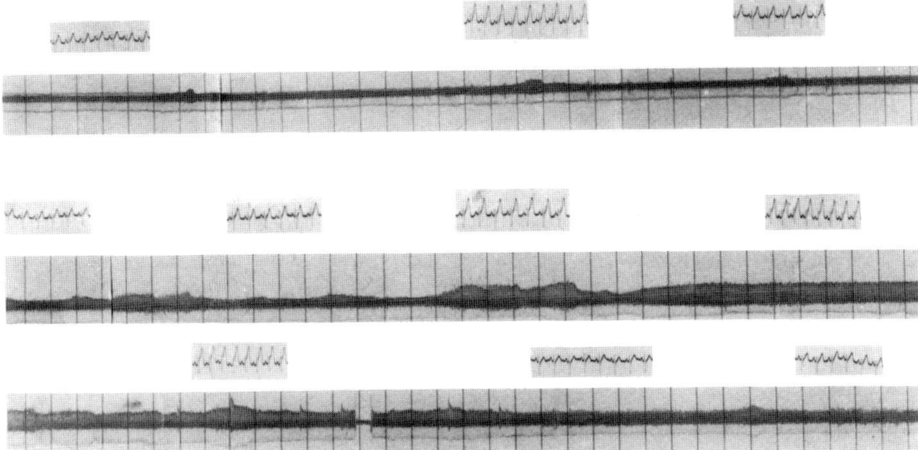

Fig. 4. Compact playback of ECG Holter monitoring. Parts of recording during 4 days before MI. Three episodes of ST segment elevation in V_3 are shown in the *upper panel*. The second day, episodes became more prolonged and less sensible to the therapy until ST elevation became persistent (*middle panel*). Return of ECG to normal following reopening of LAD by intracoronary injection of nitrates and calcium antagonists (*lower panel*). Interval between vertical lines: 3 minutes

The second case was a 52-year-old male, with previous septal MI and crescendo angina at 5 days, who showed at coronary angiography a coronary vasospasm occluding the dominant circumflex artery 1 cm proximal to a 90% stenosis during an ischemic attack, which was relieved by nitroglycerin. A second spasm (indistinguishable from the first) occurred 10 min later and was irreversible in spite of continuous nitrate infusion, morphine, and dipyridamole. The patient died 6 h later in irreversible shock. At necropsy the circumflex artery was open and a small mural thrombus in early phase of organisation was found at the level of maximal luminal reduction of the 90% stenosis of the circumflex.

The third case, a woman who was 55 years old with crescendo angina, was on Holter monitoring in CCU for 4 days before infarction and during development of MI. ECG monitoring during the first 2 days showed a high number of transient ischemic episodes. The cyclic sequence of transient ST-T changes is shown in the upper panel of Fig. 4. On the second day, ST segment elevation on the anterior leads became persistent and insensible to oral and i.v. therapy. Coronary angiography was performed and showed a complete occlusion of the middle portion of the LAD, the other vessels being normal. During angiography, nitrates and calcium antagonists were injected intracoronary with transient reopening of the vessel and a good visualization of the distal portion of the LAD. Each time the vessel reopened, an evident reduction of ST segment elevation occurred (Fig. 4). After several attempts, the vessel remained open and the ECG returned to normal. After 3 days, clear ECG signs of anterior necrosis developed with typical enzyme elevation.

These findings, although anecdotal, seem indicative of the role that functional factors (such as an increase in large coronary arterial tone, whether or not atherosclerotic lesions are present) can play in the pathogenesis of MI. The reopening of coronary arteries after the onset of MI following intracoronary nitroglycerin [12] is in accordance with the hypothesis that vascular occlusion can be provoked by vessel wall contraction.

The causes of coronary spasm and the irreversibility of the spasm remain unknown. It is likely that other factors, such as platelet aggregation and thromboxane A_2 release, could play a role in maintaining vascular contraction and producing lumen occlusion, while favoring the onset of thrombus formation which could subsequently be solved or undergo fibrous organization [11].

References

1. Baroldi G (1975) Different types of myocardial necrosis in coronary heart disease: A pathophysiologic review of their functional significance. Am Heart J 89:742–752
2. Cheng TO, Bashour T, Singh BK et al. (1972) Myocardial infarction in the absence of coronary arteriosclerosis: Result of coronary spasm (?). Am J Cardiol 30:680–682
3. Chierchia S, Brunelli C, Simonetti I et al. (1980) Sequence of events in angina at rest: Primary reduction in coronary flow. Circulation 61:759–768
4. Johnson AD, Detwiler JH (1977) Coronary spasm, variant angina, and recurrent myocardial infarctions. Circulation 55:947–950
5. Khan AH, Haywood LJ (1974) Myocardial infarction in nine patients with radiologically patent coronary arteries. N Engl J Med 291:427–431
6. Maseri A, Mimmo R, Chierchia S et al. (1975) Coronary spasm as a cause of acute myocardial ischemia in man. Chest 68:625–633
7. Maseri A, Parodi O, Severi S et al. (1976) Transient transmural reduction of myocardial blood flow, demonstrated by thallium-201 scintigraphy, as a cause of variant angina. Circulation 54:280–288
8. Maseri A, L'Abbate A, Pesola A et al. (1977) Coronary vasospasm in angina pectoris, Lancet I:713–717
9. Maseri A, L'Abbate A, Baroldi G et al. (1978) Coronary vasospasm as a possible cause of myocardial infarction. N Engl J Med 299:1271–1277
10. Maseri A, Severi S, De Nes M et al. (1978) "Variant" angina: One aspect of a continuous spectrum of vasospastic myocardial ischemia. Pathogenetic mechanisms estimate incidence and clinical and coronary arteriographic findings in 138 patients. Am J Cardiol 42:1019–1028
11. Maseri A, Chierchia S, L'Abbate A (1980) Pathogenetic mechanism underlying clinical events associated with atherosclerotic heart disease. Circulation Suppl V, 3–13
12. Oliva PB, Breckinridge JC (1977) Arteriographic evidence of coronary arterial spasm in acute myocardial infarction. Circulation 56:366–374
13. Rosemblatt A, Selzer A (1977) The nature and clinical features of myocardial infarction with normal coronary arteriogram. Circulation 55:578–580
14. Specchia G, De Servi S, Falcone C et al. (1979) Coronary arterial spasm as a cause of exercise induced ST segment elevation in patients with variant angina. Circulation 59:948–954

Myocardial Infarction and Normal Coronary Arteries: Possible Role of Spasm

R. Balcon, G. Blümchen, M. Cattell, and E. Scharf-Bornhofen [1]

Data from 7013 patients with suspected ischemic heart disease has been analyzed in an attempt to determine the incidence of myocardial infarction (MI) without demonstrable narrowing in the coronary arteries, and to determine whether there were clinical or other features that helped to clarify the etiology.

Information was collected from patients attending the Klinik Roderbirken (Leichlinger, West Germany) between 1976 and 1980 and the London Chest Hospital between 1971 and 1980. The study was retrospective and the patients were selected according to initial angiographic reports which indicated normal coronary arteries.

Of the 7013 angiograms, 800 were normal and 4.6% showed evidence of MI.

The angiograms were then independently reviewed by two observers, paying particular attention to the possible total absence of a vessel. The left ventricular angiogram was similarly evaluated and only patients with distinct hypokinesia or dyskinesia of anterior, apical, or inferior left ventricular segments were included. No patient had involvement of the whole left ventricular wall. There were 37 patients who fulfilled these criteria (Table 1), representing 1% of patients with infarction and 0.5% of the total population. They all showed additional evidence of previous MI.

Patients

The age of the patients was 19–61 years with a mean of 43 years and 12 were under the age of 40. Twenty-eight were male and nine female and 73% were cigarette smokers (average 35 cigarettes per day). Serum cholesterol values were above normal in 27% of patients and blood pressure was more than 140/90 in 57%.

All had attacks of cardiac pain lasting more than 1 h which resulted in 33 of them being admitted to hospital. All but one of these had cardiac enzymes measured, and these were elevated to more than 50% above normal in 44%. All the patients admitted to hospital underwent ECG, which was abnormal in 28 (ST-T changes in 26, Q waves in two). Twenty-seven patients underwent exercise testing and no patient developed angina, but in nine patients there was ST segment depression of more than 1.5 mm. Six of these were female. The catheterization took place within 1 year in 75% of patients and within 5 years in all except one, who was not investigated until 12 years after the event but was included because she was a well-documented case and suffered no further events during the intervening period. The

---

1 The London Chest Hospital, London, Great Britain
  and Klinik Roderbirken, Leichlingen, FRG

Table 1. Data of 37 postinfarction patients without demonstrable narrowing of the coronary arteries. LV, left ventricle; WMA, wall motion abnormality; H, hypokinesia; D, dyskinesia; A, aneurysm; AP, angina pectoris, Apic, apical; Dy, dyspnea; Ca, Calciumantagonists; V, vasodilators; DD, digitalis, diuretics

Patient	Age (years), sex	LV		Time from event to angiography					Follow up		
		WMA	Site	(months)	AP	Lipids (>250)	Cigarettes (day)	Blood pressure >140/90	Time (months)	Treatment	Outcome
1	46, F	H	Ant.	48	2	–	0	–	47	–	A
2	37, M	H	Inf.	9	3	–	25	+	0	Ca	AP
3	32, M	D	Ant.	60	3	–	1	–	53	–	AP
4	43, M	H	Ant. Apic	17	3	–	50	+	10	V	AP
5	51, M	H	Ant.	2	2	–	40	+	10	V	AP
6	42, M	H	Ant.	2	3	+	20	–	4	–	AP
7	42, F	H	Apic	6	0	–	30	+	16	CA	AP
8	42, M	H	Ant.	2	0	–	60	+	3	Ca/V	AP
9	31, M	H	Ant.	5	2	–	0	+	2	Ca/V	A
10	55, M	H	Apic	15	2	–	0	+	6	Ca	AP
11	48, F	H	Inf.	5	2	+	20	+	8	–	A
12	42, M	H	Inf.	48	0	+	0	+	6	–	A
13	52, M	H	Apic	6	3+4	–	30	+	6	–	AP
14	43, M	H	Inf.	6	0	–	0	–	10	Ca	AP
15	43, M	H	Inf.	2	0	+	15	–	10	–	A
16	39, F	H	Inf.	10	0	–	0	–	16	–	AP
17	51, M	H	Ant. Apic	5	3	–	20	+	2	–	A
18	58, F	H	Ant.	2	2	+	0	–	43	–	AP
19	43, M	H	Ant.	17	2	–	0	+	25	V	AP
20	52, F	H	Ant.	3	2	–	20	–	3	Ca/V	AP
21	53, M	H	Ant.	5	2	+	20	+	13	V	AP
22	26, M	H	Ant.	1	4	–	0	–	37	Ca/V	MI
23	26, M	D	Apic	9	2	–	30	+	3	–	A
24	27, M	H	Ant.	5	4	–	10	–	1	–	A

25	61, F	H	Inf.	5	4	+	10	−	29	Ca	AP
26	29, M	H	Ant.	1	0	+	20	−	12	−	Died
27	31, M	D	Apic	4	2+4	−	40	−	57	V	A
28	35, F	H	Apic	3	4	−	50	−	9	−	A
29	57, M	D	Apic	1	0	+	10	+	39	−	A
30	41, M	D	Apic	1	2	+	20	−	25	Ca	A
31	49, M	H	Ant.	10	4	−	30	−	40	−	A
32	33, M	H	Ant.	14	4	−	20	+	58	−	A
33	19, M	H	Inf.	3	0	−	40	−	88	−	A
34	52, M	H	Ant	1	0	−	0	+	44	Ca	MI
35	44, M	H	Ant.	6	4	−	10	+	47	−	A
36	49, M	H	Ant.	31	2+4	−	30	+	34	Ca	A
37	49, F	D	Ant. Apic	156	0	−	20	−	6	D/D	Dy

angiographic wall motion abnormality was anteroapical in 28 patients and inferior in the remaining nine and was usually hypokinetic, although six patients showed dyskinesia. The site of the ECG abnormality corresponded with the angiographic findings in the majority of cases (75%).

Coronary artery spasm was demonstrated in five patients. In all cases it involved the right coronary artery and was associated with ST segment elevation in the inferior ECG leads and the development of cardiac pain: In two cases it occurred spontaneously, one of these then progressed to documented inferior infarction with sequential ECG changes and a rise in cardiac enzymes. In the remaining three, the spasm followed intravenous ergometrine. Spasm reduced arterial diameter by 33%–100% (average 67%).

Follow-up periods were 1–88 months (average 26 months). Twenty-three of the patients were receiving treatment (10 with calcium antagonists, 12 with vasodilators, and 1 with digitalis and diuretics). Seventeen of the patients were asymptomatic, 18 had angina, and 1 dyspnea. There were two further MI and one additional patient died.

Discussion

The most obvious explanation for the phenomenon of MI in patients with apparently normal coronary arteries is that the angiographic assessment was wrong and the coronary arteries were in fact not normal, either because a stenosis had been missed or, more likely, that a branch of the coronary circulation failed to fill because of occlusion at its origin. In this series, the angiograms were reviewed at least three times by three different observers with the latter point specifically in mind, and it is therefore unlikely that misinterpretation of the angiogram was the cause in all of the patients, if indeed any. We have no data concerning abnormal hemoglobin-oxygen dissociation as suggested in some reports (Eliot and Bratt 1969), though other workers (Vokonas et al. 1970) have been unable to support this possibility.

It is recognized that women in hypercoagulable states during or after pregnancy or when taking oral contraceptives (Strauss and Diamond 1963; Egeberg and Owren 1963), may experience intravascular thrombosis and possibly MI. Of the nine women in this series, only one was taking oral contraceptives, none were pregnant or postpartum, and three were postmenopausal and not taking estrogen medication. Thus, this could not have been an important factor.

Coronary embolus with subsequent lysis or dissolution and distribution to peripheral branches is another possible explanation for this condition. However, none of the patients had atrial fibrillation or any condition indicating possible emboli formation in the left heart or pulmonary venous circulation.

Previous reports of patients with MI and normal coronary arteries have noted the relative absence of conventional risk factors, except for cigarette smoking. In our patients there was a 27% incidence of serum cholesterol above normal levels and 57% incidence of hypertension. It is not suggested that these associated factors are the cause of the infarction, since they presumably normally operate by increasing the tendency to coronary atherosclerosis. As in other series, there is a high incidence of cigarette smoking with a high consumption. A large number of possible mechanisms by which cigarette smoking can be involved with the production of myocardial ischemia have been postulated and these include increased catecholamines, increased production of carboxyhemoglobin, endothelial swelling, increased platelet stickiness and aggregation, coronary vasospasm, and reduced fibrinolysis (National Clearinghouse for Smoking and Health 1971).

It is possible that coronary thrombosis was the cause of the original infarction that was subsequently lysed. There is no evidence that this did not happen, and there was a sufficient time period between the infarction and the subsequent angiogram for it to have occurred. However, data is now available concerning angiography in the course of acute infarction followed by intravenous and intracoronary streptokinase and subsequent lysis of thrombus. In all of the data so far reported, thrombosis has been seen as complicating previously present atherosclerotic plaque, evidence of which has remained after thrombolysis (Rentrop et al. 1980; Schröder et al. 1980).

Finally, the evidence that coronary vasospasm is the major or only cause of MI is presented. One of the cases reported here was shown to have spasm in a previously angiographically normal coronary artery which progressed to later infarction. There are other reports in the literature of spasm preceding infarction in a diseased vessel (Maseri et al. 1978) and in a normal vessel (Cheng et al. 1972). It has also been implicated as the cause of infarction or sudden death in people following industrial exposure to nitroglycerine (Lange et al. 1972). Three of our patients were given ergometrine as part of a much larger study for the evaluation of angina in patients with normal or near-normal coronary arteries. These all developed a moderate degree of coronary spasm. It is not known how the remainder of the patients would have responded. Finally, approximately 25% of patients continued to have attacks of spontaneous cardiac pain at rest; again, suggesting spasm as a possible mechanism.

Most of the evidence presented here is circumstantial and it seems likely that there is no single etiological cause for the infarction in this group of patients. There may be more than one cause in all the patients. It is possible to speculate, for instance, that cigarette smoking leads to a change in the vascular endothelium or platelets which in turn adversely affects the balance between vasoactive substances derived from these two structures with subsequent vasospasm. This could itself lead to MI or could be the initiating factor, followed by thrombosis and subsequent lysis.

Since a relatively high proportion continue to have angina, it seems likely that the etiological mechanism may still be operating.

Finally, the conventional view that patients with normal coronary arteries are at no risk of MI or sudden death may need to be modified.

References

Cheng TO, Bashour T, Singh BK, Kelser GA (1972) Myocardial infarction in the absence of coronary atherosclerosis. Result of coronary artery spasm? Am J Cardiol 30:680
Egeberg O, Owren PA (1963) Oral contraception and blood coagulability. Br Med J I:220
Eliot RS, Bratt G (1969) The paradox of myocardial ischemia in young women with normal coronary arteriograms. Relation to abnormal haemoglobin-oxygen dissociation. Am J Cardiol 23:633

Lange RL, Reid MS, Tresch DD et al. (1972) Non-atheromatous ischaemic heart disease follo-
    wing withdrawal from chronic industrial nitroglycerin exposure. Circulation 46:666
Maseri A, Chierchia S, Marzilli M et al. (1978) Coronary vasospasm as a cause of acute myo-
    cardial infarction. A conclusion suggested by the study of pre-infarction angina. In: Kalten-
    bach M, Lichtlen P, Balcon R, Bussmann WD (eds) Coronary heart disease, pp. 163–175
National Clearinghouse for Smoking and Health (1971) Health consequences of smoking. US
    Dept of Health, Education and Welfare, Washington, D.C., pp 56–66
Rentrop P, Blanke H, Karsch (in press) Intra-coronary application of streptokinase and nitro-
    glycerin in unstable angina pectoris. Conference on Unstable Angina, Hannover
Schröder R, Apitzsh DE, Biamino G et al. (1980) Comparison of the effects of intra-coronary
    and systemic streptokinase infusion in acute myocardial infarction. Conference on Unsta-
    ble Angina, Hannover
Strauss HS, Diamond KL (1963) Elevation of Factor VIII during pregnancy in normal persons
    and in one with von Willebrand's disease. N Engl J Med 269:1251
Vokonas PS, Cohen PF, Klein MB et al. (1970) Haemoglobin affinity for oxygen in the anginal
    syndrome with normal coronary arteriograms. (Abstr.) Am J Cardiol 26:554

Relationship of Age and Serum Cholesterol to Platelet Survival Time in Men with Coronary Artery Disease

F. Gold and P. Steele[1]

It seems likely that platelets contribute to the pathogenesis of atherosclerotic coronary artery disease (CAD) and its complications [1–3] and platelet survival is shortened in most patients with CAD [4, 5]. Platelet survival, in relation to age, in men with CAD has not been previously studied. It is possible that younger patients with "premature atherosclerosis" have altered platelet reactivity which contributes to the early development of critical coronary artery lesions [2]. The purpose of this study was to determine whether any relationship exists between platelet survival and age in men with angiographically defined CAD. Since hyperlipidemia is an important risk factor for the CAD development [6] and can affect platelet survival time [7], serum cholesterol was also included in the analysis.

Patients and Methods

Platelet survival time was measured in 100 men with angiographically defined coronary artery disease, and normal serum triglyceride (210 mg% or less). All men had been clinically stable for at least 3 months. The age range was 25–60 years of age. Serum cholesterol in the group was 196–419 mg%. All patients had normal platelet counts.

Platelet survival was measured by labeling the platelets from about 400 ml of the patient's venous blood with 100–150 mCi ^{51}Chromium [4]. Following reinfusion of labeled platelets, blood was obtained for 7 days, and using computer-assisted least-squares analysis, a single exponent was fitted to the platelet count-rate data for determination of the half-life. In 26 normal men, platelet survival half-life averaged 3.7 days, and all had a half-life greater than 3.3 days.

Results

Average platelet survival was shortest in the younger men in this series of patients. Table 1 shows average platelet survival in the 100-patient group by age. Seven of the nine patients in the age group 25–30 years had shortened platelet survival and the average for the group was 2.2 ± 0.04 days (mean ± SEM). Men in the fourth, fifth, and sixth decades of life had group averages that were longer, but were still shortened by an average of 0.9, 0.7, and 0.5 days, respectively. Platelet survival was

1 Cardiology Division, Department of Medicine, Veterans Administration Medical Center, University of Colorado Health Sciences Center, 1055 Clermont, Denver, CO 80220, USA

shortened in 23 of the 37 patients in the 31–40-year-old group, 20 of the 43 in the 41–50-year-old group and 7 of the 11 in the 51–60-year-old group. This trend of a more shortened platelet survival in the younger age groups had an r value of 0.31 ($P < 0.01$).

When the patients were grouped according to level of serum cholesterol, a more striking relationship with platelet survival was observed. Table 2 shows that the mean platelet survival in the 21 patients with serum cholesterol greater than

Table 1. Platelet survival (half-life) in 100 men with coronary artery disease (CAD) according to age (years) groups. Normal platelet survival is 3.7 ± 0.03 days. The younger age groups have the shortest platelet survival time. Platelet survival increases with age, but is still not normal in the oldest age group

	Platelet survival (half-life)
CAD 25 – 30 (n = 9)	2.2 ± 0.04 days
31 – 40 (n = 37)	2.4 ± 0.03 days
41 – 50 (n = 3)	2.6 ± 0.05 days
51 – 60 (n = 11)	2.8 ± 0.04 days

Table 2. Relation of level of serum cholesterol and platelet survival. Platelet survival is invariably decreased in patients with cholesterol greater than 301 mg%. Note that the group with normal serum cholesterol has normal average platelet survival time

Cholesterol	Platelet survival (half-life)
≥ 301 mg% ($n = 21$)	2.1 ± 0.04 days
251 – 300 mg% ($n = 37$)	2.7 ± 0.04 days
≤ 250 mg% ($n = 42$)	3.3 ± 0.05 days

Table 3. Classification of patients by age group and serum cholesterol. Patients in the younger age groups tend to have a higher incidence of hypercholesterolemia, while older age groups have more patients with normal cholesterol levels

Age (years)	Cholesterol		
	≥ 301 mg%	251 – 300 mg%	< 250 mg%
25 – 30 ($n = 9$)	6	1	2
31 – 40 ($n = 37$)	7	19	11
41 – 50 ($n = 43$)	7	13	23
51 – 60 ($n = 11$)	1	4	6

Table 4. Summary table classifying patients according to age group, serum cholesterol, and shortened or normal platelet survival time. Note that a serum cholesterol of 301 mg% or more was invariably associated with a shortened platelet survival time in all age groups. As age increases, platelet survival is shortened in many patients with normal serum cholesterol levels

	Serum cholesterol	Age groups (years)			
		25 – 30	31 – 40	41 – 50	51 – 60
Short	$\geq$ 301 mg%	6	7	7	1
platelet	251 – 300 mg%	1	14	11	3
survival	$\leq$ 251 mg%	0	2	11	3
Normal	$\geq$ 301 mg%	0	0	0	0
platelet	251 – 300 mg%	0	5	2	1
survival	$\leq$ 251 mg%	2	9	12	3

301 mg% was 2.1 ± 0.4 days and none of these men had normal platelet survival. In the group with intermediate serum cholesterol, average platelet survival was shortened to a lesser degree and only eight of the 37 patients in this group had normal platelet survival. Of the 42 men whose serum cholesterol was normal, 26 had normal platelet survival time and the group mean was at the lower limit of normal platelet survival time. The correlation between serum cholesterol and platelet survival had an r value of 0.79 ($P < 0.01$).

These data suggest that the relationship of age and platelet survival is possibly related to serum cholesterol levels in the four groups. Table 3 shows the patients grouped by age and serum cholesterol levels. It can be seen that the incidence of intermediate or high serum cholesterol levels in each age group declines steadily with age. Of the 25–30-year-old group, 78% had elevated serum cholesterol, while a smaller incidence of 70%, 47%, and 45% was seen in the fourth, fifth, and sixth decades, respectively.

Table 4 is a summary showing age groups, serum cholesterol, and platelet survival. The only two patients in the 25–30-year group with normal platelet survival were the patients with normal serum cholesterol. As age increased, platelet survival was still invariably shortened in patients whose serum cholesterol was 301 mg% or more, but in the older age groups platelet survival was also shortened in many of the patients with normal serum cholesterol. Thus, in this series of patients, serum cholesterol appeared to be an important predictor of a shortened platelet survival in the younger age groups. In the older age groups, this relationship was less apparent.

Discussion

Platelet survival reflects the complex interaction of platelet reactivity and vascular endothelial repair [5]. A shortened platelet survival time may reflect vascular endothelial injury when platelet reactivity (adhesiveness, release, and aggregation) is normal. Alternatively, a change in platelet responsiveness to a constant level of endothelial injury would also produce a change in platelet survival; i.e., shortening if responsiveness was increased and lengthening if responsiveness was decreased. Platelet survival time is, therefore, only an indirect measurement of platelet reactivity and endothelial injury and does not provide direct information regarding the pathogenesis of endothelial injury or the dynamics of its repair.

In this series of men with CAD, the younger patients had a shorter average platelet survival time than the older patients, but there was also a greater prevalence of elevated serum cholesterol in these younger patients. In addition to its possible role in lipid-induced endothelial injury, cholesterol has been shown to alter platelet reactivity to a variety of stimuli, Carvalho and associates observed increased platelet sensitivity to aggregating agents in patients with hypercholesterolemia [8]. Shattil et al. [9] showed that platelets incubated with cholesterol-rich lipsomes acquired excess cholesterol and became significantly more sensitive to epinephrine or adenosine diphosphate-induced aggregation. Moreover, platelets which were incubated with cholesterol-poor liposomes showed a reduction in both cholesterol content an responsiveness. These in vitro data suggest that the close correlation between shortened platelet survival and high serum cholesterol in the present serie of patients may reflect enhanced platelet reactivity in part due to the high serum cholesterol.

The older patients in this series did not demonstrate a close relationship of shortened platelet survival and high cholesterol. This may reflect a greater degree of vascular endothelial injury in these older patients, without necessarily implying an alteration in platelet reactivity.

Alteration of serum lipids does alter platelet survival time in patients with coronary disease. Steele and Rainwater [7] treated 15 hyperbetalipoproteinemic men with cholestyramine at 16 g/day in divided doses for 3 months and then 24 g/day for an additional 3 months. Cholestyramine, in a dosage of 16 g/day, reduced serum cholesterol from 348 ± 7.6 to 319 ± 6.3 mg% ($P < 0.001$) in association with an increase in platelet survival (2.3 ± 0.08 days to 2.7 ± 0.07 days, $P < 0.001$). At the 24 g/day dosage cholesterol decreased slightly more, and platelet survival was increased, but neither was significantly improved over the 16 g/day dose. These results offer additional evidence for the close correlation of platelet reactivity and serum cholesterol.

It is unclear whether platelet survival time is altered by a change in serum lipids because of a decrease in arterial endothelial injury or because of a decrease in platelet responsiveness to a constant level of endothelial injury, or both mechanism in combination. Nevertheless, the results of the present study indicate that, when measuring platelet survival, the serum cholesterol must be included in the interpretation of the results. Younger men with CAD have shortened platelet survival, but they also have increased serum cholesterol.

Summary

Platelets contribute to the pathogenesis of atherosclerotic CAD and its complications. Platelet survival time is shortened in most patients with CAD. An analysis of platelet survival time in 100 men (25–60 years of age) with angiographically defined CAD and serum triglycerides of 210 mg% or less was undertaken. All men had measurements of serum cholesterol of 196–419 mg%. Younger men with CAD had average shorter platelet survival time than older men (age 25–30 2.2±0.04 days, $N=9$; normal 3.7±0.03 days; age 31–40 2.4±0.03 days, $N=37$; age 41–50 2.6±0.05 days, $N=43$; age 51–60 2.8±0.04 days, $N=11$). Serum cholesterol correlated with platelet survival ($r=0.79$) better than age ($r=0.31$) (cholesterol < 301 mg% 2.1±0.04 days, $N=21$; cholesterol 251–300 mg% 2.7±0.04 days, $N=37$; cholesterol ≦ 250 mg% 3.3±0.05 days, $N=42$).

Fifteen men with CAD, shortened platelet survival, and serum cholesterol of 301 mg% or more were teated with cholestyramine (16 and 24 g) and restudied. Cholestyramine decreased serum cholesterol (control 348±8 mg%, 16 g/day 319±6 mg, 24 g/day 310±6 mg%) and increased platelet survival (control 2.3±0.08 days, 16 g/day 2.7±0.07 days, 24 g/day 2.9±0.07 days).

Results suggest that platelet survival time is frequently shortened in men with CAD and that serum cholesterol correlates with platelet survival. Younger men with CAD have shortened platelet survival, but they also have increased serum cholesterol values. Alteration of cholesterol results in an improvement in platelet survival time.

References

1. French JE (1971) Atherogenesis and thrombosis. Semin Hematol 8:84
2. Roberts WC (1973) Does thrombosis play a major role in the development of symptom-producing atherosclerotic plaques? Circulation 48:1161
3. Harker LA, Ross R, Slichter SJ, Scott CR (1976) Homocystine-induced arteriosclerosis: The role of endothelial injury and platelet response in its genesis. J Clin Invest 58:731
4. Steele P, Battock D, Genton E (1975) Effects of clofibrate and sulfinpyrazone on platelet survival time in coronary artery disease. Circulation 52:473
5. Ritchie JL, Harker LA (1977) Platelet and fibrinogen survival in coronary atherosclerosis: Response to medical and surgical therapy. Am J Cardiol 39:595
6. Kannel WB, Castelli WP, McNamar PM (1967) The coronary profile: 12-year follow-up in the Framingham study. J Med 9:611
7. Steele P, Rainwater (1978) Effects of dietary and pharmacologic alteration of serum lipids on platelet survival time. Circulation 58:365
8. Carvalho AC, Colman RW, Lees RS (1974) Platelet function in hyperlipoproteinemia. N Engl J Med 290:434
9. Shattil SJ, Anaya-Galindo R, Bennett J et al. (1975) Platelet hypersensitivity induced by cholesterol incorporation. J Clin Invest 55:636

Risk Factors in Patients with Myocardial Infarction Under the Age of 40

J. Kaliman, H. Sinzinger, P. Probst, O. Pachinger, K. Widhalm, and F. Kaindl[1]

Results of a number of epidemiological studies have indicated that patients with elevated blood lipid levels show a higher incidence of cardiovascular disease than individuals with low or normal lipid levels (Goldstein et al. 1973; Kannel et al. 1971, 1979; Eriksson and Carlson 1974; Castelli et al. 1977; Breslow 1978).

Coronary artery disease, however, can often be detected in patients exhibiting normal serum liporotein levels. This fact can be due to accumulation of other risk factors, such as cigarette smoking or hypertension or both (Kannel et al. 1971).

On the other hand, many clinical data indicate that platelets may play an important role in the genesis of thrombosis, especially in arterial circulation, and might be involved in the development and progression of atherosclerosis (Cella et al. 1979; Burrows et al. 1978; Schernthaner et al. 1979, 1980; Sinzinger et al. 1980). In addition, platelets from patients with hyperlipoproteinemias (HLP) (Carvalho et al. 1974; Corash et al. 1976; Colman 1978; Tremoli et al. 1979) without coronary heart disease and patients surviving myocardial infarction (MI) (Szczeklik et al. 1978) have been shown to have an activated population of platelets, which has been demonstrated by a variety of platelet function tests. Of special importance in studying the in vivo behavior of platelets are a number of tests available which most probably represent most closely the in vivo function as the platelet survival (Gold and Steele, this vol. pp. 143–147), the thromboxane formation (Szczeklik et al. 1978), the malonyldialdehyde formation (Tremoli et al. 1979), and the actual levels of the platelet proteins β-thromboglobulin and platelet factor 4 (Ludlam 1979; Doyle et al. 1980). The measurement of both these proteins in human plasma is, therefore, a valuable parameter of in vivo platelet activity (Bolton et al. 1976a, b).

The aim of the present study was to investigate which risk factors could be found in young patients (less than 40 years) surviving MI.

Patients and Methods

We examined 50 patients (47 males, 3 females) 6–36 months after MI, 26–40 years of age. In all the subjects, coronary atherosclerosis was confirmed by coronary angiography. None of the patients had diabetes mellitus or hypertension, and none were taking medication for lowering blood lipid levels. Fourty-five patients were smokers before the event. Only two were obese before the infarction.

Blood samples were taken in the morning after a 12-h overnight fast. Serum was obtained after centrifugation. On the same day, determinations of total cholesterol

1 Kardiologische Universitätsklinik, Allgem. Krankenhaus der Stadt Wien, Garnisongasse 13, A-1097 Wien, Austria

and triglycerides were performed by means of full enzymatic methods using Merck and Boehringer-Mannheim reagents, respectively (Richmond 1973; Bucolo and David 1975). Quality control for cholesterol, using lipid standard sera (Precilip; Boehringer-Mannheim, FRG), resulted in a coefficient of variation of 2% –3%. External quality control was done by the WHO Lipid Reference Laboratory, Prague: The last coefficient of variation of our study was 1.8%. Estimations of lipoproteins were performed according to the US National Institutes of Health methods (Lipid Research Clinics Program).

β-thromboglobulin and platelet factor 4 levels were examined as follows: 2×5 ml blood were withdrawn by an atraumatic venipuncture without venous occlusion using a 19-gauge needle, 2.3 ml were discarded, and the remaining 2.7 ml were immediately transferred into cooled (4 °C) assay tubes containing 0.1 ml 10% NaEDTA, 0.1 ml theophylline (5.4 mg/ml), and 0.1 ml prostacyclin (33 ng/ml). The tubes were mixed by gentle inversion and cooled (4 °C) and centrifuged within 1 h at 1800 g and 4 °C for 30 min. Controls were 30 and 15 sex- and age-matched healthy people. For statistical analysis, Student's t-test was used.

Table 1. Serum lipids and lipoproteins and frequency of smoking in patients with different types of hyperproteinemia (types II a, II b, and IV)

Groups	Tot. chol.	VLDL. chol.	HDL. chol.	LDL. chol.	Trigl.	VLDL. Trigl.	Smoking Yes	No
Controls	191.7	14.5	39.8	129.3	114.8	53.6	2	13
$n=15$	± 7.2	± 1.3	± 2.6	± 7.6	⊥ 8.4	± 6.9		
II a	300.0	29.2	30.9	231.3	141.1	61.7	8	2
$n=10\ (20\%)$	± 15.0	± 4.1	± 2.9	± 15.4	± 10.5	± 5.9		(6)
II b	302.9	52.4	31.7	214.0	335.1	152.8	10	0
$n=10\ (20\%)$	± 16.9	± 10.4	± 2.7	± 9.6	± 64.5	± 23.0		(8)
IV	229.3	49.0	31.7	137.6	446.6	237.3	8	2
$n=10\ (20\%)$	± 9.2	± 7.5	± 1.4	± 12.7	± 118.8	± 66.8		(5)

$\bar{X}\pm SEM$

Table 2. Serum lipids and lipoproteins and frequency of smoking in patients with normal lipid values

Groups	Tot. chol.	VLDL. chol.	HDL. chol.	LDL. chol.	Trigl.	VLDL Trigl.	Smoking Yes	No
Controls	191.7	14.5	39.8	129.3	114.8	53.6	2	13
$n=15$	± 7.2	± 1.3	± 2.6	±ö 7.6	± 8.4	± 6.9		
Patients with	195.4	22.6	37.6	125.9	119.2	56.5	19	1
normal lipids	± 8.5	± 2.6	± 2.7	± 6.6	± 9.2	± 5.9		(13)
$n=20\ (40\%)$								
	NS	$P<0.01$	NS	NS	NS	NS		

Table 3. β-TG and platelet factor 4 in patients with three different types of hyperlipoproteinemia

Groups	β-TG	PF$_4$	Smoking	
			Yes	No
Controls $n = 30$	57.2 $\pm$ 10.4	20.4 $\pm$ 3.8	6	24
II a II b IV $n = 30$	103.8 $\pm$ 15.8	55.7 $\pm$ 9.7	26	4 (19)
	$P < 0.02$	$P < 0.002$		

$\bar{X} \pm$ SEM

Table 4. β-TG and platelet factor 4 in patients with normal lipid values

Groups	β-TG	PF$_4$	Smoking	
			Yes	No
Controls $n = 30$	57.2 $\pm$ 10.4	20.4 $\pm$ 3.8	6	24
Patients with normal lipids $n = 20$	91.1 $\pm$ 16.8	34.7 $\pm$ 6.7	19	1 (13)
	NS	NS		

$\bar{X} \pm$ SEM

Table 5. Indices of HDL/Chol, HDL/LDL, and LDL/HDL in patients with different types of hyperlipoproteinemia

Groups	HDL Chol	HDL LDL	LDL HDL
Controls $n = 15$	0.21 $\pm$ 0.01	0.33 $\pm$ 0.03	3.51 $\pm$ 0.3
II a $n = 10$	0.10 $\pm$ 0.01	0.14 $\pm$ 0.01	7.9 $\pm$ 0.9
II b $n = 10$	0.11 $\pm$ 0.01	0.15 $\pm$ 0.02	7.2 $\pm$ 0.75
VI $n = 10$	0.14 $\pm$ 0.006	0.25* $\pm$ 0.03	4.43 $\pm$ 0.5
Patients with normal lipids $n = 20$	0.19* $\pm$ 0.01	0.31* $\pm$ 0.02	3.71* $\pm$ 0.3

* NS; $\bar{X} \pm$ SEM

Results

The patients were grouped according the type of HLP (ten patients type II a HLP, ten patients type II b HLP, and ten patients type IV HLP). Twenty patients (40%) had normal lipoprotein levels. The serum lipids and lipoproteins are given, as well as smoking habits, in Table 1. It seems noteworthy that the serum lipids of MI patients without HLP had comparable blood lipid values and lipoproteins, with the exception of the VLDL cholesterol levels (Table 2) being significantly different ($P < 0.01$). The actual values of platelet proteins were extremely high in comparison to a control group which was treated in the same way in the outpatient clinic. The values between the HLP patients and the controls were both statistically significant (Table 3). Surprisingly, the platelet protein levels between controls and MI patients without HLP also showed different mean values. However, the difference was due to the high variation, which was not statistically significant (Table 4). The value of various indices such as HDL-LDL cholesterol. LDL-HDL cholesterol and the HDL-cholesterol are given in Table 5. The most important finding seems to be that

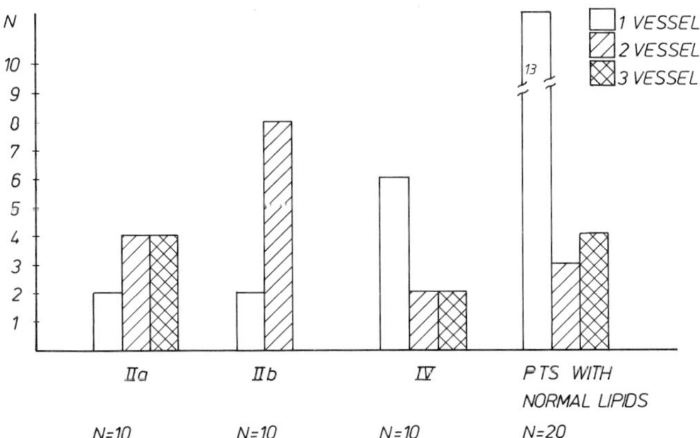

Fig. 1. Vessel involvement (*1, 2, 3*) in different HLP groups (Fredrickson)

those patients with normal lipids and lipoprotein profiles mainly had a single-vessel disease whereas, especially in type II a and II b HLP patients, the percentage of two- and three-vessel disease was dominant, being more severe in type II a than II b (Fig. 1).

Discussion

Results of many investigations have demonstrated the close association between HLP and angiographically proven coronary artery disease (Zampogna et al. 1980;

Wieland et al. 1980; Naito et al. to be published; Okabe 1979; Gohlke et al. 1980a; Barboriak et al. 1974, 1979). Though this study represents only a somewhat superficial analysis of parameters and does not take into account the laboratory findings before the event of MI, it seems noteworthy that three important risk factors can be detected very easily.

One of the most important generally accepted risk factors for the development of coronary heart disease is cigarette smoking. 90% of our patients were cigarette smokers before MI. In 19 of the 50 patients, smoking was the only one risk factor present. Gohlke et al. (1980b) reported the same percentage with a comparable patient group, and were able to show that those patients who continued smoking after MI had the highest progression rate, whereas those who stopped had the highest regression as proven by coronary angiography. Whether this is a direct effect, or an influence mediated via an activated platelet population which is known to occur in heavy smokers is not clear.

Surprisingly, the platelet protein values are extremely high in comparison to the control group (Table 4). Comparing the patients with an older age group suffering from MI, the values are also much higher. These findings are in concordance with data reported by Ritter et al. (1980) as to platelet factor 4 which was, in their study, much higher than in older MI patients. Ritter et al. (1980) concluded that the platelets might probably be involved much more intensively in MI at young age. Concerning the actual level of platelet proteins, it has to be stressed that the values found for outpatients are always much higher than for hospitalized patients, due to their physical activity coming to the clinic, etc. However, this influence can be ignored, as both the patient and control group were examined in the same way.

The great importance of a lipoprotein profile in the etiology of coronary artery disease can be demonstrated by the high frequency of HLP (60%) in our patients, which were distributed in thirds into the groups IIa, IIb, and IV, respectively, according to the Fredrickson classification. Among the so-called normolipemic patients, many had decreased HDL cholesterol concentration. The finding that those patients without HLP had vessel involvement to a significantly lesser degree (Fig. 1) is consistent with data reported by Moore et al. (1979), where an increase in HLP led to an increase in vessel disease.

The fact that 22 of our patients were smokers with HLP, 19 were smokers alone, and 22 had a positive family history points out the special mosaic of risk pattern in MI at young age.

Attention will be drawn in the future to follow-up of the patients by annual control, and by dietary, and drug intervention if necessary. Especially the children of these patients will be controlled for the existence of HLP.

Beside the well-known multifactorial etiology and individual variability, our findings in a population of 50 patients at young age show the important role of smoking, HLP and activated platelet function in the evolution of coronary artery disease, especially in younger individuals.

Summary

In 50 patients (47 males, 3 females) with MI below the age of 40 years, 6–36 months after the event plasma lipids and lipoprotein profile, platelet proteins (β-thromboglobulin and platelet factor 4) were examined. The patients were grouped according to the type of HLP: Ten patients had type II a HLP, ten type II b, and ten type IV. In 20 patients (40%) a normal lipoprotein profile was found. The platelet proteins were higher in MI survivors with HLP than those without HLP. Single-vessel disease was the dominating feature in patients without HLP, whereas patients with type II a und II b mainly had a two- or three-vessel disease. These findings, as well as the fact that 90% were smokers before MI, demonstrate an image of the special mosaic of risk factors in patients with MI at young age.

Acknowledgements. The expert technical help of Andrea Gall during this study is kindly acknowledged.

References

Barboriak JJ, Rimm AA, Anderson AJ et al. (1974) Coronary artery occlusion and blood lipids. Am Heart J 87:716–721

Barboriak JJ, Anderson AJ, Rimm AA, King JF (1979) High density lipoprotein cholesterol and coronary artery occlusion. Metabolism 28:735–738

Bolton AE, Ludlam CA, Moore S et al. (1976a) Three approaches to the radioimmunoassay of human β-thromboglobulin. Br J Haematol 33:233–238

Bolton AE, Ludlam CA, Pepper DS et al. (1976b) A radioimmunoassay for platelet factor 4. Thromb Res 8:51–58

Breslow L (1978) Risk factor intervention for health maintenance. Science 200:908–912

Bucolo G, David H (1975) Quantitative determination of serum triglycerides by the use of enzymes. Clin Chim Acta 59:271–275

Burrows AW, Chavin SI, Hockaday TDR (1978) Plasma β-thromboglobulin concentrations in diabetes mellitus. Lancet I:235–236

Carvalho ACA, Colman RW, Lees RS (1974) Platelet function in hyperlipoproteinemia. N Engl J Med 290:434–438

Castelli WP, Doyle JT, Gordon T et al. (1977) HDL cholesterol and other lipids in coronary heart disease. Circulation 55:767–772

Cella G, Zahavi J, DeHaas HA, Kakkar VV (1979) β-Thromboglobulin platelet production time and platelet function in vascular disease. Br J Haematol 43:127–136

Colman RW (1978) Platelet function in hyperbetalipoproteinemia. Thromb Haemost 39:284–293

Corash L, Schaefer E, Poindexter E, Andersen J (1976) Platelet function and survival in familial hypercholesterolemia. Circulation 117:53

Doyle DJ, Chesterman CN, Cade JE et al. (1980) Plasma concentrations of platelet-specific proteins correlated with platelet survival. Blood 55:82–84

Eriksson M, Carlson LA (1974) Lipoproteins in myocardial infarction. In: Schettler G, Weizel A (eds) Atherosclerosis III. Springer, Berlin Heidelberg New York, p 838

Gohlke H, Gohlke-Bärwolf C, Stürzenhofecker P et al. (1980a) Der transmurale Herzinfarkt unter 40 Jahren – Korrelation von angiographischen Befunden mit Risikofaktoren und Anamnese bei 619 Patienten. Z Kardiol 69:724

Gohlke H, Stürzenhofecker P, Görnandt L et al. (1980b) Progression und Regression der koronaren Herzerkrankung im chronischen Infarktstadium bei Patienten unter 40 Jahren. Schweiz Med Wochenschr 110:1663–1665

Goldstein JL, Hazzard WR, Schrott HG et al. (1973) Hyperlipidemia in coronary heart disease. J Clin Invest 52:1533

Kannel WB, Castelli WP, Gordon T (1971) Serum cholesterol, lipoproteins and the risk of coronary heart disease: The Framingham study. Ann Intern Med 74:1–12

Kannel WB, Castelli WP, Gordon T (1979) Cholesterol in the prediction of atherosclerotic disease. Ann Intern Med 90:85–91

Ludlam CA (1979) Evidence for the platelet specificity of β-thromboglobulin and studies on its plasma concentration in healthy individuals. Br J Haematol 41:271–278

Moore RB, Long JM, Matts JP et al. (1979) Plasma lipoproteins and coronary arteriography in subjects in the program on the surgical control of the hyperlipidemias. Atherosclerosis 32:101–119

Naito HK, Greenstreet R, David JA, Sheldon WL, Shirey EK, Lewis RC, Proudfit WL, Gerrity RG (1981) HDL cholesterol concentration and severity of coronary atherosclerosis determined by cine-angiography. Artery (in press)

Okabe M (1979) The high occurrence of low density lipoprotein subfractions in coronary heart disease. Jpn Circ J 43:1059–1071

Pometta D, Micheli H (1979) Atherosclerose coronarienne et lipoproteines seriques. Schweiz Med Wochenschr 109:1926–1930

Richmond W (1973) Preparation and properties of an cholesterol oxidase from Nocardia SP and its application to the enzymatic assay of total cholesterol in serum. Clin Chem 19:1350–1356

Ritter B, Budde U, Etzel F, Roskamm H (1980) Plättchenfaktor 4 bei Patienten mit jugendlichem Herzinfarkt. Z Kardiol 69:724

Schernthaner G, Mühlhauser I, Silberbauer K (1979) β-thromboglobulin lowered by dipyridamole in diabetes. Lancet II:748

Schernthaner G, Sinzinger H, Silberbauer K, Freyler H (1980) Altered platelet function in diabetes mellitus. Decrease of prostacyclin, analysis of plasma β-thromboglobulin and platelet factor 4 according to state of metabolic control and diabetic microangiopathic stages. In: Tesi M (ed) 1st International Colloquium of Angiology, Academic Press, New York London, p 352

Sinzinger H, Kaliman J, Silberbauer K, Schernthaner G (1980) In vivo und in vitro Plättchenaktivität bei Patienten mit peripherer arterieller Verschlußkrankheit. Proc Thromb 421–425

Szczeklik A, Gryglewski RJ, Musial J et al. (1978) Thromboxane generation and platelet aggregation in survivals of myocardial infarction. Thromb Haemost 40:66–74

Tremoli E, Maderna P, Sirtori M, Sirtori CR (1979) Platelet aggregation and malondialdehyde formation in type II a hypercholesterolemic patients. Haemostasis 39:284–293

Wieland H, Seidel D, Wiegand V, Kreuzer H (1980) Serum lipoproteins and coronary artery disease. Comparison of the lipoprotein profile with the results of coronary angiography. Atherosclerosis 36:269–280

Zampogna A, Luria MH, Manubens SJ, Luria MA (1980) Relationship between lipids and occlusive coronary artery disease. Arch Intern Med 140:1067–1069

Zimmer F, Riebeling V, Benke B et al. (1980) Das LDL-HDL-Verhältnis bei Patienten mit Koronarsklerose. Z Kardiol 69:149–153

Mechanism and Prevention Possibilities in Coronary Thrombosis

G. V. R. Born[1]

If it is accepted that many myocardial infarctions (MI) are caused, in younger as in older patients, by coronary thrombosis (Davies et al. 1979), modern analysis is providing evidence (see Born 1979) that it depends on complex haemodynamic interactions between atherosclerotic lesions and blood constituents, primarily the platelets. These interactions have implications, both positive and negative, for prevention and treatment. Platelet aggregation as the immediate cause of arterial thrombosis is the basis for the world-wide interest in and large-scale trials of platelet-inhibiting agents as potential anti-thrombotic drugs. In principle, one approach to the prevention of arterial thrombosis should be through drugs capable of inhibiting platelet aggregation. Rapidly increasing biochemical and pharmacological knowledge about platelets has revealed potent inhibitors of aggregation with different modes of action. Encouraging results have been obtained recently with models of extra-corporeal circulation, e.g. artificial kidneys in which the thrombotic deposition of platelets can be prevented by adenosine (Richardson et al. 1976) or by prostacyclin (prostaglandin I_2) (Bunting et al. personal communcation). It was on the basis of their platelet-inhibiting activities that three established drugs, acetylsalicylic acid (aspirin), dipyridamole (persantin) and sulphinpyrazone (anturane) have been undergoing extensive trials in different well-defined clinical situations arising in consequence of arterial thromboses. Results so far have left considerable uncertainties. All these drugs have actions on many other systems in the body, so that any therapeutic effectiveness need not be due to their actions on platelets. Another approach to the prevention of arterial thrombosis may be through membrane-stabilising drugs, such as chlorpromazine (Seeman 1972) which apparently diminish the interactions between erythrocytes and platelets (Born et al. 1976; Born 1979; Born and Wehmeier 1979).

References

The Anturane Reinfarction Trial Research Group (1978) N Engl J Med 298:289
Born, GVR (1979a) Letter. Lancet I:822
Born GVR (1979b) Plenary lecture to VIII World Congress of Cardiology, Tokyo, September 1978. Excerpta Medica, Amsterdam
Born GVR, Wehmeier A (1979) Nature 282:212
Born GVR, Bergqvist D, Arfors KE (1976) Nature 259:233
Davies MJ, Fulton WFM, Robertson WB (1979) J Pathol 127:99
Richardson PD, Galletti PM, Born GVR (1976) Trans Am Soc Artif Intern Organs 22:22
Seeman P (1972) Pharmacol Rev 24:583

---

1 Department of Pharmacology, King's College, Strand, London WC2R 2LS, UK

Intracoronary Fibrinolysis in Acute Myocardial Infarction in Young Patients

W. Rutsch and H. Schmutzler [1]

A decrease in the mortality rate among patients hospitalized with acute myocardial infarction can only be expected from therapeutic measures which reduce the area of necrotic tissue. Restitution of coronary flow and myocardial reperfusion before irreparable cell damage occurs would appear to be the best way of achieving this goal. Intracoronary infusion of fibrinolytic substances such as streptokinase provides high local concentrations and allows recanalization of coronary thrombosis while avoiding hemorrhagic complications.

Kordenat [1] reported on animal experiments in 1971, and Ganz [2] has recently described thrombolysis by means of streptokinase infusion in coronary arteries occluded by thrombosis resulting from placement of copper wires in the vessels.

We followed a standardized procedure for recanalization in 50 patients with evolving myocardial infarction. They were included in the study if the following criteria were met:

1. Short history of anginal pain
2. Exact definition of onset of anginal pain
3. Onset and admission less than 3 h
4. Presence of one of the following objective criteria of coronary artery occlusion in addition to chest pain
   a) ST elevation in the ECG
   b) Akinesia demonstrated in the 2D-Echocardiogram
5. Normal serum creatine phosphokinase (CPK) values
6. Normal coagulation studies
7. No history of reanimation with external cardiac resuscitation
8. No history of injury to a major vessel (unsuccessful attempt at canalization of the subclavian artery, for example)
9. No generalized arteriosclerosis
10. Consent to coronary bypass surgery.

The primary symptom was persistent therapy resistent angina pectoris. Time of onset of angina was determined as exactly as possible, and the interval from onset of pain until diagnosis was 3 h or less. ST segment elevation was the preferred criterion of myocardial ischemia, but disorders of regional wall motion in the 2-dimensional echocardiogram were also used, and the patients were included in the study after demonstration of akinesia. CPK values were in the normal range. Patients with a history of infarction were excluded since preexistent disorders of regional wall motion would have made accurate evaluation of therapeutic effect extremely difficult

1 Klinikum Charlottenburg, Kardiologische Abteilung, Freie Universität Berlin, Spandauer Damm 130, 1000 Berlin 19

in this group. The usual contraindications to streptokinase were observed, and patients with coagulopathy were excluded from the study. Ventriculography was performed and repeated 60 min after successful recanalization as well as 3 weeks later, in order to demonstrate and quantify the disorder of regional wall motion. The right and left coronary arteries were demonstrated with the Judkins technique in order to document coronary artery occlusion and to evaluate the severity of coronary heart disease. Intracoronary infusion of 3000 U/min was performed via a Judkins catheter. Recanalization was usually accompanied by arrhythmias, rapid changes in ST elevation, and characteristic increases in CPK levels with a peak value at 7.2 ± 3.3 h after recanalization and 12.0 ± 3.3 h after onset of angina pectoris (Fig. 1).

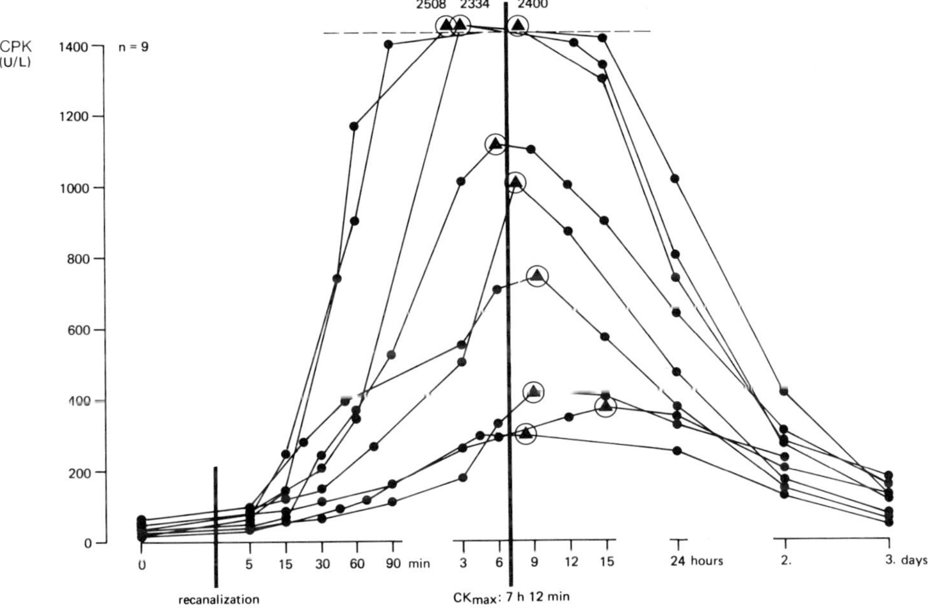

Fig. 1. Changes in CPK levels after recanalization in patients with myocardial infarction

A soft-tipped guide wire was used in an attempt at mechanical perforation of the occluding thrombus in 7 of 50 patients included in the study (Fig. 2), with successful recanalization in three of the seven patients. The remaining 43 patients received intracoronary streptokinase infusion alone. Of these patients, 39 demonstrated total occlusion of a coronary vessel during the stage of evolving infarction, while four others had subtotal occlusion. Streptokinase produced little change in the latter, while adequate recanalization and restitution of myocardial perfusion was obtained in 34 patients with total occlusion. We divided the patients into two age groups in order to evaluate age-specific differences in the evolution of infarction and possible influences of age on results of intracoronary infusion with thrombolytic substances (Table 1). Group I comprised 11 patients with a mean age of 38.5 ± 1.5 years, and group II included 28 patients with a mean age of 58.7 ± 9.5 years. Sex distribu-

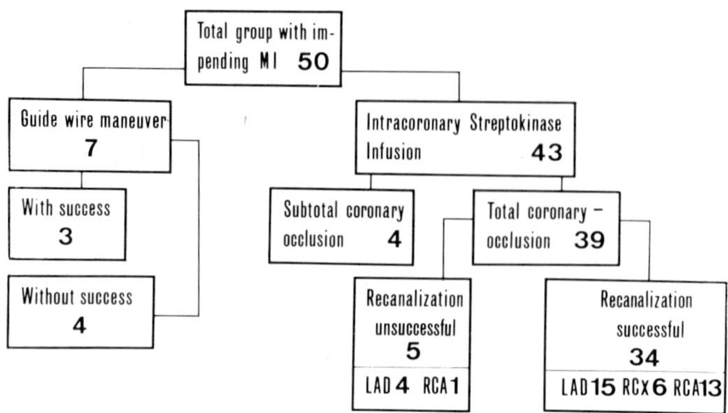

Fig. 2. Treatment given to 50 patients with impending MI. LAD, left anterior descending; RCA, right coronary artery; RCX, ramus circumflexus

tion was not uniform. 70% of patients in the younger group were male; 59% of group II were males and 41% females.

Severity of coronary heart disease and location of the vascular occlusion also varied between the two groups. Of the younger patients, 60% had one vessel disease, 20% two vessel disease, and 20% three vessel disease. In the older group 47% had one vessel disease, 47% two vessel disease, and 6% three vessel disease. The low proportion of three vessel disease in the older age group may be explained by the fact that our study excluded patients with previous infarction or a history of severe angina pectoris. Location of vascular occlusion also varied with age. Of the cases in group I, 50% had occlusion in the left anterior descending artery, 10% in the circum-

Table 1. Evaluation of myocardial infarction in two age groups

	Group I ($<$ 40 yrs)	Group II ($>$ 40 yrs)
Age (yrs)	38.5 ± 1.5	58.7 ± 9.5
Sex %		
Female	30	41
Male	70	59
Recanalization %		
Successful	90	77
Unsuccessful	10	23
Site of occlusion %		
LAD	50	29
RCX	10	13
RCA	40	58
Residual stenosis %		
After thrombolysis	77	83 n.s.
3rd week control	61	78 $P<0.05$

LAD, left anterior descending; RCX, ramus circumflexus; RCA, right coronary artery.

flex artery, and 40% in the right coronary artery. Occlusions of the right coronary artery were more common in the older age group – in 58% of cases – followed by occlusion of the left anterior descending artery in 29% of cases and occlusion of the circumflex artery in 13% of group II. Success in thrombolytic therapy of evolving infarction is related to the cause of occlusion. If one is able to draw conclusions on the etiology of infarction, then one must also be able to speculate on age-specific differences in the development of coronary artery occlusion. Our studies have shown that thrombotic material plays a more significant part in coronary artery occlusion in younger patients than in the older age group. Degree of stenosis due to an arteriosclerotic plaque and the amount of streptokinase required for thrombolysis prove that thrombosis is the major factor in coronary artery occlusion in younger patients. Coronary artery recanalization with streptokinase was successful in 90% of cases in the younger group of patients and in 77% of the older group. In other words, occlusion was not related to thrombosis in one of ten patients in group I, and one-quarter of the older patients had a cause other than thrombosis. Degree of stenosis after thrombolysis was $76.9 \pm 13.4\%$ in the younger group and $83.11 \pm 13.9\%$ in group II. Follow-up studies 3 weeks after occlusion showed a further reduction in stenosis in both groups with a more significant reduction in group I to $61.3 \pm 18.9\%$ as compared to $77.8 \pm 28.4\%$ in group II. These differences are highly significant in statistical terms. The period from onset of angina until the start of streptokinase infusion was approximately the same in both groups (Table 2). Therefore it is possible to draw indirect conclusions on size of the thrombus from the duration of therapy and total dose necessary for recanalization. The interval from onset of angina until start of streptokinase infusion averaged 175 min in group I and 154 min in group II. The streptokinase dosage was the same in all cases, i.e., 3000 U/min. Recanalization was achieved after 57.7 ± 25.2 min in group I and after 42.8 ± 22.9 min in group II. As a result, the total dose of streptokinase in group I was considerably higher – $225\,000 \pm 107\,700$ U – than in group II, where total dosage averaged $135\,000 \pm 63\,500$ U. The differences were highly significant.

It is more difficult to assess the influence of recanalization on myocardial function in cases of evolving infarction because very little is known about myocardial function in the natural history of myocardial infarction in man. Location of the occlusion certainly plays a major role. Definitive statements can be made only after relevant data have been gathered in a large number of patients. Given these qualifications, a comparison of ventricle volume and ejection fraction before recanalization

Table 2. Therapy of myocardial infarction in two age groups

	Group I (<40 yrs)	Group II (>40 yrs)	
Period from onset of angina until the the start of SK infusion	172.0 ± 35	154.0 ± 28	min n.s.
Time requirement for recanalization	57.7 ± 25.2	42.8 ± 22.9 min	$P < 0.05$
Amount of SK required for thrombolysis	$225\,000 \pm 107\,700$	$135\,000 \pm 63\,500$ U	$P < 0.005$

SK, streptokinase

Table 3. End-diastolic volume and ejection factor in two age groups with myocardial infarction

	Group I (<40 yrs)	Group II (>40 yrs)
EDVI ml/m²	n.s.	
After thrombolysis	93.6 ± 12.8 ⟶	80.9 ± 29.7
3rd week control	78.6 ± 10.4 ⟶	63.1 ± 19.0
	$P<0.005$	$P<0.01$ $P<0.005$
EF %		
After thrombolysis	53.6 ± 12.7 ⟶	52.0 ± 12.5
3rd week control	54.2 ± 17.5 ⟶ n.s.	57.6 ± 14.2
	n.s.	n.s.

EDVI, end-diastolic volume; EF, ejection factor

and 3 weeks later is instructive. End-diastolic volume in group I was 93.6 ± 9.5 ml/m² before recanalization, considerably greater than the 80.9 ± 24.7 ml/m² found in group II (Table 3). Successful recanalization was followed by a clear decrease in volume at 3 weeks, especially in the older patients, whose end-diastolic volume decreased to 63.1 ± 19.0 ml/m², as compared to 78.6 ± 10.4 ml/m² in group I. Ejection fraction (EF) was almost identical in both groups before recanalization with 53.6 ± 12.7% in group I and 52.0 ± 12.5% in group II. EF was basically unchanged in group I at 54.2 ± 17.5% and slightly improved in group II with 57.6 ± 14.2%. A possible interpretation for these differences is to be found in the development of collateral circulation in older patients with coronary artery disease and regions of diminished perfusion. These patients may be better adapted with no means of coping with the sudden decrease in perfusion.

Summary

1. Results of intracoronary streptokinase infusion in acute coronary artery occlusion suggest that in younger patients thrombotic occlusion is a more important factor than arteriosclerotic changes. A smaller degree of stenosis after complete thrombolysis, further regression of the stenosis with time, longer duration of thrombolysis, and higher total streptokinase dose may be interpreted as indirect evidence of the greater importance of the thrombus.
2. Recanalization during evolving myocardial infarction produces less improvement in myocardial function in younger patients, possibly as a result of less complete adaptation to acute coronary artery occlusion.

References

1. Kordenat RK, Kezdi P (1972) Experimental intracoronary thrombosis and selective in situ lysis by catheter technique. Am J Cardiol 30:640
2. Ganz W (1979) Experimental intracoronary lysis by means of streptokinase infusion in animal experiments. German Society of Cardiology, Cologne

Beta-Blocker Treatment in the Chronic Phase of Myocardial Infarction in Young Age Groups

C. Wilhelmsson, A. Vedin, R. Bergstrand, and L. Wilhelmsen[1]

Treatment of myocardial infarction (MI) patients with beta-blockers both during the acute and long-term phases has aroused a growing interest. Independent studies have demonstrated that alprenolol and practolol prevent sudden deaths during the long-term course after MI (Wilhelmsson et al. 1974; Multicenter International Study 1975; Ahlmark and Saetre 1976; Andersen et al. 1979). The question remains whether all patients should be treated or if the treatment should be restricted to certain ages or other categories.

The purpose of this presentation is to review current knowledge regarding chronic beta-blockade in an effort to apply the relevant information to young patients.

Natural History

The prognosis for young patients is different from that of older patients (Bergstrand et al. this vol.). Several studies have demonstrated better long-term surival among young patients (Helmers 1974; Pole et al. 1976; Kovacsics et al. 1977). However, in some centers, higher mortality rates are also sometimes found (World Health Organisation 1976).

During hospitalization, young patients may have signs of more extensive infarctions, which differentiate them from older patients. Thus, they have higher enzyme peaks, higher frequency Q waves, and a higher frequency of ventricular fibrillation (Bergstrand et al. to be published). Despite the high prevalence of factors tending to worsen prognosis absolute mortality remains low, but there is considerable excess mortality in relation to healthy contemporaries (Vedin et al. 1975 b; Helmers and Lundman 1979). Several other factors have also been shown to influence the long-term course after discharge from the hospital (Wilhelmsson et al. 1975; Vedin et al. 1977). In this context, it is important that younger patients stop or lessen cigarette smoking after MI (Bergstrand et al. pp. 23–28). This may at least partly explain why the reinfarction rate is as high among young patients as among older ones (Bergstrand et al. this vol.).

The usual systems for prognostication after MI available are not sufficiently defined for young patients. Furthermore, the risk of a nonfatal recurrence is not related to the same risk factors and nonfatal reinfarction has proved difficult to predict.

---

1 Department of Medicine, University of Göteborg, Östra Hospital, S-416 85 Göteborg, Sweden

Completed Prospective Studies

Several studies have been completed and some have shown inconclusive findings, as reviewed and discussed previously (Vedin and Wilhelmsson 1979, 1981). A list of completed conclusive and positive studies is presented in Table 1.

Table 1. Completed, positive prospective long-term studies with beta-blockers

Authors	Year	Compound (mg/day)	No. of patients	
			Total	< 50 years of age
Wilhelmsson et al.	1974	Alprenolol (400)	230	0
Multicentre International	1975	Practolol (400)	3 038	817
Ahlmark et al.	1974	Alprenolol (400)	159	26
Andersen et al.	1979	Alprenolol (400)	282	55

Positive findings were first reported in a randomized prospective study of 230 patients, 57–67 years of age, randomly allocated to placebo or alprenolol separately in four different risk strata (Wilhelmsson et al. 1974; Vedin et al. 1975 a). It was possible to define a subgroup with a benign prognosis and, consequently, other groups with a more malignant course. Treatment started during posthospitalization week 1 and was maintained until death, reinfarction, or the end of 2 years. The daily dose of alprenolol was 400 mg. The number of sudden deaths was significantly reduced, but though the overall mortality was reduced by 50% this reduction did not reach statistical significance: The same individuals made up the difference between the groups both in sudden deaths and total deaths. Thus, the sudden death reduction also implied a meaningful reduction of total mortality. In order to demonstrate a significant reduction of overall mortality, larger numbers would have been required. Concomitant treatment was administered according to standardized criteria. The frequency of digitalis treatment and use of diuretics was high. However, the patients were representative of all the MI cases in the same age group in the area and all pretrial exclusions have been detailed.

With some reservations, due to the small number, the findings indicate that alprenolol was capable of reducing sudden deaths in the long-term course after MI. Supportive evidence was later presented in an open study (Ahlmark and Saetre 1976) using the same drug, dose, and duration of treatment in which similar results were obtained. A retrospective analysis of this study suggests that the patients in the treatment and control groups were comparable.

Data showing that another beta-blocker, practolol (400 mg/day), reduced sudden deaths after MI were obtained in the Multicentre International Study (1975, 1977). In this study 3000 patients were randomized. The duration of treatment was up to 2 years. A reduction of not only sudden deaths, but also total mortality was demonstrated and there was also a trend towards reduction of the nonfatal reinfarction rate. The major criticism of this study is that it is impossible to define the patients included in the study, since the pretrial exclusions were not counted or characterized.

Furthermore, the retrospective analysis (Multicentre International Study 1975, 1977) has overemphasized defining groups where practolol is particularly useful. This analyses seem to indicate that patients with anterior infarcts and low diastolic entry pressures did better with practolol than placebo. This analysis has attracted unfortunate attention, since it has become clear that bradyarrhythmias in patients with inferior infarction, who were admitted to the study early in the course of their disease, were responsible for the lack of early difference between treatments with respect to different sites of infarction. When the later results are analyzed, site of infarction is unimportant.

Finally, a Danish study (Andersen et al. 1979) has used alprenolol in a 1-year study where all patients with a suspected or proven MI regardless of age were included. A beta-blocker or placebo was immediately injected in the emergency room of the hospital. The oral dose was 400 mg daily. After 1 year a significant reduction of mortality was clearly shown in all randomized patients under the age of 65. No effect on short-term mortality could be demonstrated. No adverse effects were found in patients who did not develop a MI. There was no significant difference between the two treatment groups in patients above 65 years of age. However, in patients with unstable circulation, acute alprenolol administration seemed contraindicated.

In conclusion, the studies presented support the concept that practolol and alprenolol reduce long-term mortality after MI. The mechanism of action is not yet defined. It is not clear whether antiarrhythmic actions, effects on myocardial metabolism, or both are responsible for the outcome. The pathogenesis of the lethal arrhythmias themselves is virtually unknown.

It has not been established whether all patients need to be treated or treatment can be reserved for some selected groups. The optimal dose has not been found and it is not clear when treatment should ideally begin, or how long it should be maintained.

The evidence of a lowered reinfarction rate after beta-blockade is more controversial than the evidence for a mortality reduction. No study has focused particularly on the effects of beta-blockade among patients 50 years of age and younger. In the completed studies few patients below 40 and only 898 patients below 50 have been involved (Table 1). Close to 20000 patients are presently involved in ongoing or recently completed trials (Table 2). However, the total numbers of young patients in each of these studies is low and, in connection with low mortality, it is unlikely that conclusive data regarding the effects of beta-blockade and mortality in young patients will be obtained. However, if the studies had been homogeneous in terms of design, patient selection, and confounding factors, it would be possible to pool the results, provided that different beta-blockers produced the same effects. None of these conditions are fulfilled and therefore pooling data from different studies will produce no reliable results concerning young patients.

Table 2. Some ongoing prospective secondary preventive trials with beta-blockers

Center	Compound	No. of patients	Prognostic stratification	Acute intravenous injection
Multicenter, France	Acebutalol	550	–	–
Stockholm, Sweden	Metoprolol	250	+	–
Amsterdam, The Netherlands	Metoprolol	500	+	–
Gothenburg, Sweden	Metoprolol	600	+	+
Multicenter, USA	Metoprolol	3 000	–	–
Multicenter, UK	Oxprenolol	1 100	–	–
Multicenter, West Germany	Oxprenolol	4 000	–	–
Multicenter, Sweden-Australia	Pindolol	500	+	–
Multicenter, UK	Propranolol	500	–	–
Multicenter, USA	Propranolol	4 200	–	–
Oslo, Norway	Propranolol	700	+	–
Multicenter, North England	Sotalol	1 600	–	–
Multicenter, Norway	Timolol	1 800	+	–
Total		19 000		

An important unresolved question relates to the differences in the drugs tested. The available beta-blockers vary regarding $beta_1$ and $beta_2$ affinity, intrinsic sympathomimetic activity (ISA), and membrane-stabilizing activity. At present, there is nothing to suggest that one ancillary property of beta-blockers is clinically more useful than another. The crucial properties may yet have to be defined.

The drugs in the different studies have been selected on a fairly arbitrary basis. However, the fact that several different drugs are being studied is undoubtedly useful. If the next presented study with timolol or sotalol or metoprolol all show a convincing benefit from treatment, then it will be reasonable to assume that many beta-blockers are interchangeable in this respect. A convincing benefit from one drug, but not from another, may give a clue as to the mechanism of action.

Conventional indications for beta-blockers, in addition to the prophylactic indication, are found among many patients. In a Gothenburg patient series of cases below 40 years of age, 55% had hypertension and 50% had angina pectoris. Assuming an even distribution of hypertension among angina patients, and vice versa, 70% of all patients have a conventional indication for treatment with a beta-blocker.

Conclusion

There is no clinical or experimental finding indicating that young patients show a different response pattern compared to older patients. The high frequency of conventional indications for chronic beta-blockade after MI reduces the number of patients with a single prophylactic indication.

Young patients with MI are exposed to excessive risks of reinfarction and death in relation to healthy contemporaries and should, therefore, be treated.

References

Ahlmark G, Saetre H (1976) Long-term treatment with beta-blockers after myocardial infarction. Eur J Clin Pharmacol 10:77–83

Andersen M, Bechsgaard P, Fredriksen J et al. (1979) The effect of alprenolol on mortality among patients with definite or suspected acute myocardial infarction. Lancet II:865–868

Bergstrand R, Vedin A, Wilhelmsson C, Wilhelmsen L (to be published) Incidence and prognosis of acute myocardial infarction among men below age 40 in Göteborg, Sweden. Eur Heart J (accepted for publication)

Helmers C (1974) Short and long-term prognostic indices in acute myocardial infarction. Acta Med Scand [Suppl] 555

Helmers C, Lundman T (1979) Early and sudden deaths after myocardial infarction. Acta Med Scand 205:3–9

Kovacsics H, Kovacsics A, Petersen I et al. (1977) Langzeitschicksal nach Myokardinfarkt bei Männern unter 40 Jahren. Verh Dtsch Ges Kreislaufforsch 43:280

A Multicentre International Study (1975) Improvement in prognosis of myocardial infarction by long-term beta-adrenoceptor blockade using practolol. Br Med J II:735–740

A Multicentre International Study (1977) Reduction in mortality after myocardial infarction with long-term beta-adrenoceptor blockade. Br Med J II:419–421

Pole DJ, Thompson PL, Woodings TL et al. (1976) Acute myocardial infarction: One-year follow-up of 1138 cases from the Perth Community Coronary Register. Aust NZ J Med 6:437–440

Vedin A, Wilhelmsson C (1979) A review of current beta-blocker trials in the world. Heart Bull 10:180–182

Vedin A, Wilhelmsson C (1981) Secondary prevention trials: A review of beta-blocker trials

Vedin A, Wilhelmsson C, Werkö L (1975 a) Alprenolol after myocardial infarction. Acta Med Scand [Suppl] 575

Vedin A, Wilhelmsson C, Elmfeldt D et al. (1975 b) Deaths and non-fatal reinfarctions during 2-years follow-up after myocardial infarction. Acta Med Scand 198:353–364

Vedin A, Wilhelmsen L, Wedel H et al. (1977) Prediction of cardiovascular deaths and non-fatal reinfarctions after myocardial infarction. Acta Med Scand 201:309–316

Wilhelmsson C, Vedin A, Wilhelmsen L et al. (1974) Reduction of sudden deaths after myocardial infarction by treatment with alprenolol. Lancet II:1157–1160

Wilhelmsson C, Vedin A, Elmfeldt D et al. (1975) Smoking and myocardial infarction. Lancet I:415–420

World Health Organization, Regional Office for Europe (1976) Myocardial Infarction Community Registers. Public Health in Europe, Copenhagen

Prevention of Sudden Death in Young Patients: The Role of Antiarrhythmic Therapy

L. SEIPEL and G. BREITHARDT[1]

Sudden death in young patients is associated with different forms of cardiac disease (Table 1). It has been described in various congenital heart malformations and in patients with the Wolff-Parkinson-White (WPW) and QT syndrome. However, in most instances, various forms of cardiomyopathy and coronary artery disease have been found at autopsy. Due to the topic of this symposium, the special problems in patients with WPW and QT syndrome will be excluded from the following paper.

Table 1. Sudden death in young patients

Congenital heart disease	Cardiomyopathy
Mitral valve prolapse	Coronary artery
Cardiac tumor	– Malformation
Ventricular dysplasia (right)	– Myocardial bridges
Preexcitation syndrome	– Spasm
QT syndrome	– Stenosis

Table 2. Ventricular tachycardia (VT) and fibrillation (VF)

Triggering mechanism ⟶	ECG
Ventricular premature beats	Exercise test
	Holter monitoring
Basic requirement ⟶	Ventricular pacing
Ventricular instability	Late potentialis
Reentrance pathway	

In most instances, sudden cardiac death is due to ventricular tachycardia (VT) or fibrillation (VF) [17]. The well-known precursors of this final event are ventricular premature beats (VPB) [3, 7, 9, 15, 22, 31]. A typical example in a young patient with congestive cardiomyopathy is shown in Fig. 1. However, the basic requirement for the initiation of VF-VT by VPB are abnormalities of conduction and refractoriness setting the stage for intraventricular reentry or the "instability" of the myocardium due to the underlying heart disease (Table 2). Other factors like the autonomic nervous system, can also influence the fibrillation threshold [22]. As a consequence, antiarrhythmic therapy can have two different goals; suppression of VPB and/or normalization of ventricular instability.

---

1 Medizinische Klinik und Poliklinik, Klinik B, Moorenstr. 4, 4000 Düsseldorf, FRG

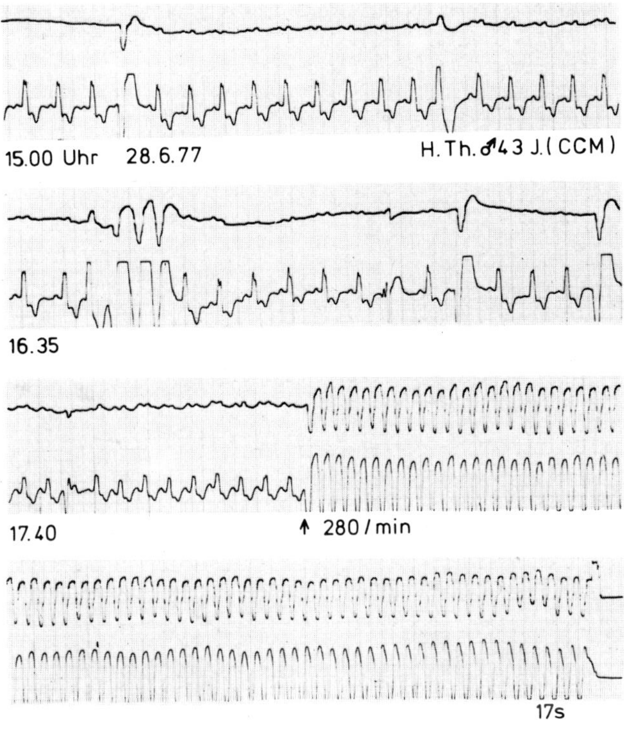

Fig. 1. Sudden death out of hospital in a young patient with congestive cardiomyopathy during Holter monitoring. After the occurrence of multifocal ventricular premature beats (VPB) and short ventricular series a VPB initiates the final ventricular tachycardia (VT). We assume that the transportation mechanism of the tape recorder was stopped when the patient fell down on the street

Unfortunately, in the studies published so far, it could not be demonstrated that antiarrhythmic therapy can reduce the incidence of sudden death in endangered patients [6, 8, 13, 18, 20, 21, 29, 34]. That does not mean that these drugs, in principle, cannot prevent VF-VT. The failure could be due to different factors shown in Table 3, which were not controlled in most of these studies. Chamberlain et al. [6] demonstrated that under standard antiarrhythmic therapy 30%–40% of the patients had subtherapeutic plasma levels. Some preliminary studies in a selected group of

Table 3. Antiarrhythmic therapy: Causes for "drug failure"

1. Inefficacy of the drug

2. Insufficient plasma levels due to
 – Low resorption
 – Rapid elimination (e. g., fast and slow acetylation; induction of enzymes)

3. Incorrect dosage intervals

4. Untreated basic disease

5. Noncompliance of the patient

Table 4. Reduction of sudden death in a group of endangered patients by controlled anti-arrhythmic therapy. Lown and Graboys [23]

Group I	Dose-adjusted antiarrhythmic therapy controlled by exercise tests and monitoring (26 patients follow-up 17 months): Two sudden deaths (8%)
Group II	Conventional antiarrhythmic therapy (17 patients, follow-up 14.8 months): Ten sudden deaths (59%)

patients with documented VF-VT demonstrated that antiarrhythmic therapy can reduce the recurrence of these tachyarrhythmias if the therapy is controlled by exercise tests and monitoring, or if the influence on ventricular "vulnerability" is assessed by electrophysiological techniques. In addition, the measurement of drug plasma levels used seems to be of great importance.

Lown and Graboys [23] treated patients with documented VF-VT after successful resuscitation. In a randomized manner one group of patients recieved standard antiarrhythmic therapy, whereas in the other group the effectiveness of the antiarrhythmic therapy was controlled by exercise tests and monitoring. In the latter group, dose was adjusted and combinations of different drugs were given until ventricular arrhythmias were suppressed or significantly reduced in the ECG. During a relatively short follow-up the incidence of sudden death was significantly lower in the group of patients under controlled treatment (Table 4). That demonstrates the usefulness of exercise test and monitoring in predicting antiarrhythmic efficacy during follow-up. However, some studies have shown that even 24-h recordings are not an ideal tool for controlling antiarrhythmic therapy because of the great spontaneous variability of the arrhythmias [1, 14, 25, 26, 35, 36]. An example is shown in Fig. 2. In this patient with VPB, the first 24-h recordings during the control period and under therapy with the new antiarrhythmic drug tocainide seem to prove an antiarrhythmic effect of the drug. However, further Holter recordings during follow-up showed that this effect was only due to the spontaneous variability of the frequency of the ectopic beats and the drug was actually not effective.

Myerburg et al. [27] treated a similar group of highly endangered patients with documented VF-VT with quinidine and procainamide. In addition to Holter monitoring, they measured plasma levels of the drugs. They demonstrated that in patients with constant therapeutic plasma levels there was no recurrence of the arrhythmia during follow-up, in contrast to the high incidence of VF-VT in the group

Table 5. Significance of plasma level for rate of recurrence of VT or VF during treatment with quinidine or procainamide during 12 months. Myerburg et al. [27]

Plasma level	n	Recurrence of VT-VF	VES/ h
Therapeutic	6	0	104[a]
Subtherapeutic	10	8	184[a]

[a] NS

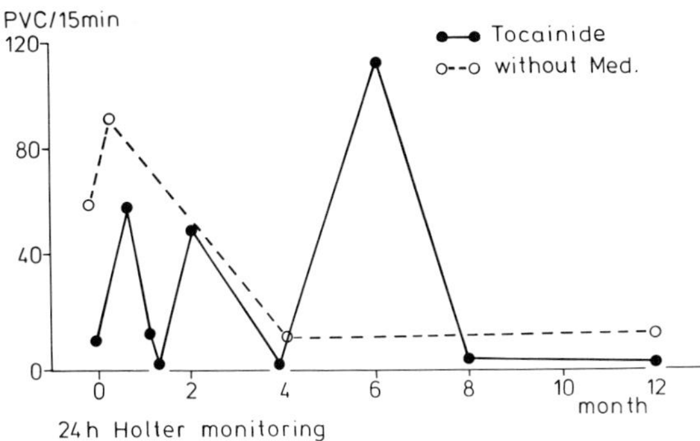

Fig. 2. Spontaneous variation of the incidence of ventricular premature beats (VPB) with and without antiarrhythmic therapy in a series of tape recordings during follow-up of the patient (modified from Winkle [35])

with subtherapeutic plasma concentrations. There were no significant differences in number of VPB during Holter recordings within these two groups (Table 5). Therefore, the authors recommend routine measurement of plasma levels in addition to ECG recordings during antiarrhythmic therapy. The only explanation for these findings is that quinidine and procainamide in therapeutic concentrations did influence ventricular instability without influencing the occurrence of VPB.

Meanwhile, the influence of antiarrhythmic drugs on ventricular instability can be tested directly in the laboratory by means of electrophysiological techniques. The same type of programmed ventricular stimulation is used by many groups to control antiarrhythmic therapy in selected groups of patients [2, 5, 10–12, 16, 24, 30–33, 37]. Our study protocol is chematically shown in Fig. 3. Using this protocol we were able to demonstrate an abnormal ventricular vulnerability, i.e., the induction of series of ventricular echo beats with or without degeneration in VF or the induction of a stable VT in about 95% of our patients with documented VF-VT [4]. The same sensitivity of this technique was found by the Josephson group [19], whereas other investigators observed a lower incidence of abnormal responses in patients resuscitated after cardiac arrest [27]. The procedure is repeated under different antiarrhythmic regiments so as to find a drug or drug combination effective in supressing the abnormal ventricular response (Figs. 4, 5). In any given patient, it was impossible to predict the effect of a drug as the same drug could suppress abnormal responses in one patient while no influence of even enhancing ventricular instability in another

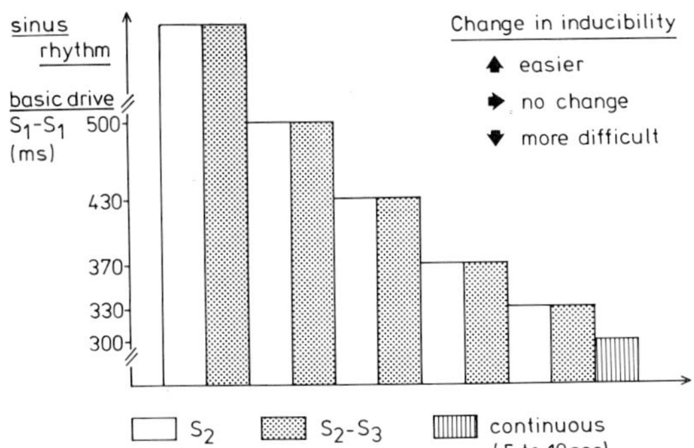

Fig. 3. Stimulation protocol for control of antiarrhythmic drug therapy in patients with documented VF-VT

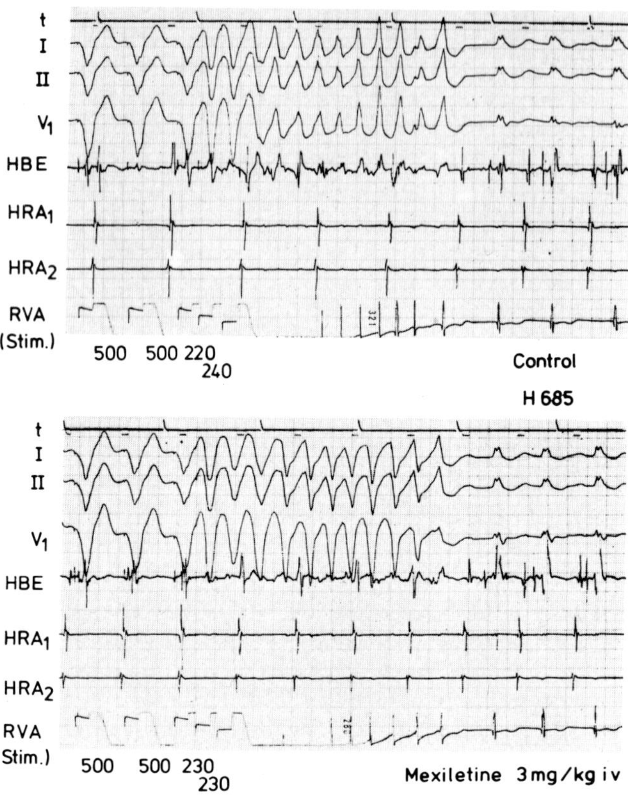

Fig. 4. Abnormal ventricular response during programmed pacing. At a basic drive of 120 bpm (cycle length 500 ms) two premature beats are introduced followed by a series of multiform ventricular echo beats (*upper tracing*). Mexilitine was not able to prevent the occurrence of echo beats in this case. Abbreviations are as follows: *t* = time scale 1000 ms; *I, II, V1* = surface ECG; *HBE* = His-bundle electrogram; *HRA* = high right atrial electrogram; *RVA* = right ventricular apical recording or stimulation (stimulus artefact)

one (Fig. 6). Figure 7 shows the outcome of our patients with documented VF-VT 80 weeks after serial drug testing. In those patients in whom we could find a medication effective in altering the abnormal ventricular response, VT occurred only in one patient. In all patients in whom ventricular instability could not be influenced during testing, VF-VT recurred under standard antiarrhythmic therapy within 20 weeks [5]. Similar results in selected groups of patients have been reported by the investigators mentioned above. It is noteworthy that in our series and in others [12], there was no strong correlation between the results of the electrophysiologic testing and the effect of the drugs on spontaneous VPB in the same patient. Based on these preliminary results we feel that programmed ventricular stimulation is very useful in identifying patients with abnormal repetitive response who are prone to sudden death and in predicting antiarrhythmic efficacy, as far as the prevention of VF-VT is concerned.

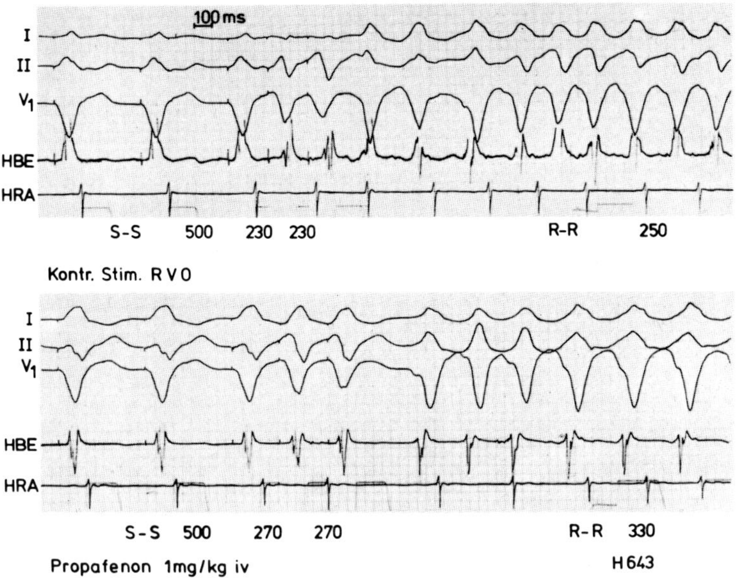

Fig. 5. Initiation of a stable ventricular tachycardia by programmed stimulation (*upper tracing*), which is terminated by overdrive. After application of propafenone the tachycardia can be reinitiated

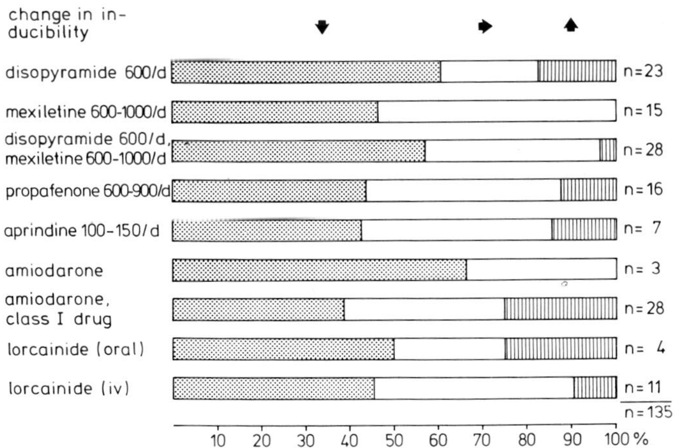

Fig. 6. Effect of various antiarrhythmic drugs on inducibility of VF-VT in 45 patients. *Arrows* indicate change in inducibility (see Fig. 3)

In summary, antiarrhythmic drugs in principle seem useful in preventing sudden death among the endangered group of patients. However, antiarrhythmic therapy can only be of value if therapeutic plasma levels are achieved and if effectiveness is controlled by exercise test and monitoring. In addition, we feel that electrophysiological techniques are an important clinical tool in predicting the effectiveness of a therapeutic regimen during follow-up.

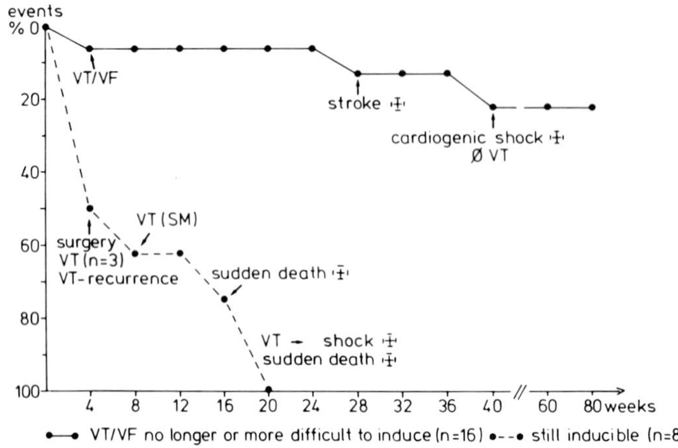

Fig. 7. Follow-up of patients with documented VF-VT during antiarrhythmic therapy

References

1. Andresen D, Tietze U, Leitner ER von et al. (1980) Spontanvariabilität tachykarder Rhythmusstörungen. Z Kardiol 69:214
2. Benditt DG, Pritchett ELC, Wallace AG, Gallagher JJ (1979) Recurrent ventricular tachycardia in man: Evaluation of disopyramide therapy by intracardiac electrical stimulation. Eur J Cardiol 9:255
3. Bigger JT, Dresdale RJ, Heissenbuttel RH et al. (1977) Ventricular arrhythmias in ischemic heart disease: Mechanism, prevalence, significance, and management. Prog Cardiovasc Dis 19:255
4. Breithardt G, Seipel L, Loogen F (1980) Der akute Herztod. Bedeutung elektrophysiologischer Stimulationsverfahren. Verh Dtsch Ges Herz Kreislaufforsch 46:38
5. Breithardt G, Seipel L, Abendroth RR, Loogen F (1980) Serial electrophysiological testing of antiarrhythmic drug efficacy in patients with recurrent ventricular tachycardia. Eur Heart J 1:11
6. Chamberlain DA, Jewitt DE, Julian DG et al. (1980) Oral mexiletine in high-risk patients after myocardial infarction. Lancet II:1324
7. Chiang BN, Perlman LV, Ostrander LD, Epstein FH (1969) Relationship of premature systoles to coronary heart disease and sudden death in the Tecumseh epidemiologic study. Ann Intern Med 70:1159
8. Collaborative Group (1971) Phenytoin after recovery from myocardial infarction. Controlled trial in 568 patients. Lancet II:1055
9. Coronary Drug Project (Blackburn H) (1973) Prognostic importance of premature beats following myocardial infarction. JAMA 223:1116
10. Dhatt MS, Akhtar M, Reddy CP et al. (1977) Modification and abolition of reentry within the His-Purkinje system in man by diphenylhydantoin. Circulation 56:720
11. Fisher JD, Cohen HL, Mehra R et al. (1977) Cardiac pacing and pacemakers. II. Serial electrophysiologic-pharmacologic testing for control of recurrent tachyarrhythmias. Am Heart J 93:658
12. Greenspan AM, Horowitz LN, Spielman SR, Josephson ME (1980) Large dose Procainamide therapy for ventricular tachyarrhythmia. Am J Cardiol 46:453
13. Hagemeijer F, Durme JP van, Lubsen J et al. (1979) The Ghent-Rotterdam aprindine study: Antiarrhythmic prophylaxis after myocardial infarction. In: Mason DT, Neri Serneri GG, Oliver MF (eds) Florence international meeting on myocardial infarction. Exerpta Medica, Amsterdam, p 964
14. Harrison DC, Fitzgerald JW, Winkle RA (1978) Contribution of amulatory electrocardiographic monitoring to antiarrhythmic management. Am J Cardiol 41:996

15. Hinkle LE, Argyros DC, Hayes JC et al. (1977) Pathogenesis of an unexpected sudden death: Role of early cycle ventricular premature contractions. Am J Cardiol 39:873

16. Horowitz LN, Josephson ME, Farshidi A et al. (1978) Recurrent sustained ventricular tachycardia. 3. Role of the electrophysiologic study in selection of antiarrhythmic regimens. Circulation 58:986

17. Iseri LT, Humphrey SB, Siner EJ (1978) Prehospital brady-asystolic cardiac arrest. Ann Intern Med 88:741

18. Jackson NC, Metcalfe MJ, Wade C et al. (1980) Comparison between oral mexiletine, disopyramide, and placebo used prophylactically after acute myocardial infarction. (Abstr.) Br Heart J 43:717

19. Josephson ME, Horowitz LN, Spielman SR, Greenspan AM (1980) Electrophysiologic and hemodynamic studies in patients resuscitated from cardiac arrest. Am J Cardiol 46:948

20. Klein W, Harpf H (1979) Ergebnisse einer Langzeitstudie über die Arrhythmiebehandlung von Koronarkranken mit einem Betarezeptorenblocker und Ajmalinbitartrat. In: Antoni H, Bender F, Gerlach E, Schlepper M (eds) Schattauer, Stuttgart, p 381

21. Kosowsky BD, Taylor J, Lown B, Ritchie RF (1973) Long-term use of procaine amide following acute myocardial infarction. Circulation 47:1204

22. Lown B (1979) Sudden cardiac death: The major challenge confronting contemporary cardiology. Am J Cardiol 43:313

23. Lown B, Graboys TB (1977) Management of patients with malignant ventricular arrhythmias. Am J Cardiol 39:910

24. Mason JW, Winkle RA (1978) Electrode catheter arrhythmia induction in the selection and assessment of antiarrhythmic drug therapy for recurrent ventricular tachycardia. Circulation 58:971

25. Michelson EL, Morganroth J (1980) Spontaneous variability of complex ventricular arrhythmias detected by long term electrocardiographic recording. Circulation 61:690

26. Morgenroth J, Michelson EL, Horowitz LN et al. (1978) Limitations of routine long-term ambulatory electrocardiographic monitoring to assess ventricular ectopic frequency. Circulation 58:408

27. Myerburg RJ, Sung RJ, Conde CA et al. (1977) Intracardiac electrophysiologic studies in patients resuscitated from unexpected cardiac arrest outside the hospital. Am J Cardiol 39:275

28. Myerburg RJ, Conde C, Sheps DS et al. (1979) Antiarrhythmic drug therapy in survivors of prehospital cardiac arrest: Comparison of effects on chronic ventricular arrhythmias and recurrent cardiac arrest. Circulation 59:855

29. Peter T, Ross D, Duffield A et al. (1978) Effect on survival after myocardial infarction of long-term treatment with phenytoin. Br Heart J 40:1356

30. Reddy CP, Damato AN, Akhtar M et al. (1977) Effect of procainamide on reentry within the His-Purkinje system in man. Am J Cardiol 40:957

31. Ruberman W, Weinblatt E, Goldberg JD et al. (1977) Ventricular premature beats and mortality after myocardial infarction. N Eng J Med 297:750

32. Schaeffer AH, Greene HL, Reid RR (1978) Suppression of the repetitive ventricular response: An index of long-term antiarrhythmic effectiveness of aprindine for ventricular tachycardia in man. Am J Cardiol 42:1007

33. Seipel L, Breithardt G (1978) Electrophysiological effects of mexiletine in man: Influence on stimulus-induced ventricular arrhythmias. In: Sandoe E, Julian DC, Bell JW (eds) Management of ventricular tachycardia: Role of mexiletine. Exerpta Medica, Amsterdam, p 219

34. Vajda FJE, Prineas RJ, Lovell RRH, Sloman JG (1973) The possible effect of long-term high plasma levels of phenytoin on mortality after acute myocardial infarction. Eur J Clin Pharmacol 5:138

35. Winkle RA (1978) Antiarrhythmic drug effect mimicked by spontaneous variability of ventricular ectopy. Circulation 57:1116

36. Winkle RA (1980) Ambulatory electrocardiography and the diagnosis, evaluation, and treatment of chronic ventricular arrhythmias. Prog Cardiovasc Dis 23:99

37. Wu D, Wyndham CR, Denes P et al. (1977) Chronic electrophysiological study in patients with recurrent paroxysmal tachycardia: A new method for developing successful oral antiarrhythmic therapy. In: Kulbertus HE (ed) Re-entrant arrhytmias. MTP, Lancaster, p 294

Occupational Situation in Postinfarction Patients Under the Age of 40

L. Samek, M. Spinder, F. Müller, P. Betz, K. Schnellbacher, and H. Roskamm[1]

The return to work after myocardial infarction (MI) is dependent on many factors: Severity of the disease, work demands, motivation, physician's recommendation, duration of disability and the economic situation seem to be the most important determinants [1–9]. It was the goal of our study to evaluate the influence of some of these factors in postinfarction patients under the age of 40.

Patients

From January, 1973, to December, 1979, 746 men with a proven transmural MI and who were under the age of 40 were admitted to our clinic. The average age at the time of MI was 35.7, at the time of admission it was 36.5 years. At 6 months to 7 years later (mean 3.5 years), we sent an employment questionnaire to these patients, to which 2.8% did not respond and 658 responded (9% had died) (Fig. 1).

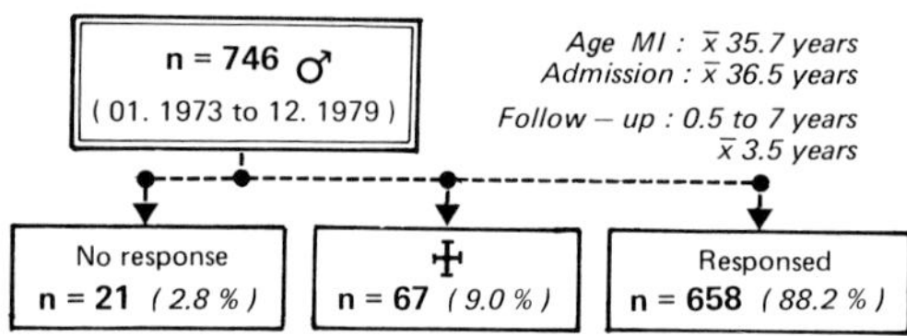

Fig. 1. Patients with transmural MI under the age of 40

The patients had undergone comprehensive rehabilitation including coronary bypass surgery in 6.4%. Coronary angiography was performed in 74% of the patients.

Results

On the average, at 3.5 years after hospitalization, 72% of the patients had *returned to work*, though 6% of these were currently unemployed. This latter figure is twice as high as that of the general working population in southwest Germany at that time. Thirteen percent were currently ill and 15% were retired (Fig. 2).

---

1 Rehabilitationszentrum, Südring 15, 7812 Bad Krozingen, FRG

The ratio between those who returned to work and those who did not, remained unchanged during follow-up. The ratio between those who were currently ill and those who were retired changed significantly. After the first year, only 4% of the patients were retired. This number increased in the sixth year to 21%. The reason for the low retirement figure during the first 2 postinfarction years is at least partially due to retirement regulations and proceedings in West Germany, which normally become operative after 1.5 years of sick leave.

Figure 3 shows the relationship between the *level of education and work status* after MI. There is a significant relationship between educational level and the number of patients who returned to work. The lowest number (61%) was found in the group with elementary school education, the highest number (85%) in the group with university degrees.

A relationship between educational level and frequency of retirement also exists, although maximum work tolerance and heart volume (HV) per kg body weight (an indicator of myocardial damage) do not differ significantly within the four groups (Fig. 3).

The study group was further divided into four subgroups according to *occupational position* before MI (Fig. 4): 57% blue-collar workers; 26% white-collar workers; 7% civil servants; and 10% self-employed. The numbers are similar to those of the

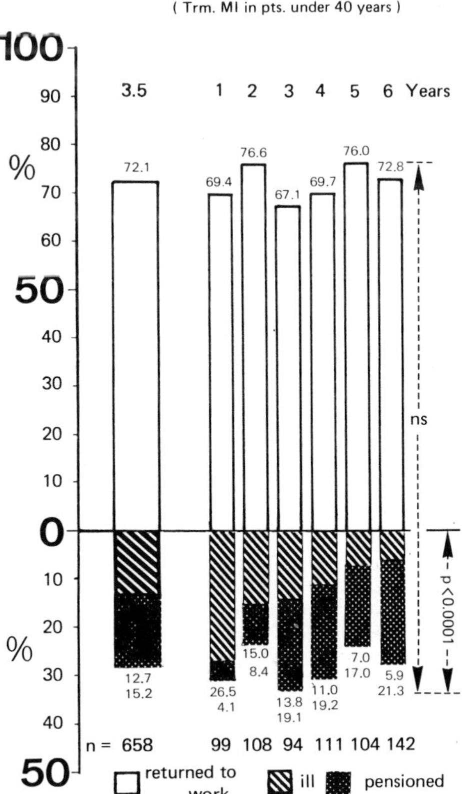

Fig. 2. Return to work and disability after MI during a follow-up. The frequency of patients who returned to work remained unchanged over 6 years. The number of retirements significantly increased during this time period

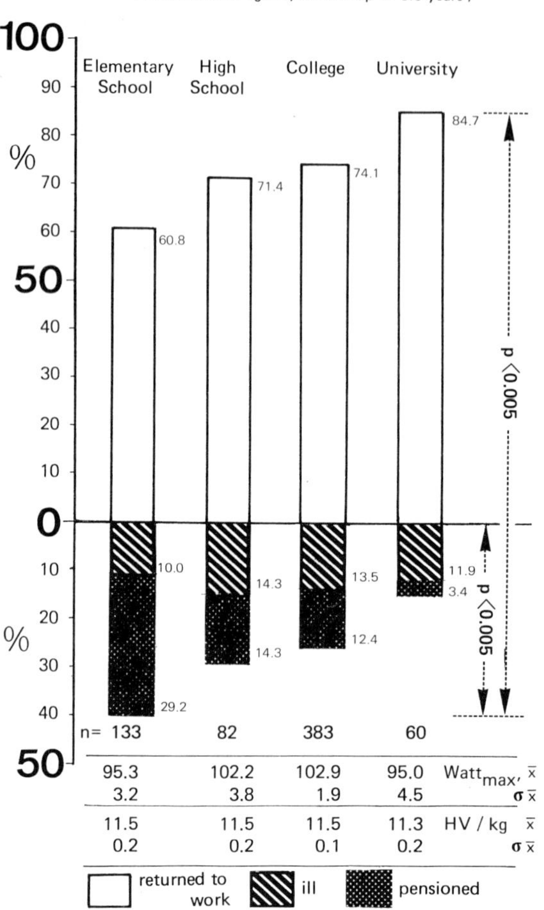

Fig. 3. Level of education and return to work. Higher educational level is related to a greater number of patients returning to work and a smaller number of those retired. Maximal work capacity and heart volume/kg did not differ in the four educational level groups. Abbreviations are as follows: W_{max} = maximal work load during exercise on a bicycle ergometer in supine position; HV/kg = heart volume per kilogram body weight

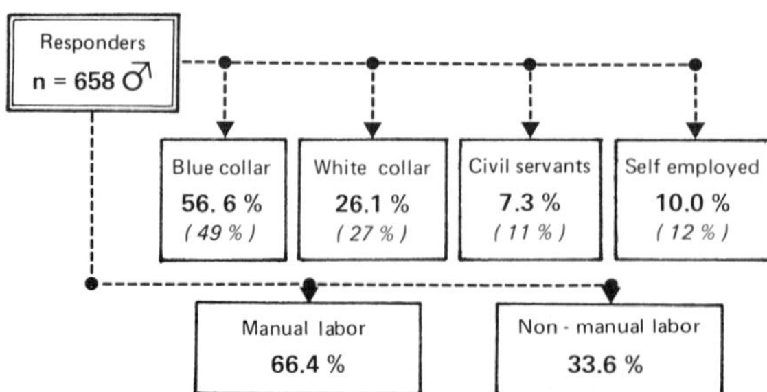

Fig. 4. Occupational position and work intensity. The numbers in the brackets represent the population average for West Germany in 1977: There is no substantional difference between the general population and our study group. "Nonmanual labor" means occupations without a substantial amount of physical activity

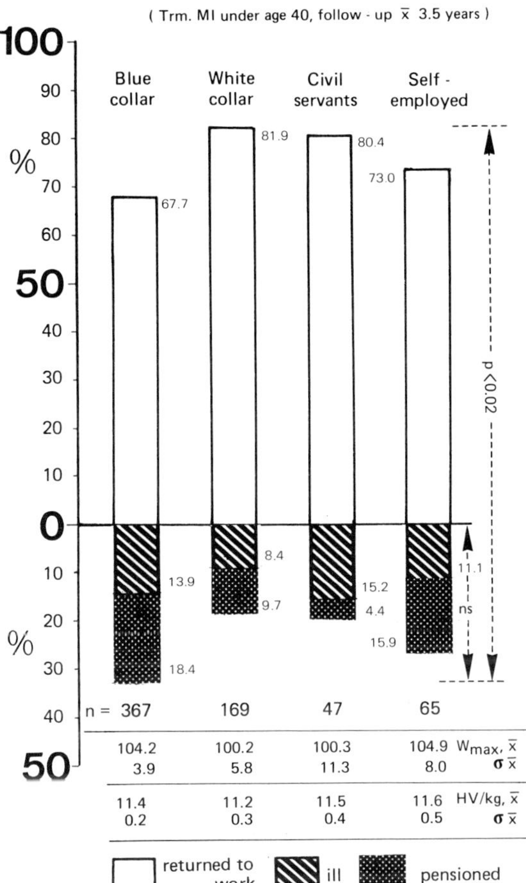

Fig. 5. Occupational position before MI and return to work. Of the blue-collar workers the number of patients returning to work is lowest. For abbreviations see Fig. 3

general working population in West Germany (49% blue-collar workers, 27% white-collar workers, 11% civil servants, 12% self-employed).

Of the white-collar workers, 82% returned to work, 80% of the civil servants, and 73% self-employed (Fig. 5). The lowest figure was found in the blue-collar workers (68%). Again, maximum work capacity and HV/kg did not differ in the four groups.

Furthermore, the entire group was divided into the two subgroups *manual laborers and nonmanual laborers* (Fig. 6). Persons were considered nonmanual laborers if there was no substantial amount of physical activity connected to their job (peak values less than 13 ml/kg/min oxygen uptake). Of the manual laborers, 67% returned to work while, in the group of nonmanual laborers, a significantly higher number (81%) returned.

In the group of manual laborers there is a close relationship between *maximum work capacity*, tested on a bicycle ergometer in the supine position at an average 9 months after MI, and return to work. Of patients with a maximum work capacity of 50 W or less, only 40% returned to work. Return-to-work frequency increases significantly with increase of work capacity: Of patients with a work capacity of more

L. Samek et al.

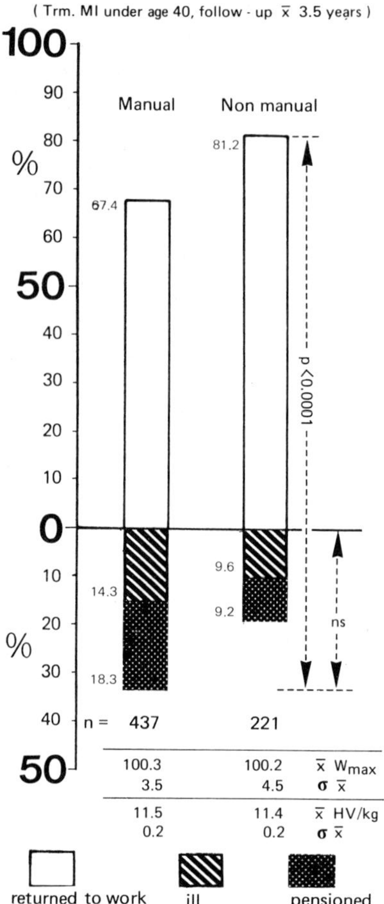

Fig. 6. Manual and nonmanual labor and return to work. There is a significant difference between the two groups. For abbreviations see Fig. 3

than 125 W, 82% returned to work. On the other hand, the number of persons retired decreases significantly with increased work capacity: Of patients with a work capacity of 50 W or less, 44% had retired but only 1% of those with a work capacity of more than 125 W (Fig. 7).

In nonmanual laborers the relationship between return to work and work capacity was not so close (Fig. 8). Even of patients whose work capacity was 50 W or less, 74% returned to work, compared to 40% of the manual laborers.

Figure 9 shows the relationship of the *number of more than 50% stenosed vessels* and return to work. In the manual labor group, those with three-vessel disease have a lower return-to-work frequency than those with no- or one-vessel disease. In the three-vessel disease group, the number of persons retired is very high, with 45% (Fig. 9). In the nonmanual labor group this relationship also exists (Fig. 10).

Heart volume per kg (calculated from simple X-ray pictures in two projections) is an acceptable indicator of myocardial damage. With increasing heart volume the number of patients who returned to work decreased. With an HV increase greater than 3 SD from that of the normal population (HV/kg greater than 13.6), the number of manual workers who returned to work was as low as 43%, while 40% were retired (Fig. 11).

In the nonmanual labor group the relationship between return to work and HV is not significant. Even in the largest HV group, 75% of the patients returned to work, compared to only 43% in the manual labor group with the same HV (Fig. 12). This means that in the nonmanual laborers, the degree of myocardial damage was not as significant a return-to-work-influencing factor as in manual laborers.

Figure 13 shows the extent to which our *recommendations for return to work* were followed by the patients. Of the group to whom we had recommended return to the same work, 62% had actually resumed the same work as before MI, even after an average of 3.5 years. Fifteen percent were performing less strenuous work compared to their preinfarction status. Of the group recommended to retire, 46% did so. Of these patients, 22 of 26 (85%) were manual laborers and 21 of 26 (81%) had a work capacity

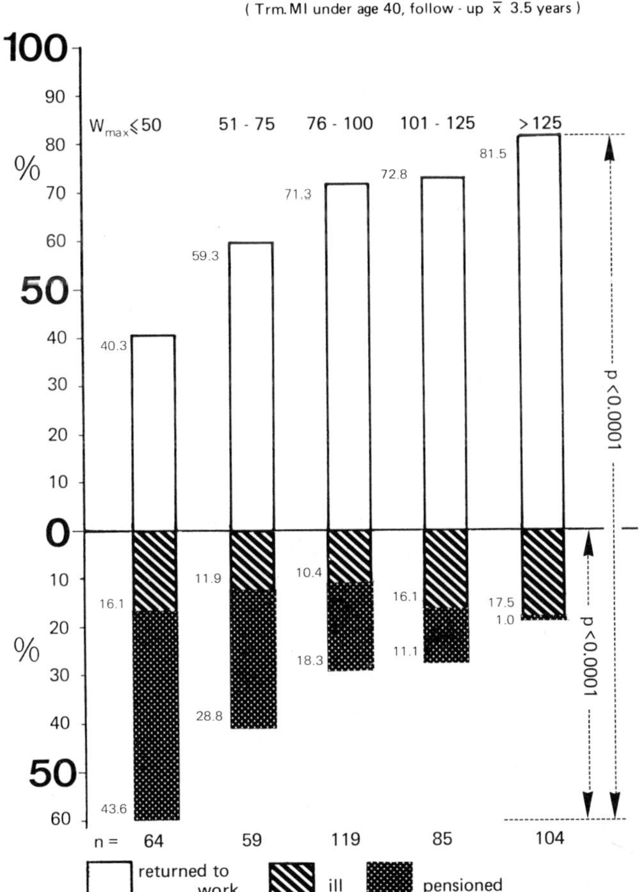

Fig. 7. Maximal work load (W_{max}) in manual laborers and return to work. Retirement and return to work is related to W_{max}

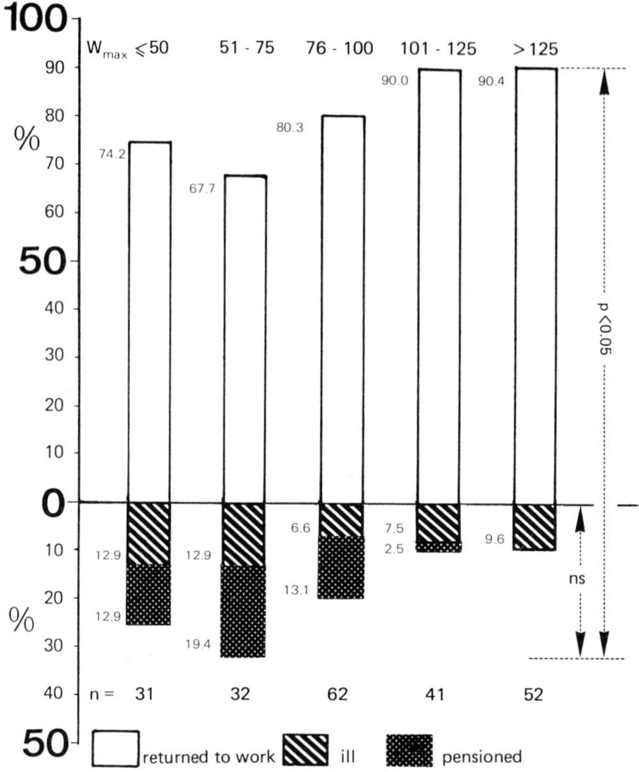

Fig. 8. Maximal work load (W_{max}) in nonmanual laborers and return to work. Return to work is only slightly related to W_{max}

of 50 W or less. Fourteen of 26 (54%) had an enlarged HV/kg (over 13.6), and 14 of 21 (67%) had multivessel disease and moderate or severe left ventricular dysfunction. It should be emphasized that 27% of the patients in this group had died during follow-up. This figure is significantly higher than in all other groups.

Discussion

MI at young age seems to be a very suitable model for a study of the influences of coronary heart disease on return to work, since these young patients are not afflicted with other factors, e.g., old age and age-related symptoms and diseases, which may also have a bearing on return to work.

Our results can be considered representative for the following reasons:

1. All postinfarction patients under age 40 were included in the study irrespective of symptoms and findings. Those who had coronary angiography are also represen-

tative because this procedure had been recommended to all patients, again regardless of symptoms and findings, and 74% of the patients had agreed.
2. The distribution of our patients into the different occupational groups is similar to that of the general working population in West Germany (Fig. 4).
3. Furthermore, these patients had undergone comprehensive rehabilitation, including medical, psychological, vocational and, if needed, surgical treatment.

As already mentioned, return to work is dependent on several conditions which can be grouped into the categories of (1) factors related to the severity of the disease (2), factors related to the physical demands of work, and (3) psychosocial factors.

Factors Related to Severity of Disease. In some studies, return-to-work in coronary heart disease patients was found to be independent of factors related to the severity

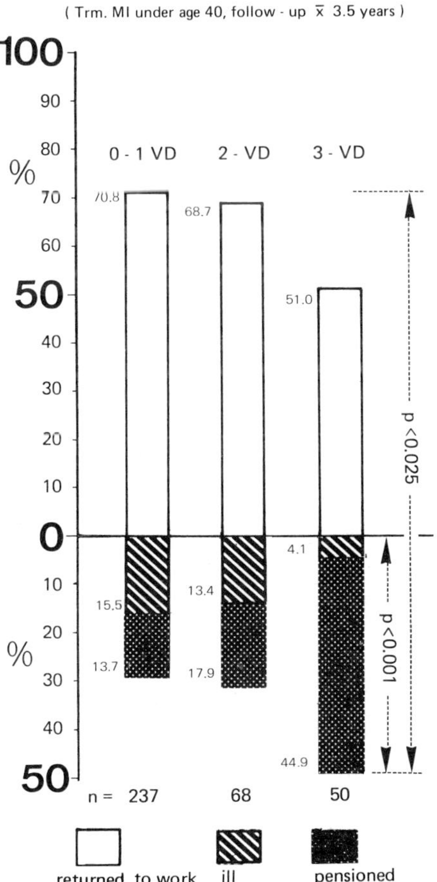

Fig. 9. Number of vessels diseased (VD) (> 50% stenosis) in manual laborers and return to work, a significant correlation was demonstrated

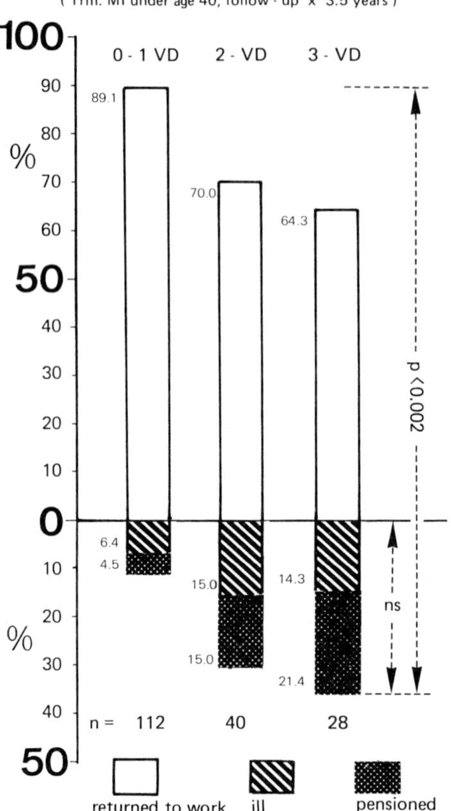

Fig. 10. Number of vessels diseased (VD) (> 50% stenosis) in nonmanual laborers and return to work. A significant correlation was demonstrated

of the disease [2, 3]. If this is not the case in our study, it is probably because of our comprehensive rehabilitation which tries to bring all patients, in whom medical conditions permit, back to work, Patients who were recommended for retirement had very severe damage, i.e., 81% of them had a work capacity of only 50 W or less, 54% had enlarged hearts, and 67% had multivessel disease.

Medical criteria influencing return to work were work capacity, HV/kg body weight, and number of diseased vessels. These are in part interrelated. Angina pectoris as a limiting factor is not often found in these young patients, thus, decreased work capacity mainly reflects the status of the left ventricle. All three factors are related to prognosis [10–13], and this knowledge probably influenced our recommendations. Of those who were recommended to retire, 27% had died during the follow-up. We do not think that these patients died as a consequence of retirement, but because of their severe disease.

Factors Related to the Physical Demands of Work. For patients who were manual laborers, return-to-work frequency was significantly lower than for those who were nonmanual laborers. This is in agreement with studies on coronary heart disease patients in general [7, 8, 14–16]. In some manual labor patients, retirement because of the physical demands of the job seems unjustified. Many general practitioners as well as patients, at least in our country, still feel that physical exercise or work may be harmful even for patients with only moderately damaged ventricles. We also believe that severe left ventricular dysfunction is an indication for retirement recommendation.

It is generally accepted, that healthy persons are able to perform (during 8 h) one-third of their maximum work capacity [17]. In angina pectoris patients, the allowable level of performance during 8 h can be so high as to correspond to one-half of their maximum work capacity with peaks close to the maximum [18].

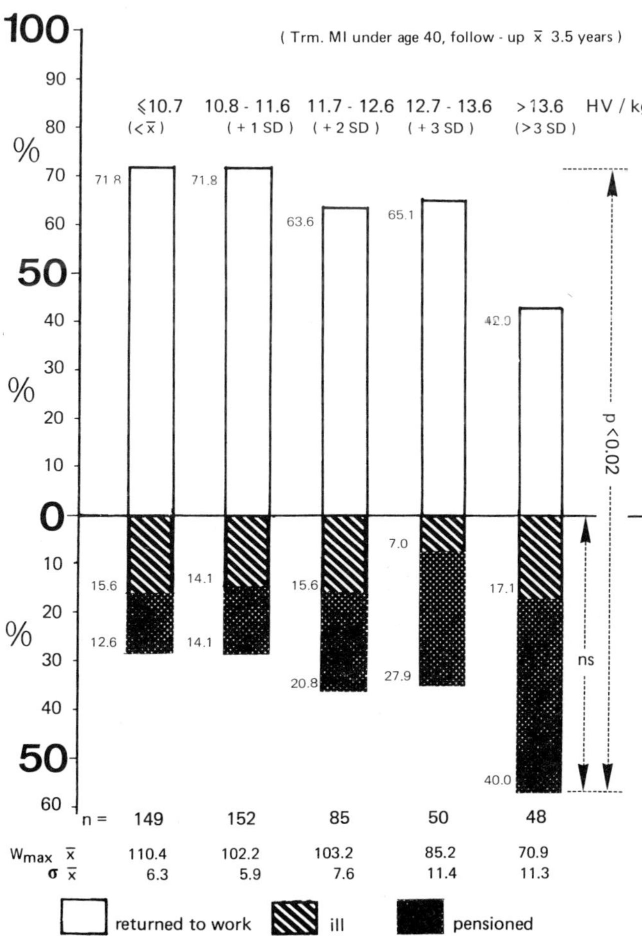

Fig. 11. Relative heart volume (HV) in manual laborers and return to work. A significant correlation was demonstrated

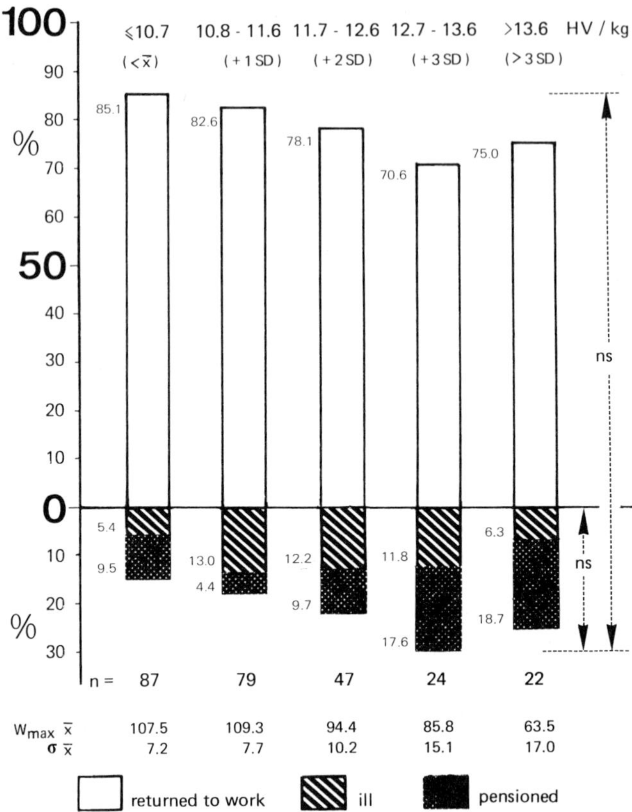

Fig. 12. Relative heart volume (HV) in nonmanual laborers and return to work. A significant correlation was not demonstrated

Psychosocial Factors. A significant relationship between educational level and number of patients who returned to work was found in this study. This is in agreement with results found in coronary heart disease patients in general [5, 19, 20]. The relationship is, of course, at least partially influenced by the extent of manual work done in the different educational levels.

Other factors influencing return to work, like job satisfaction and duration of inactivity [21], were not examined in this study.

Summary

In 746 men with a transmural MI before the age of 40, return to work was studied during a follow-up period of 6 months to 7 years (median 3.5 years). The main results were:

1. The 72% of patients who returned to work, remained practically constant during the follow-up period.

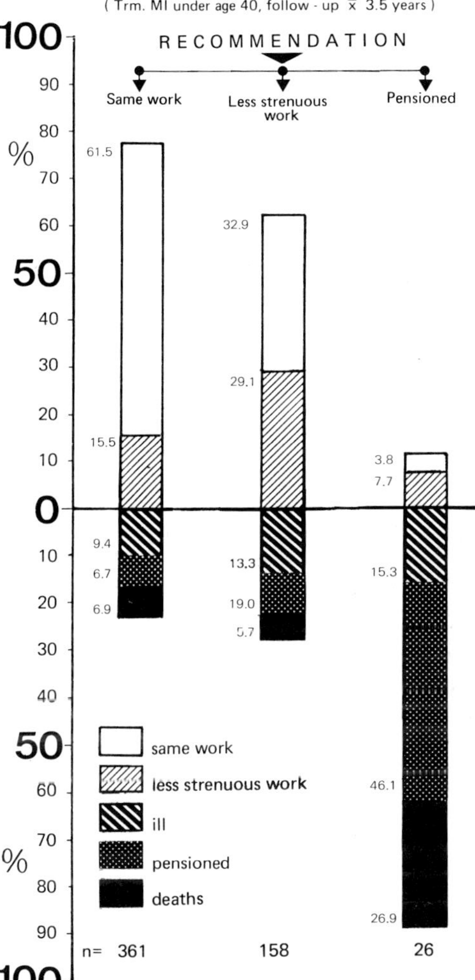

Fig. 13. The extent that our recommendations to return to work were followed by the patients, e.g., in the group in which we recommended returning to the same work (*left*), 61.5% of patients, even 3.5 years later, performed the same work. In the group in which we recommended retirement (*right*) 46.1% were retired and 26.9% had died

2. Return to work was related to the following: the degree of manual labor before MI ($P < 0.001$); educational level ($P < 0.005$); and the occupational position before MI ($P < 0.02$).

3. Return to work was also related to work tolerance (manual laborers $P < 0.001$, nonmanual laborers $P < 0.05$), the number of vessels diseased (manual laborers $P < 0.025$, nonmanual laborers ($P < 0.002$), and the HV/kg (manual laborers only $P < 0.002$).

Acknowledgements. This work was supported by grants of the BMA and BMFT (Bundesministerium für Arbeit und Sozialordnung and Bundesministerium für Forschung und Technologie).

References

1. Angster H (1974) Herzinfarkt und adäquater Arbeitsplatz, ein wichtiges Nachsorgeproblem. MMW 116:2007–2012
2. Benesch L, Neuhaus KL, Rivas-Martin J, Loogen F (1979) Clinical results and return to work after coronary heart surgery. In: Roskamm H, Schmuziger M (eds) Coronary heart surgery: A rehabilitation measure. Springer, Berlin Heidelberg New York, pp 379–384
3. Blümchen G, Scharf-Bornhofen E, Brandt D et al. (1979) Clinical results and social implications in patients after coronary bypass surgery. In: Roskamm H, Schmuziger M (eds) Coronary heart surgery. A rehabilitation measure. Springer, Berlin Heidelberg New York, pp 375–378
4. Cay EL, Vetter N, Philip A, Dugard P (1973) Return to work after a heart attack. J Psychosomat Res 17:231–243
5. Gleichmann U, Fassbender D (1977) Probleme der Früh- und Spätrehabilitation nach Herzinfarkt. In: Schettler G, Horsch A, Mörl H, Orth H, Weizel A (eds) Der Herzinfarkt. Internationales Symposion in Wien 1977. Schattauer, Stuttgart New York, pp 518–529
6. Halhuber MJ, Leppert M (1973) Zur Wiederaufnahme der Arbeit nach Herzinfarkt. Therapiewoche 23/34:2753–2756
7. Kellermann JJ, Modan B, Levy M et al. (1968) Return to work after myocardial infarction. Geriatrics 23:151–156
8. Schnellbacher K, Heidecker K, Samek L et al (1980) Arbeitsfähigkeit nach aorto-koronarer Bypass-Operation bei 420 Patienten ≦ 55 Jahre. Z Kardiol 69:200
9. Wilhelmsson C, Vedin A, Elmfeldt D et al. (1976) Symptoms, disablement and treatment during 2 years after myocardial infarction. Scand J Rehabil Med 8:85–90
10. Matzdorff F (1975) Herzinfarkt. Prävention und Rehabilitation. Urban & Schwarzenberg, Munich Berlin Wien, p 72
11. Parker JO (1978) Prognosis in coronary artery disease: Arteriographic, ventriculographic and hemodynamic factors. Cleveland Clin Q 45:145–146
12. Bruschke, AVG (1978) Ten-year follow-up of 601 nonsurgical cases of angiographically documented coronary disease: Angiographic correlations. Cleve Clin Q 45:143–144
13. Samek L, Roskamm H, Haakshors W (1979) Beziehungen zwischen Rhythmusstörungen, Herzgröße, Ventrikelfunktion und Herztod bei jugendlichen Herzinfarktpatienten. Z Kardiol 68:121, 650
14. Wallwork J, Potter B, Caves PK (1978) Return to work after coronary artery surgery for angina. Br Med J 16:1680–1681
15. Love JW (1980) Employment status after coronary bypass operations and some cost considerations. Thorac Cardiovasc Surg 80:68–72
16. Kubicek F (1977) Ambulante Langzeitrehabilitation in der Infarktspätphase. In: Schettler G, Horsch A, Mörl H, Orth H, Weizel A (eds) Der Herzinfarkt. Internationales Symposion in Wien 1977. Schattauer, Stuttgart New York, pp 551–566
17. Bonjer FH (1968) Physical working capacity and energy expenditure. In: Denolin H et al. (eds) Ergometry in cardiology. Report of a symposium, Freiburg i. Br. 8–11 February 1967. Boehringer, Mannheim, pp 23–30
18. Salhadin P, Degre S, van Elst P, Denolin H (1975) From physical capacity to fitness to work in coronary patients. Acta Cardiol (Brux) 30:79–83
19. Schiller E, Baker J (1976) Return to work after a myocardial infarction: Evaluation of planned rehabilitation and of a predictive rating scale. Med J Aust 1:859–862
20. Barnes GK, Ray MJ, Oberman A, Kouchoukos NT (1977) Changes in working status of patients following coronary bypass surgery. JAMA 238:1259–1262
21. David P (1979) Contributing factors preventing return to work of cardiac surgery patients. In: Roskamm H, Schmuziger M (eds) Coronary heart surgery. A rehabilitation measure. Springer, Berlin Heidelberg New York, pp 370–374

Psychological and Vocational Aspects in Postinfarction Patients Below the Age of 40

W. Langosch, G. Brodner, and U. Michallik-Herbein[1]

Postinfarction patients below the age of 40 are especially in need of comprehensive rehabilitation because the infarction endangers their professional career and the social status of the family. Furthermore, it can be expected that living with a chronic disease causes considerable psychological problems. For older postinfarction patients, psychological deterioration some months after hospitalization is well documented [1–5].

In postinfarction patients under 40 there is unfortunately no empirical data about occupational and social problems for the period after hospitalization when they have resumed their jobs readily available.

Therefore, it was the purpose of our study to investigate the following questions:

1. What are the immediate and long-term consequences of myocardial infarction (MI) under 40 years of age on psychological findings and life habits?
2. How do these postinfarction patients react to job stressors and is this behavior different from other chronically ill patients?
3. What is their vocational status after having resumed their jobs?

Patients and Methods

The psychological and vocational data of three groups of male patients (all under 40) were recorded (Table 1): MI patients under 40, 6 months after MI (sample 1); patients who had suffered from a transmural MI 3.5 years ago at an age under 40 years (sample 2): and patients under the age of 40 who were suffering from Bechterew's arthritis for several years (control group for sample 2) (sample B).

Nearly all MI patients under 40 who were admitted to our clinic immediately after MI (between July, 1978, and June, 1980) consented to participate in the study (sample 1). From the patients who were readmitted 3.5 years after MI, for cardiac checkup, several were lost to the study because they did not stay in the hospital long enough (sample 2).

For the control group (sample B) we selected patients with Bechterew's arthritis because they were chronically ill, but without coronary heart disease; psychosomatic factors are not supposed to be operative in the course or development of Bechterew's arthritis; and the patients are (like MI patients) strongly achievement oriented. The sample B patients, on the average, had been suffering from Bechterew's arthritis since 1968. The intensity of the rheumatic pain was measured on a 3-point scale and 12% felt only slight pain, 50% felt moderate pain, and 38% felt intense pain. Progres-

1 Rehabilitationszentrum, Südring 15, 7812 Bad Krozingen FRG

Table 1. Numbers of patients investigated

	Sample 1 6 months after MI n	Sample 2 42 months after MI n	Sample B Bekhterev's arthritis n
First test (hospital)	123	70	42
Second test (at home)	52	33	–

sion of the disease was evaluated on a 4-point scale and 63% of the patients be-
longed into class 2, and 62% fell to class 3.

Those patients of the MI groups who had been tested the previous year were re-
tested with a limited set of psychological and occupational inventories. The questionnaires were completed at home.

The statistical methods used for analysis were as follows:

Student's t-test for independent groups; two-way analysis of variance with respect to
the factors groups and terms;
Pearson-Bravais correlation coefficient; and
factor analysis (mean component analysis with VARIMAX rotation), the selection
of the factor solution being based on
   a noticeable decline in eigen values,
   a small increase in the fraction of clarified variance,
   and
   an improved psychological interpretation.

Results

MI groups did not differ in sociographic variables, such as education, number of
children, residential district, period of professional activity, number of job changes,
continuity of professional advancement, effort to gain a better professional qualifi-
cation, number of years employment at the present firm, income, and social status
of the patient and of his father. Therefore, they can be regarded as subsamples of
the same population of postinfarction patients, i.e., differences in the dependent
psychological and vocational variables are attributed to the independent variable
different duration of illness.

The first test, performed during the hospitalization period, did not reveal significantly different psychological and life style variable scores for the two MI groups
(Student's t-test for independent groups). According to the results of separate factor
analyses of the psychological data of both groups, however, this similiarity of personality structure is limited (Table 2). Factors in common were achievement-behavior
and social withdrawal. They differed with respect to two other factors: Sample I

Table 2. Factor structure of personality dimensions for two groups of postinfarction patients below the age of 40

	Sample 1 ($n = 123$)[a]	Sample 2 ($n = 70$)[b]
Factor 1	Depressed/irritated behavior	Impulsive/impatient behavior
Factor 2	Achievement behavior	Achievement behavior
Factor 3	Social withdrawal	Psychophysical complaints
Factor 4	Physical complaints	Social withdrawal

[a] $SD^2 = 51\%$ of variance are clarified
[b] $SD^2 = 59\%$ of variance are clarified

showed a depressed, irritated behavior and sample 2 showed accentuated impulsivity and impatience. While sample 1 complained mostly of pain and cardiac symptoms, sample 2 had psychophysiological complaints.

Between sample 2 and sample B we found many psychological differences (Table 3). The ratings, performed by an experienced clinical psychologist, revealed that sample 2 patients were significantly more disturbed in several psychological aspects (Student's t-test for independent groups). The results correspond to differences in personality variables (significant on the 5% level) (Table 4).

The factor analysis shows dissimilarity of personality structure in these two groups (Table 5).

The particular difficulties of sample 2 concern interpersonal relationships: They did not use achievement behavior to master their physical restrictions as sample B did, and sample 2 was impulsive and impatient, while sample B tended to be insecure and irritated.

An analysis of vocational data was only performed for those MI patients and Bechterew's arthritis patients whose occupational activities turned out to be very similar in the hierarchical cluster analysis.

In the group of MI patients, job stressors were frequently related to insufficient approval of professional activities, while in sample B they were related to insuffi-

Table 3. Differences of psychological data in different groups of chronically ill patients (mean $\pm$ SD)

Variables[a]	Sample 2	Sample B	P[b]
Dissimulating	2.63 ± 1.62	1.90 ± 1.05	0.02
Inhibited	1.63 ± 1.00	1.21 ± 0.56	0.05
Depressive	2.09 ± 1.01	1.47 ± 0.99	0.01
Excitable	2.37 ± 1.13	1.52 ± 0.86	0.00
Mood labile	1.69 ± 0.96	1.28 ± 0.59	0.03
Family problems	1.96 ± 1.33	1.19 ± 0.55	0.01
Diet problems	1.43 ± 1.01	1.00 ± 0.00	0.04
Neurotic symptoms	1.70 ± 1.07	1.23 ± 0.57	0.03
Sleep disturbances	1.50 ± 1.12	2.31 ± 0.78	0.00

[a] Rating scale from 1 (not present) to 5 (very intensive, very often present)
[b] Student's t-test for independent samples

Table 4. Differences of personality dimensions of different groups of chronically ill patients (mean ± SD)

Variables	Sample 2	Sample B	P^a
Nervousness	6.00±4.31	2.89±2.98	0.04
Excitability	4.62±2.63	2.71±2.08	0.00
Dominance	4.26±2.15	2.74±2.05	0.00
Emotional lability	4.94±2.76	3.29±2.15	0.02
Cardiac complaints	14.74±6.17	10.87±3.26	0.00
Hypochondriacal behavior	21.33±5.97	17.95±5.42	0.02
Pain	14.10±4.75	17.34±4.00	0.00
Subjective stress tolerance	24.75±6.03	29.03±3.74	0.01

[a] Student's t-test for independent samples

Table 5. Factor structure of personality dimensions for two different groups of chronically ill patients

	Sample 1[a]	Sample 2[b]
Factor 1	Impulsive/impatient behavior	Insecure/irritated behavior
Factor 2	Achievement behavior	Achievement behavior as a reaction to physical restrictions
Factor 3	Psychophysical complaints	Social anxiety
Factor 4	Social withdrawal	hypochondriacal behavior, time urgency, and impatience

[a] $SD^2 = 59\%$ of variance are clarified
[b] $SD^2 = 55\%$ of variance are clarified

Table 6. Frequency of single job stressors for postinfarction patients ($n = 30$) and a control group of Bechterew's arthritis patients (sample B) ($n = 30$)

Stressor	Sample 2 (%) MI	Sample B (%)
Multifunctional-task demands	97	86
Insecure decisions	83	63
Vigilance	97	72
Noise	53	30
No control of work success	77	90
Overtime work	63	80
Additional engagements	27	38
Too much controlled	13	21
No influence on sequence of operation	33	52
Lack of information	23	47
Demands of improved knowledge	97	73
Necessary overtime work not appreciated	57	41
Lack of communication	27	3

Table 7. Correlations between job stressors and job stress in MI and Bechterew's arthritis patients (sample B) (correlation coefficient $r \geqq 35$ in one sample)

Variables	Sample 2 ($n = 30$)	Sample B ($n = 30$)
Interruptions	0.59	0.10
Services	0.55	0.10
Understaffing	0.70	0.44
Terms	0.24	0.60
Insecure decisions	0.07	0.38
No control of work success	0.32	0.46
Vigilance	0.36	0.62
Working time	0.06	0.47
Stressful environment	0.16	0.84
Threat of accident	0.07	0.59
Way to work	0.37	0.89

Table 8. Correlation between job stressors and overall job satisfaction in MI and Bechterew's arthritis patients (sample B)

Stressors	Sample 2 ($n = 30$)	Sample B ($n = 30$)
Multifunctional-task demands	+0.45	−0.19
No control of work success	+0.46	−0.14
Services	+0.17	−0.59
Working time	+0.37	−0.02
Stressful environment	+0.37	+0.08

Table 9. Interactions of the factors groups and terms in a two-way analysis of variance

Variables	Sample 1 ($n = 50$)		Sample 2 ($n = 30$)		
	Test 1 (mean)	Test a (mean)	Test 1 (mean)	Test 2 (mean)	P
Hypochondriacal behavior	17.10	21.12	20.10	20.43	0.00
Job involvement	21.32	20.55	18.93	20.04	0.07
Job competition	19.30	18.26	16.26	17.30	0.14
Job responsibility	25.83	24.31	24.96	26.52	0.00
Social desireability	12.78	12.20	13.47	13.87	0.03
Inhibition	3.75	4.08	3.91	3.35	0.08
Presence of occupational problems[a]	1.66	1.52	1.44	1.59	0.05
Self-rated degree of fitness on the job[b]	3.83	3.11	3.39	3.21	0.09
Alcoholic units[c] during the last 12 months	10.94	34.50	30.07	35.57	0.01

[a] No/yes = 1/2

[b] Not at all fit (1) to very much fit (5)

[c] Scale of alcoholic units: 1 l beer/week 1 point; ½ l wine/week 1 point; 4 cl brandy/week 0.2 points

Table 10. Follow-up data of postinfarction patients (18 months after MI)

Variables	Mean	No. of patients
Support from the family[a]	3.60	52
Regard given to the disease on the job[a]	2.20	45
Time pressure[b]	1.69	42
Insecurity in decisions, responsibility, etc.[b]	1.80	35
Tension[b]	1.88	32
Stressful environment[b]	1.88	34
Overtime[b]	1.41	27
Interpersonal problems[b]	1.79	34
Secondary job[b]	1.80	30

[a] Not at all (1) to very much (5)
[b] Reduced (1), unchanged (2), or increased (3) as compared to the time before infarction

cient control of activities. The correlation coefficients between stressors and self-rated job stress were, in general, lower in MI patients than in sample B (Tables 6,7).

The scores for overall job satisfaction and several components of job satisfaction were higher in the MI group, and the correlation between stressors and overall job satisfaction was positive. In sample B the correlation coefficients are mainly negative (Table 8).

At 1 year after hospitalization the results of a two-way analysis of variance with the factors groups and terms showed significant deterioration of many psychological data in both MI groups. Only the psychological scales for achievement behavior and interpersonal problems showed no significant differences from data collected during the first hospitalization. In accordance with these results, the patients themselves reported many negative changes in their daily life; difficulties falling asleep, sleep is interrupted, requiring more sleep, and feeling less rested in the morning and less fit on the job. They admit that their way of life tends to be as it was before MI. On some scales, especially in variables concerning achievement behavior, the significant interaction effect between the factors groups and terms shows a different trend for sample 1 and sample 2 patients (Table 9).

For sample 1 patients the scores of the scales job-involvement and job-responsibility decrease, while when compared to the results of the first investigation they increase for sample 2. The variables job competition, presence of occupational problems, and self-rated degree of fitness on the job show a similar trend.

One year after discharge from the hospital and 18 months after MI sample 1 patients stated that they received reasonable support from their families in trying to adapt to the disease and to handle the new situation, while on the job little regard is given to their disease (Table 10).

Therefore, the results obtained by investigation correspond with the patients' statements that most job stressors have not diminished since the time before MI.

Discussion

Starting from the data obtained during hospitalization, the most striking difference between sample 1 and 2 patients is the dissimilarity in their personality structure. Being confronted with chronic disease has entailed a qualitative change in the personality structure of these patients.

If the potentially confounding effect of different test settings is eliminated, however, the quantitative psychological differences between the postinfarction patients, independent of the duration of the disease, are small. Therefore, the psychological deterioration found before in older MI patients is not only due to the longer duration of the disease, but also to different test settings (most of these patients had their first test in the hospital and the second at home) [1–5].

This hypothesis is supported by the results of the retest, which showed that the patients were inclined to reveal psychological problems when confronted with daily problems and difficulties. This was true for both MI groups, i.e., also for those MI patients who had been readmitted to the hospital for cardiac checkups. Thus, these results show that, even 3 years after MI the patients are unable to accept the fact that they are chronically ill. The hope that the results of the checkup might be excellent represses the negative experiences and brings about an unrealistically optimistic attitude toward the future. This hypotheses could explain the fact that MI patients are inclined to dissimulate or to deny psychological problems during hospitalization [6].

The significant interaction effect of achievement-behavior variables shows that, during the first years after MI, patients succeed in trying to reduce achievement behavior, but in the long run return to their former life habits, especially to their former patterns of occupational striving, even if they still feel less fit on the job.

The comparison of sample 2 and sample B patients reveals a higher emotional lability in MI patients. In several psychological aspects they are also more conspicious than Bechterew's arthritis patients and, in addition, the personality structures of the two patient groups are quite dissimilar.

These results are in contrast to the statement of Stocksmeier [7, 8], who claims that all patients with a chronic disease suffer from a "psychic syndrome of the chronic patient" that is independent of the somatic diagnosis. In conclusion, it can be said that though chronically ill patients have some psychological traits in common, different types of different somatic disease seem to be associated with specific psychological problems.

The results of the job analysis indicate that for MI patients many job stressors are not necessarily associated with exhaustion or physical complaints, as is true for the control group. It is possible that MI patients consciously ignore mild symptoms of fatigue or that they have an elevated exhaustion threshold. Furthermore, positive correlation coefficients between job stressors and overall job satisfaction in the MI group seem to prove that MI patients have a positive attitude toward job stressors. They seem to like a challenging environment. Therefore, job dissatisfaction is not a characteristic of MI patients as formerly reported by House [9]. It can be assumed that, for MI patients, job dissatisfaction is the result of high occupational demands which exceed the patients' efficiency over a long period and, finally, result in a kind of depressive syndrome. This hypothesis is in agreement with the statement of Appels [10], that vital exhaustion and depression are precursors of MI. The results also agree with the hypothesis of Glass that individuals with type-A behavior are not only infarction-prone [11] and reinfarction-prone [12], but also have an increased tendency for "control ability" [13]. Individuals who regard most of their occupational demands as a challenge they are fond of coping with, and who are insensitive to mild symptoms of fatigue, not only meet some requirements necessary for successful control of their environment, but also increase the MI risk.

Finally, it can be deduced from the patients' statements that most job stressors have not diminished in intensity as compared to the situation before the MI, and that the observed increase of achievement behavior is at least in part a consequence of the work load they are confronted with immediately after having resumed their jobs. The unchanged pattern of external stimuli persuades the patients to pursue their desire for control ability and, therefore, to again use achievement behavior as a means to effectively control their occupational environment.

Conclusions

1. In the long run, MI has a disturbing effect on psychological condition. Postinfarction patients under 40 are psychologically clearly more conspicious than a control group of chronically ill patients without coronary heart disease.
2. During hospitalization, postinfarction patients tend to dissimulate psychological problems as well as difficulties concerning their life habits.
3. Postinfarction patients have a way of coping with job stressors that is not recommended for chronically ill persons.
4. Postinfarction patients claim that in their professional environment little regard is given to their disease and that the intensity of most job stressors has not been reduced since before the MI.

Acknowledgments. This work was supported by grants of the BMA and BMFT (Bundesministerium für Arbeit und Sozialforschung and Bundesministerium für Forschung und Technologie). The authors are especially grateful to Dr. H. J. Albrecht and Dipl. Psych. H. Köhler, Rheumaklinik Oberammergau, for expert advice. The authors also feel especially obliged to Dipl. math. F. Foerster, Forschungsgruppe Psychophysiologie, Universität Freiburg, for statistical analysis.

References

1. Croog SH, Levine S (1977) The heart patient recovers. Human Science, New York, London
2. Langosch W, Brodner G (1979) Ergebnisse einer psychologischen Verlaufsstudie an Herzinfarktpatienten. Z Klin Psychol 8:256–269
3. Langosch W (1980) Ergebnisse psychologischer Verlaufsstudien bei Herzinfarktpatienten (Ein- und Drei-Jahres-Katamnese). In: Langosch W (ed) Psychosoziale Probleme und psychotherapeutische Interventionsmöglichkeiten bei Herzinfarktpatienten. Minerva, Munich, pp 99–114
4. Mayou R, Foster A, Williamson B (1978) Psychosocial adjustment in patients 1 year after myocardial infarction. J Psychosom Res 22:447–453
5. Medert-Dornscheidt G, Myrtek U (1977) Ergebnisse einer Zwei-Jahres-Katamnese an Patienten eines Heilverfahrens. Rehabilitation (Bonn) 16:207–217

6. Hackett TP, Weisman AD (1969) Denial as a factor in patients with heart disease and cancer. Ann NY Acad Sci 164:802–817
7. Stocksmeier U (1976) Medical and psychological aspects of coronary heart disease. In: Stocksmeier U (ed) Psychological approach to the rehabilitation of coronary patients. Springer, Berlin Heidelberg New York, pp 9–19
8. Stocksmeier U (1981) Medizin-psychologische Aspekte koronarer Herzkrankheit. In: Stocksmeier U, Hermes G (eds) Psychologie in der Rehabilitation. Schindele, Rheinstetten, pp 41–52
9. House JS (1974) Occupational stress and coronary heart disease: A review and theoretical integration. J Health Soc Behav 15:12–27
10. Appels A (1980) Vitale Erschöpfung und Depression als Vorboten des Herzinfarkt. In: Langosch W (ed) Psychosoziale Probleme und psychotherapeutische Interventionsmöglichkeiten bei Herzinfarktpatienten. Minerva, Munich, pp 33–46
11. Brand RJ, Rosenman RH, Scholtz RJ, Friedman MC (1976) Multivariate prediction of coronary heart disease in the Western Collaborative Group Study compared to the findings of the Framingham study. Circulation 53:348–355
12. Jenkins CD, Zyzanski SJ, Rosenman RH (1976) Risk of new myocaridal infarction in middle-aged men with manifest heart disease. Circulation 53:342–347
13. Glass D (1977) Stress, behaviour patterns and coronary heart disease. Am Sci 65:177–187

Risk Reduction and Coronary Progression
and Regression in Humans

R. Selvester, M. Sanmarco, and R. Blessey [1]

In various prospective studies [1–7] a sedentary overweight subject had an increased risk of new coronary events ranging up to 1.5. These studies have been done by occupational stratification into sedentary, active, strenuous, and very strenuous levels. A number of studies have been attempted in primary prevention of coronary artery disease by multiple risk factor intervention trials, and early results are beginning to appear [8, 9]. A number of secondary prevention trials are under way and have shown a consistent reduction in mortality from recurrent infarction in the active exercising subjects, when compared to less active controls, and a significant change in the incidence of new coronary events [10–14].

We have been doing serial angiograms in a group of patients with angina and/or a prior myocardial infarct (MI) [15]. This has the distinct advantage over epidemiological studies of looking at the target organ (the coronary arteries) directly instead of the more indirect end points of new events, documented infarction, or mortality, which are the secondary effects on the end organ. It has the disadvantage that the target population being studied is not the apparently healthy population, but the patient who has already suffered some direct consequence of serious disease.

Patients and Methods

Several years ago a four-way randomized study of patients with symptomatic angina and/or MI was started. Patients meeting inclusion criteria and who accepted the program were randomized into four groups: surgery + low-level exercise; surgery + high-level exercise; medicine + low-level exercise; medicine + high-level exercise. All were managed by a multidisciplinary cardiac rehabilitation team consisting of physicians, rehabilitation nurses, physical therapists, occupational therapists, a psychologist, a psychiatric social worker, and a nutritionist. All four groups of patients were exposed individually and in groups to an intense risk-reduction program, including diet counseling (low animal fat, prudent diet), weight reduction, aggressive control of blood pressure and arrhythmias, cessation of smoking, and a supervised progressive exercise program. For this study those randomized into low-level exercise groups were maintained at heart rates that do not produce fitness training effects. They were encouraged to exercise at least 30 min three times a week at pulse rates at or below 110 bpm. Those randomized into high-level exercise groups progressed, under supervision, to fitness levels of exercise training. Specifically, to be called high-level trained in this study, patients were exercising at least three times a week

1 Division of Internal Medicine, Section of Cardiology, University of Southern California School of Medicine, Rancho Los Amigos Campus, Downey, CA 90242, USA

at 75% or more of their maximum heart rate for 30 min or more. Most exercised five or six times a week at this level.

Patients with left main artery disease and what we labeled left main equivalent disease were excluded from randomization and were advised to have surgery. Of the patients with left main artery lesions, 20% themselves decided not to have surgery. Of those with left main equivalent disease, 40% decided against surgery. Patients with poor ventricular function (ejection fraction less than 35%) were also excluded.

All patients accepted into the protocol signed informed consent forms at onset for serial angiograms at entry, 18 months, and 4 years.

From the beginning there was significant noncompliance and crossover that we could not control in spite of intense team effort. Forty percent were noncompliers, 30% were fair, and 30% were good to excellent compliers. Self-selection was, in fact, the modus operandi.

In this paper we report serial angiographic studies at an average of 21 months in 104 medically managed patients previously reported [15] and 84 undergoing saphenous vein bypass grafting. Twenty-nine medically managed patients and 15 postbypass patients became good compliers to the program, including the achievement of fitness levels of exercise training during the interval between angiograms.

Ventriculograms were recorded at right and left anterior oblique projections. Left ventricular volumes and ejection fractions (EF) were calculated by the method of Sandler and Dodge, as modified in our laboratory. Selective cine coronary angiograms were recorded on 35-mm film using the Judkins technique and were recorded in at least five projections in the left coronary artery and three in the right.

All films were reviewed independently by two experienced angiographers. Drawings were made of the right and left coronary artery and its branches at right anterior oblique and left anterior oblique projections. Location and extent of narrowing was marked on each drawing. Each local obstructive coronary lesion was graded as to the percent of narrowing of cross-sectional area deemed present. Differences of less than 10% were considered insignificant and the average of the two numbers was used in the analysis: Of all identified lesions, 85% fell into this category. Differences in readings of more than 10% narrowing were resolved during a conference between the two primary reviewers. Five sets of films, where one set or the other was deemed technically unsatisfactory for adequate comparison, were rejected. For the purpose of this analysis, an increase of 30% or more or progression to total occlusion as a consensus reading in serial angiograms was considered as true progression.

Results

Change was observed in only 2 of 195 vessels showing total occlusion and, therefore, they were considered "nonprogressible" and were excluded from tabulation. Significant progression was seen in only 3 of 107 normal vessels in the medically managed patients. These vessels were also considered "nonprogressible" and excluded from tabulation. Curiously, progression occurred in 15 of 80 previously normal vessels in patients who had under gone surgery, and these were tabulated along with 332 vessels in both groups showing 50% or more occlusion but less than 100% occlusion (defined as "progressible" vessels).

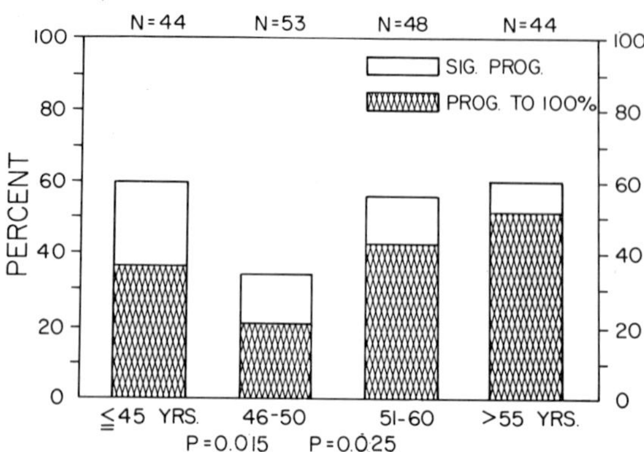

Fig. 1. Coronary progression as a function of age

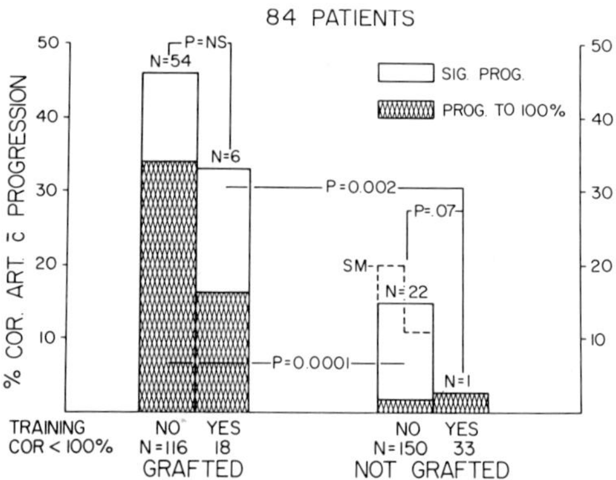

Fig. 2. Coronary progression in 84 patients undergoing saphenous vein bypass grafting. The two left-hand bars represent progression in vessels proximal to the grafts and the two on the right represent progression in the nongrafted vessels

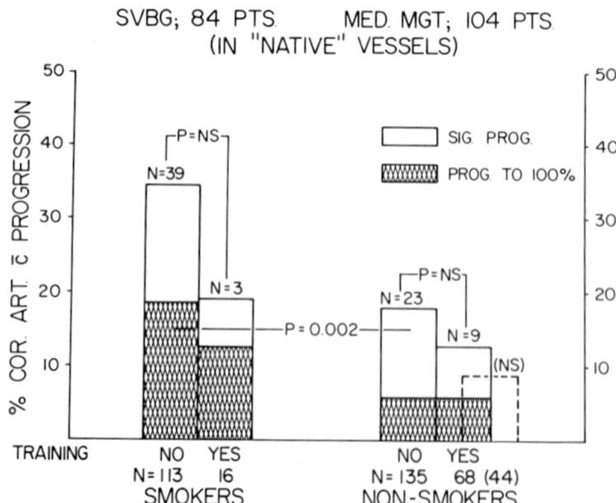

Fig. 3. Coronary progression in the "native" (nongrafted) vessels in all 188 patients studied. Four groups are tabulated: Smokers who were not training during the interval between serial angiograms; those who were training during this interval; nonsmokers who were not training; and nonsmokers who were training. The *dotted-line bar* to the right represents coronary progression in subjects achieving high levels of physical fitness. N on this graph represents the number of "progressible" vessels

Overall, coronary progression was found to be related to age in a bimodal fashion. When examined by half-decades, the lowest progression rate was in 53 patients in the half-decade from 46–50 years of age with a significant increase in older age groups ($P<0.025$). Subjects ($N=44$) 45 years of age and younger had a significantly higher progression rate ($P<0.015$). These data are shown in Fig. 1.

Coronary progression in the vessels proximal to bypass graft (Fig. 2) was fourfold greater than in nongrafted vessels ($P<0.001$). The 37 patients from the medical or surgical group who became good compliers to a risk-reduction program and maintained fitness levels of training in the interval between serial angiograms, had a four fold overall decrease in coronary progression ($P<0.001$). These results are summarized in Fig. 3.

In stepwise multivariant regression analysis, young age at onset of infarction and smoking consistently emerged as the most important variables. Cessation of smoking decreased the risk of progression by a factor of 2. Sedentary lifestyle, obesity, and hypertension were highly correlated. When taken together, fitness levels of training, weight reduction, and control of hypertension reduced the risk of coronary progression another two fold.

Conclusions

The following conclusions from this data seem justified:

1. All patients with left main disease and those with two- and three-vessel disease, with angina, *two or more* progressible vessels, and good ventricular function, especially if they have been refractory to medical management, will have significant relief of symptoms and improved exercise tolerance from bypass surgery. Surgery alone may be a temporary reprieve, *not a pardon.* They will experience significantly more functional improvement if they comply with a high-level exercise program, adopt a low-fat diet, lose weight, and stop smoking. They will also enjoy significantly less progression in the native ungrafted vessels and fewer new coronary events.

2. Medically managed patients and those undergoing saphenous vein bypass grafting who remain sedentary, continue to smoke, and are, in general, noncompliers to risk-reduction lifestyle changes can expect progression in the native circulation at the alarming rate of 21% per major "progressible" vessel per year. Ten percent of these vessels per year progress to 100% occlusion and angiographically visible infarct. Seven percent of these major "progressible" vessel per year will experience clinical infarct. This progression rate is significantly higher in the younger patient (below 45 years).

3. A comprehensive Risk Reduction Coronary Rehabilitation Program which includes high-level (and we emphasize high level) fitness training not only produces major improvements in fuctional capacity and significantly increased high-density lipoproteins, but it reduces the risk in both postbypass and medically managed patients nearly fourfold from 21% progression per major "progressible" vessel per year to 5.7%, from 10% to 2.5% for progression to 100% occlusion with visible angiographic infarct, and from 7% to 1.7% for new clinical infarct.

This requires a major change in lifestyle for the vast majority of patients. One which can enhance both the quality of life in addition to significantly decreasing the rate of new MI. Such a lifestyle change is even more important to the younger patient (under 45 years) with a recent MI who would, without infarction, have had every reason to expect that his most productive 3 or 4 decades were yet ahead of him. From this data it appears that they still can be, but it will require a clear-cut change in living patterns; a redefinition, in our view, of "THE GOOD LIFE". *This is as much a social problem as a medical one.*

References

1. Kannel WB, Dawber TR, Kagan M et al. (1961) Factors or risk in the development of heart disease: Six-year follow-up experience. The Framingham study. Ann Intern Med 55:33–50
2. Kannel WB, Sorlie P, McNamara PM (1971) The relation of physical activity to the risk of coronary disease: The Framingham study. In: Clarksen OA, Malborg AO (eds) Coronary heart disease and physical fitness. University Park Press, Baltimore, pp 256–272
3. Chapman JM, Massey FJ (1964) The inter-relationship of serum cholesterol, hypertension, body weight and risk of coronary artery disease: Results of the first ten-year follow-up in Los Angeles Heart Study. J Chronic Dis 17:922–999
4. Epstein FH, Ostrander LD, Johnson BC et al. (1965) Epidemiological studies of cardiovascular disease in a total community – Tecumseh, Michigan. Ann Intern Med 62:1170–1187
5. Morris JN, Adams C, Chave SPW et al. (1973) Vigorous exercise in leisure time and the incidence of coronary heart disease. Lancet I:333–339
6. Paffenbarger RS Jr (1975) Work activity and coronary heart mortality. N Engl J Med 292:545–550
7. Rabkin DE, Mathewson AL, Hsu P (1977) Relation of body weight to development of ischemic heart disease in a cohort of young North American men after a 26-year observation period. The Manitoba study. Am J Cardiol 39:452–550
8. Farrand ME et al. (1980) Nutrition in the multiple risk factor intervention trial (MRFIT). J Am Diet Assoc 76/4:347–351
9. Hjermann I (1980) Smoking and diet intervention in healthy coronary high-risk men. Methods plus 5-year follow-up of risk factors in a randomized trial. The Oslo study. J Oslo City Hosp 30/1:3–17
10. Hellerstein HJ, Horsten TR, Goldberg A et al. (1967) The influence of active conditioning upon subjects with coronary artery disease. Can Med Assoc J 96:901–903
11. Brunner D Meshulman N (1969) Prevention of recurrent myocardial infarction by physical exercise. Isr J Med Sci 5:783–785
12. The National exercise and Heart Disease Project Staff (1980) Effects of a prescribed supervised exercise program on mortality and cardiovascular morbidity in myocardial infarction subjects: a randomized clinical trial. Cardiovas Dis Epidemiol Newsletter 28:55
13. Kallio V, Hamalainen H, Hakkila J, Luurila OJ (1979) Reduction in sudden deaths by a multifactiorial intervention programme after acute myocardial infarction. Lancet II:1091
14. Shephard RJ (1979) Recurrence of myocardial infarction in an exercising population. Br Heart J 42:133
15. Selvester R, Camp J, Sanmarco M (1978) Effects of exercise training on progression of documented coronary arteriosclerosis in men. Ann NY Acad Sci 301:495

Myocardial Revascularization in Patients Under 40 Years of Age

H. J. Radtke[1], C. Hahn, H. Roskamm, and M. Schmuziger[2]

Aortocoronary bypass grafting today plays a fixed role in the therapeutic approach to coronary artery disease. That it improves quality of life by increased angina-free working tolerance [1, 5, 7, 9] is certain, and even prolongation of life is considered proven [3, 10, 14] in special forms of coronary artery sclerosis.

Of special interest are patients under 40 years of age [4, 13, 15] with regard to risk factors, natural history of the disease, and medical or operative therapeutic possibilities [6, 8]. The following is a report on our experience with coronary revascularization in patients under the age of 40 years.

Patients and Methods

Between 1973 and December, 1980, 1552 patients from our institution underwent coronary revascularization (Fig. 1). 72 or 4.64% of those (3 women, 69 men) were under 40. One patient was 24, another 25, 13 patients were 30–34, and 57 patients were 35–39 years old. The angina-free and maximal exercise tolerance was assessed using a bicycle ergometer and a Swan-Gantz catheter with the patient in a supine position. A complete follow-up was attempted 1 year postoperatively and since 1978, 8 weeks postoperatively with yearly exercise-tolerance testing. The number of risk factors was evaluated by information from patients and laboratory data.

Results

The main risk factors (Fig. 2) were smoking (90.5%), overweight (98.5%), hyperlipidemia (94%), and hypercholesterolemia (89%). Hypertension, hyperuricemia, and a family history of coronary disease were encountered frequently, whereas diabetes did not play a significant role in this patient group [6, 8, 13, 15]. Of the 72 patients, 57 already had preoperative infarctions with mildly impaired left ventricular function in 50%, moderate impairment in 19%, severe impairment in 5%, and only 26% with normal left ventricular function.

At angiography only six patients had single-vessel disease (Fig. 3) with a very proximal lesion (proximal to the first septal branch) of the left anterior descending artery (LAD) which caused severe symptoms. Twenty-four patients had double-vessels disease, with right coronary artery disease in addition to the LAD lesions

1 *Present address:* Römerbergklinik der BVA, 7542 Schömberg
2 Rehabilitationszentrum, Südring 15, 7812 Bad Krozingen, FRG and Clinique médico-chirurgical de Genolier, Switzerland

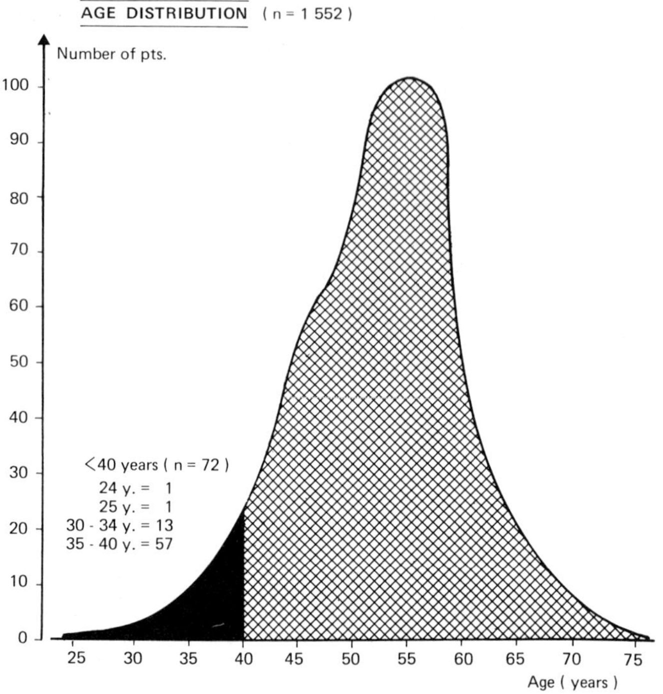

Fig. 1. Age distribution of all operated patients between 1973 and December, 1980

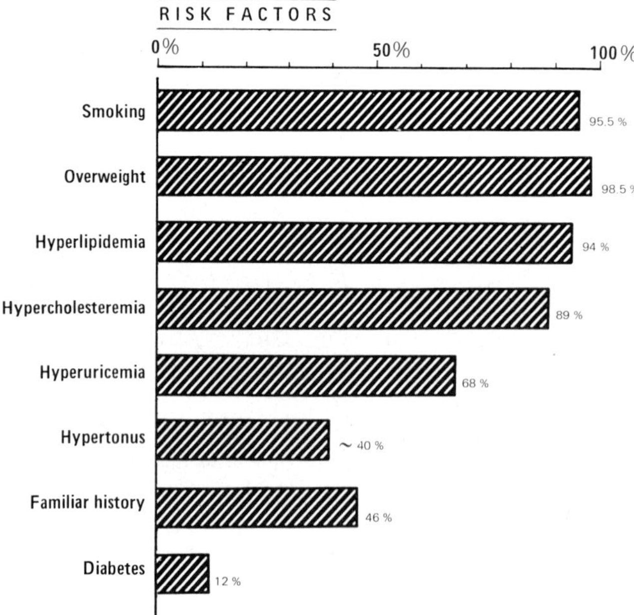

Fig. 2. Risk factors in 72 patients under age 40

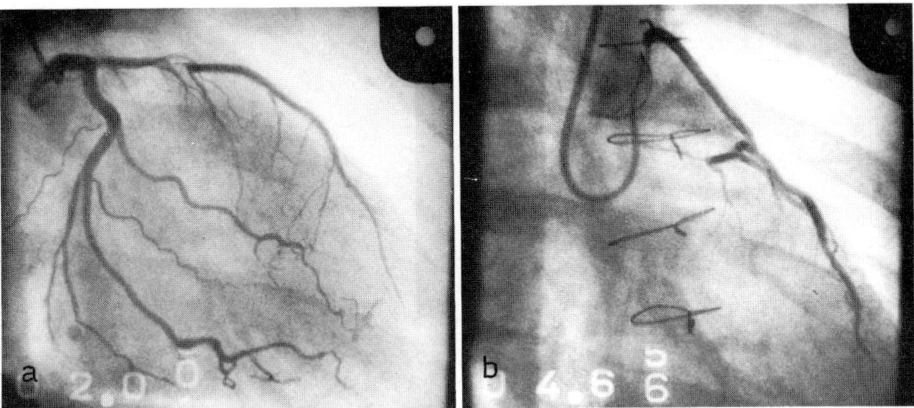

Fig. 3. a Subtotal LAD stenosis proximal to the first septal branch and **b** the same patient with coronary graft

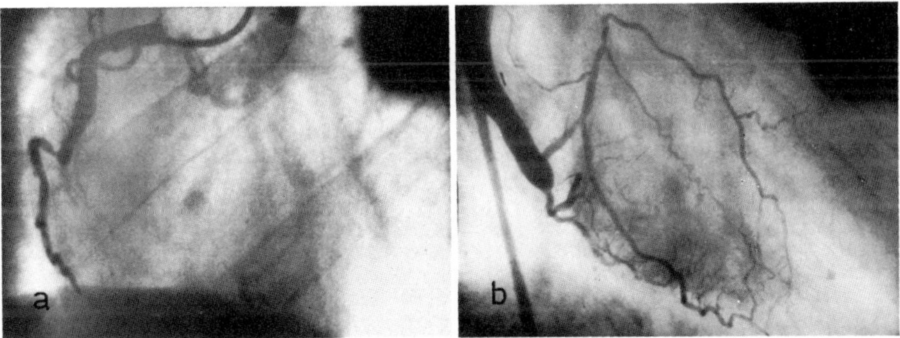

Fig. 4. a In addition to the LAD stenosis, total occlusion of the right coronary artery (RCA) and **b** the same patient with bypass to the RCA

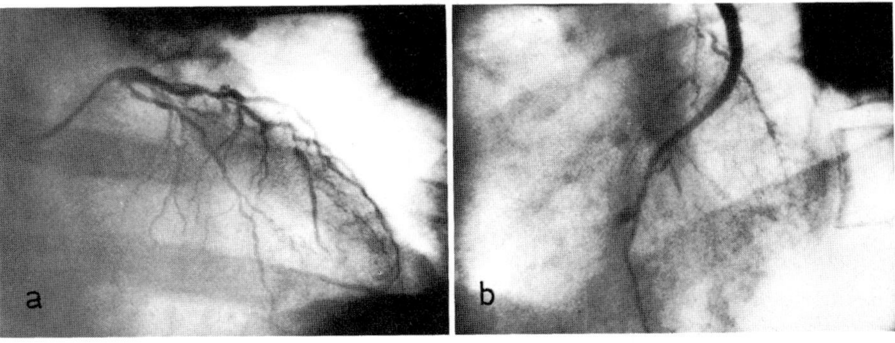

Fig. 5. a Diffuse triple-vessel disease (LAD and circumflex area with left main stem stenosis) and **b** the same patient with bypass to LAD and diagonal branch

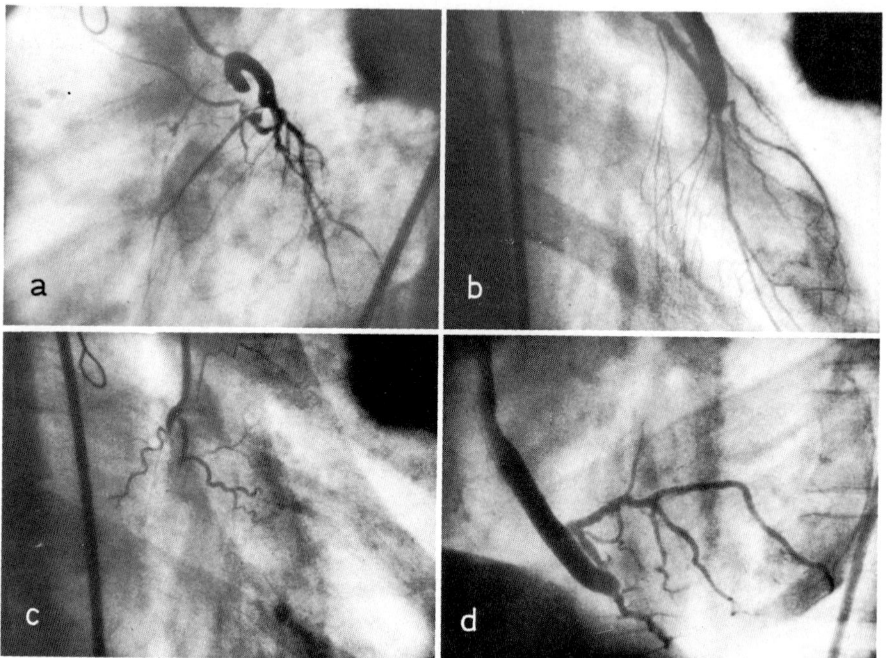

Fig. 6a–d. Massive and diffuse, actually inoperable (LAD and circumflex area) **a,** the same patient with bypass to the LAD **b,** the same patient with additional total occlusion of the RCA **c,** and the same patient with bypass to the RCA **d**

(Fig. 4). The remaining 42 patients had triple-vessel disease, mostly with massive and diffuse disease of the peripheral vessels (Fig. 5). According to the usual criteria, some of them had been refused for revascularization (Fig. 6) and only their youth and disabling angina at low exercise tolerance (25–50 W) without hope of improvement through medical therapy, which ruled out vocational rehabilitation, prompted us to operate on them.

210 anastomoses, i.e., 2.91 grafts per patient, were performed. We lost one patient because of low cardiac output with renal failure 10 days postoperatively (operative mortality rate 1.38%). Another patient died 1 year postoperatively from an acute myocardial infarction (MI). The postmortem, however, showed both grafts to be patent. A third patient sustained a reinfarction 4 months postoperatively, however he had not reduced any of his risk factors (smoking, hypercholesterolemia, hyperlipidemia, hyperuricemia) and increased from 30 kg above normal weight preoperatively to 40 kg above normal postoperatively. He is now (4 years postoperatively) retired, but his angina-free exercise tolerance increased from 25 W preoperatively to 125 W postoperatively, and then fell to 75 W after the reinfarction (total increase 50 W).

Another six patients sustained a perioperative MI, diagnosed by ECG changes and specific enzyme rises, for an infarction rate of 8.3%. One patient now has a 75 W tolerance with angina, as preoperatively, and is retired, one patient suffers from congestive heart failure in spite of three patent grafts of four performed and he is disabled. The other four were enlargements of old preoperative infarctions without complications or hemodynamic impairment.

Of the 72 patients, 59 were restudied. The other 13 were from other institutions (three patients), refused (three patients), or were only operated during November and December, 1980 (seven patients). At coronary reangiography, 115 of 154 performed anastomoses were patent (patency rate 74.6%) (Fig. 7). Complete revasculari-

In all 72 patients performed grafts 210
        = 2.91 grafts / patient

In contr. 59 patients perform. gr. 154
        = 2.61 grafts / patient

Patent grafts in 59 patients grafts 115
        = 1.95 grafts / patient

PATENCY RATE 74.6%

Fig. 7. Number of performed, restudied, and patent grafts

zation (all grafts patent) was achieved in 51%. Satisfactory revascularization (50% or more performed grafts patent) was achieved in 37%, giving a total of 88% satisfactory results (Fig. 8). In 7% (four patients) all grafts were occluded and in 5% (three patients) an unsatisfactory result (less than 50% performed grafts patent) was achieved. In the group of satisfactory revascularizations are nine patients with just two grafts performed, of which one is occluded graft. These patients belong to our earlier experience, whereas our more recent policy is towards more complete revascularization, i.e., more grafts per patient. The classification of satisfactory results derives from increased angina-free exercise tolerance.

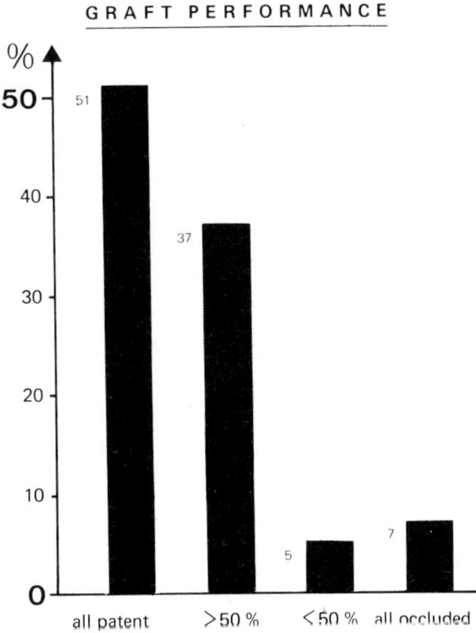

Fig. 8. Graft performance in patients at follow-up

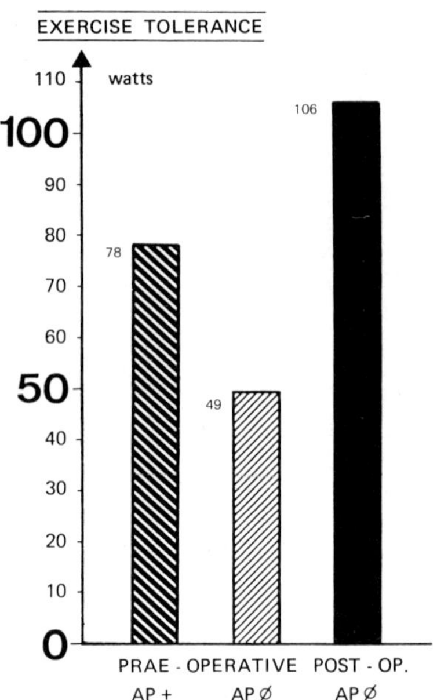

Filg. 9. Mean exercise tolerance preoperatively with and without angina (AP) and postoperatively without angina

Preoperative mean maximum exercise tolerance under medication was 78 W with angina (Fig. 9). The mean angina-free exercise tolerance was only 49 W. The mean angina-free exercise tolerance increased postoperatively to 106 W, i.e., by 57 W (116%). With this increase it is understandable that all but eight patients, (86.4%) are fit to work, which they would have been unable to do because of disabling angina even with maximal medical therapy. Some patients, however, had to be trained for physically less demanding jobs.

Conclusions

These results show that coronary artery surgery in this age group can be done with low mortality rates and low morbidity, even with unfavorable distal coronary vessels [9, 10]. As expected with this aggressive form of atherosclerosis, the overall patency rate is lower than in the rest of our patients (84%–86%). But, in spite of the higher occlusion rate, postoperative exercise tolerance and the percentage of patients who are now back at work are both higher than usual [2, 11, 12]. So, like others [6, 8], we feel encouraged in our policy of aortocoronary bypass surgery in the rehabilitation process of patients under 40 with almost inoperable coronary vessels and disabling angina. It seems to be a positive answer to the question of whether to be "written off", sitting in a wheelchair, or to lead a normal life.

References

1. Anderson, RP, Rahimtoola SH, Bonchek LI, Starr A (1974) The prognosis of patients with coronary artery disease after coronary bypass operation: Time-related progress of 532 patients with disabling angina pectoris. Circulation 50:274

2. Barnes GK, Ray MJ, Oberman A, Kouchoukos NT (1977) Changes in working status of patients following coronary bypass surgery. JAMA 238:1259–1262
3. Cohn LH, Collins JJ Jr (1974) Improved long-term survival following coronary artery bypass. Circulation [Suppl III] 50:66
4. Engel HJ, Page HL, Campbell B (1974) Coronary artery disease in young women. JAMA 230:1531–1534
5. Hatcher CR, Jones EL, King SB et al. (1975) The surgical treatment of unstable angina pectoris. Ann Surg 181:754
6. Kelly TF, Craver JM, Jones EL, Hatcher CR (1978) Coronary revascularization in patients 40 years and younger: Surgical experience and long-term follow-up. Am Surg 44:675–678
7. Kouchoukos NT, Kirklin JW, Oberman A (1974) An appraisal of coronary bypass grafting. Circulation 50:11–16
8. Laks H, Kaiser GC, Barner HB et al. (1978) Coronary revascularization under age 40 years. Am J Cardiol 41:584
9. Lawrie GM, Morris GC, Howell JF, Ogura JW (1977) Results of coronary artery bypass more than 5 years after operation in 434 patients. Am J Cardiol 40:665
10. Lawrie GM, Morris GC, Howell JF et al. (1978) Improved survival beyond 5 years in 1108 patients undergoing coronary bypass. Am J Cardiol 41:355
11. Oberman A, Kouchoukos NT (1979) Working status of patients following coronary bypass surgery. Am Heart J 98:132–133
12. Rimm AA, Barboriak JJ, Anderson AJ, Simon JS (1976) Changes in occupation after aortocoronary vein-bypass operation. JAMA 236:361–364
13. Roth O, Berki A, Wolff GD (1967) Long-range observation in 53 young patients with myocardial infarction. Am J Cardiol 19:331–338
14. Sheldon WC (1977) Effect of bypass graft surgery on survival: A 6–10 year follow-up study of 741 patients. In: The first decade of bypass graft surgery for coronary artery disease: An international symposium (Syllabus) Cleveland Clinic Foundation, Cleveland, p 127
15. Walker WJ, Gregoratos MG (1967) Myocardial infarction in young men. Am J Cardiol 19:339

Long-Term Results of Ventricular Aneurysm Repair in Patients Under 45 Years of Age

P. S. Diamond, L. Kowalczyk, R. Pifarre, and R. M. Gunnar[1]

Myocardial infarction (MI) is increasingly a cause of morbidity and mortality among the younger adult population. Left ventricular aneurysm formation occurs in approximately 5%–15% of such patients (Schlichter et al. 1954). Recent interest focused on coronary bypass in the younger population has not specifically addressed the results of aneurysm repair (Laks et al. 1978). In view of this, we decided to review our experience in patients 45 years of age or younger who underwent aneurysm repair at our institution during the past 10 years. Thirty-two patients met criteria to be included in this study, and it is our purpose to report the presenting characteristics of these patients and late follow-up of their survival and functional recovery.

Patients and Methods

Between January, 1970, and December, 1980, 4186 coronary artery bypass operations were performed at L.U.M.C. During this same period, 266 aneurysm repairs were also performed: Two of those repairs were performed in children with congenital aneurysms and these patients were excluded from this study. Of the remaining 264 patients, 32 patients were age 45 or under. Thirty patients had aneurysms of arteriosclerotic origin, while in two patients the aneurysm was secondary to chest wall trauma. These 32 patients comprised the study group.

All patients' charts were reviewed, and follow-up was obtained either from these records or direct contact with each patient or the patient's physician.

All patients underwent cardiac catheterization, coronary angiography, and left ventriculography. Patients were followed up over a variable length of time, with a mean follow-up period of 61 months. Operative reports and pathology results were reviewed. Location of the aneurysm was specified in all patients, as was the number of diseased vessels bypassed. Presence or absence of thrombus in the aneurysm was noted in the operative report.

Preoperative N.Y.H.A. functional classification was compared to the clinical classification in the late postoperative period in each patient by review of the clinical notes. The specific reasons for surgery were tabulated. All cardiovascular complications in surviving and nonsurviving patients were tabulated and the specific cause of death was ascertained in all nonsurvivors.

---

1 Departments of Medicine and Surgery, Sections of Cardiology and Cardio-Thoracic Surgery, Loyola University Stritch School of Medicine, 2160 South First Avenue, Maywood, IL 60153, USA

All patients were followed up for a minimum of 6 months, but long-term follow-up in two patients was incomplete, although of these two, one patient was followed up for 6 months and one for 12 months. There were no preoperative embolic episodes, and none of these patients required valve replacement or repair.

Results

The 32 patients 45 years of age or under who underwent aneurysm repair represented 13.7% of the total group of patients who underwent aneurysm repair at our institution over the specified 10-year period. There were 29 males and three females, for a male to female predominance of 9.7:1. Of those 30 patients who had suffered previous infarction, the majority (70%) underwent aneurysm repair within 1 year of that infarction. In the two patients with trauma, one aneurysm was due to blunt trauma and the other a consequence of coronary artery laceration.

The reason for surgery was congestive heart failure in 16 patients, including the two patients with traumatic aneurysm, angina pectoris in 11 patients, and uncontrolled ventricular arrhythmias in five (Table 1). Preoperatively, 26 (81%) of the patients were in functional class III or IV by N.Y.H.A. criteria (Table 2). The site of aneurysm involved the anterior and/or apical regions of the left ventricle in the majority of cases (Table 3). At the time of surgery, three patients had only repair of aneurysm, while 29 patients had aneurysm repair plus a variable number of coronary

Table 1 Primary reason for surgery

	No. of patients	Survived	Died	Survival (%)
Congestive heart failure	16	13	3	81
Angina	11	11	0	100
Arrhythmia	5	2	3	40

Table 2. NYHA classification

	Preoperatively	Postoperatively
Survivors		
Class I	0	21
Class II	6	5
Class III	18	0
Class IV	2	0
Nonsurvivors		
Class I	0	0
Class II	0	0
Class III	5	5
Class IV	1	1

Table 3. Site of aneurysm

	No.
Anterolateral + apical	9
Anteroapical	7
Anterolateral	4
Apical	6
Posterior	6
Total	32

Table 4. Surgical procedure

	No.
Aneurysm repair alone	3 (9.4%)
Aneurysm repair + ACBP[a] × 1	13 (40.7%)
Aneurysm repair + ACBP × 2	12 (37.5%)
Aneurysm repair + ACBP × 3	3 (9.4%)
Aneurysm repair + ACBP × 4	1 (3.0%)
Total	32

[a] Aortocoronary bypass surgerey

artery bypasses (Table 4). The left anterior descending (LAD) was the most common artery to be bypassed, but the right coronary artery, obtuse marginal, and diagonal were also frequently bypassed. A total of 48 bypasses were performed (Table 5). All patients survived the initial operative procedure, but one patient died in the perioperative period (6 days) (operative mortality 3%). The remaining 31 patients were followed up for a mean of 60.7 months (6–103 months). Of this group, there were five late deaths, for an overal mortality of 19% in the entire study group.

Survivors. Twenty-four patients were available for long-term follow-up in December, 1980, and two patients were lost to follow-up after 6–12 months though both were alive at the time of last contact. Twenty-four patients followed-up to the present time are in N.Y.H.A. class I or II, with 19 in class I. The two patients lost to follow-up were both in class I at last contact (Table 2). The two patients with traumatic aneurysms are presently class I. Twenty-four of the patients available for long-term follow-up have survived for at least 1 year, and the longest survival times are now over 8 years since their aneurysm repair (four patients).

Late complications have occured in eight patients (Table 6). Late MI occurred in two patients and cerebrovascular accident occurred in two. One of these latter two patients suffered two infarctions as well as cardiopulmonary arrest and cerebrovascular accident, but he is currently class II with minimal neurologic sequelae. Ventricular arrhythmias have occurred in three patients, but are currently controlled by antiarrhythmic agents. Two patients underwent a second surgical procedure: In both of these patients, one bypass graft had occluded requiring a second bypass, and in one of them a recurrent aneurysm also required resection. Both patients are now class II. In both patients with cerebrovascular accidents, no cardiac source of embolization was documented. In the remaining patients, no thromboembolic episodes have occurred, although one patient developed a superficial thromphlebitis. Atrial arrhythmias have not been a problem in the late follow-up period. Almost all patients remain normotensive without antihypertension therapy.

Nonsurvivors. The one perioperative death was a result of uncontrolled ventricular arrhythmias with hemodynamic deterioration secondary to the dysrhythmia. In the other five remaining nonsurvivors, mean length of survival was 63 months

Table 5. Site of coronary artery bypass

Vessel	No.
Left anterior descending	17
Right coronary	11
Obtuse marginal	10
Diagonal	6
Circumflex	1
Ramus intermedius	1
Internal mammary implant	1
Posterior descending	1
Total	48

Table 6. Late complications in eight survivors

	No.
Ventricular arrhythmias	3
MI	3
Cerebrovascular accident	2
Sudden death	1
Atrial arrhythmias	1
Phlebitis (Superficial)	1
Sternal Fistula	1

(36–77 months) (Table 7). All of these patients remained in class III postoperatively. Of these five patients, congestive heart failure was a contributing cause of death in all and was the primary cause in three. One patient died as a direct result of a new MI and one patient died suddenly. Two of the patients who died of congestive failure also had pulmonary emboli documented during their final hospital admission. Of the six nonsurvivors, congestive heart failure was the main indication for surgery in three and uncontrolled ventricular arrhythmias in three. Two patients had aneurysm repair alone, two patients had single bypasses, and two patients had double bypasses. The LAD coronary artery was bypassed in three nonsurvivors.

Discussion

Atherosclerotic coronary artery disease is the major cause of left ventricular aneurysm formation in the adult population, with an incidence of 3.5%–38% in patients with acute MI (Abrams et al. 1963; Davis and Ebert 1972; Dubnow et al. 1963; Schlichter et al. 1954). Early autopsy studies by Schlichter et al. (1954) determined that 5-year survival in medically treated patients was 12%. Later autopsy

Table 7. Cause of death in nonsurvivors

	Postoperative survival
1. Perioperative ventricular arrhythmias[a]	6 days
2. Acute MI ventricular tachycardia (during recatheterization for ventricular tachycardia)[a]	61 months
3. Sudden death (Class III, angina, premortem)[a]	64 months
4. Cardiogenic shock, pulmonary embolus	36 months
5. CHF	77 months
6. CHF, pulmonary embolus	76 months

[a] Patients operated upon for arrhythmia

studies have been in general agreement with this finding (Cabin and Roberts 1980). As a consequence of this dismal prognosis, efforts since 1958 have focused on surgical repair to improve the long-term survival of patients with post-MI aneurysms (Cooley et al. 1958).

Follow-up time after surgical repair with or without additional coronary artery bypass has been variable, but, in general, 2-year survival approaches 80%, while 5-year survival is approximately 60% (Burton et al. 1979).

None of these studies have directly investigated the early and late aspects of ventricular aneurysm in the younger adult age group. Shaw et al (1978) identified 11 patients, age 45 or under, in their study. We have not noticed that aneurysm formation is unusual after MI in the younger patient, and were surprised how few of these patients we actually subjected to surgery.

It may be that the younger patient, frequently with first infarction, can compensate for the aneurysm because of the good remaining myocardium. If such patients have single-vessel disease, they would probably not be considered for bypass even with some post-infarction angina because the bypassed vessel would go mainly to scar tissue. We thought our low incidence of aneurysm repair in young patients might be confined to our population, but of the 169 patients in the Burton et al. (1979) report of the Stanford experience with left ventricular aneurysm repair, only seven patients were under 40 years of age, and only 12 patients at ages 40–45 and 45 years (11% under age 46) (Shumway, personal communication). This compares well with the 32 of 264 (12%) of our patients operated upon with aneurysms who were 45 years old or younger. In the autopsy report of Schlichter et al. (1954), only 10% of patients were under 45 years of age; and in the series of Cabin and Roberts (1980), only 3 of 28 patients (11%) were in this age group.

In our group of patients, the long-term survival of 81% is somewhat higher than reported for aneurysm repair in all age groups. In addition, perioperative mortality was only 3%. Although Shaw et al. (1978) reported a similar value of 4.5% mortality and we have previously reported 6.5% mortality for all age groups (Moran et al. 1976), many investigators have reported an operative mortality of 9%–25%, with an average of approximately 12%. The lower mortality in our series and that of Shaw et al. (1978) may have special significance when surgical intervention is considered for this age group. Although none of our patients required septal defect repair or mitral valve replacement, all other aspects of the patient group were comparable to previous studies. Cooperman et al. (1975) and Hutchinson et al. (1978) found that increased age carried a higher mortality, but studies by Shaw et al. (1978) determined that age did not alter long-term survival. The results of our study, when compared to previous reports, suggest that patients 45 years of age or under may have a longer survival after aneurysm repair than older patients undergoing similar aneurysm repair. The data presented here becomes more significant because of the length of follow-up.

Surgery for malignant arrhythmias was associated with the worst prognosis, while patients operated upon for symptoms of angina alone had a 100% survival. Congestive heart failure was the most common reason for surgery and was a contributing cause of death in most nonsurvivors. All of these findings are in agreement with other studies, although the absence of mortality in the angina group is both anusual and very encouraging, especially since most of those patients are now in functional class I. The 9.7:1 preponderance of males in this study remains unexplained, but suggests that younger adult males who sustain MI at age 45 or under have a greater risk of developing a ventricular aneurysm than females in that same age group.

At the time of current functional evaluation, all survivors are in N.Y.H.A. class I or II. The patients who did not survive until most recent follow-up had all remained class III postoperatively, and this confirms the findings of others that poor left ventricular function postoperatively is associated with high mortality and can be predicted from the poor left ventricular function present preoperatively. Relatively few serious complications occurred late in the course of the patients who survived, although "sudden death" in one patient and MI in two patients had potentially catastrophic consequences.

Thromboembolic complications have been reported in up to 52% of patients with aneurysms treated medically (Schlichter et al. 1954), while reports of surgically treated patients have reported a low incidence of thromboembolism. In our group, thromboembolic phenomenon were documented in only two patients, both of whom were in the terminal stage of their disease when this occurred. Only 12 patients had thrombus present in the aneurysm at the time of surgical repair, which is a somewhat lower incidence than in previous reports, and may have been a factor in the low occurrence of thromboembolic phenomenon in this group.

Conclusion

It appears that left ventricular aneurysm requiring surgical repair is uncommon in the age group 45 years or less, but patients who undergo aneurysm repair in this age group have a low surgical mortality, and if congestive heart failure is absent in the postoperative period, chances of 5-year survival are excellent. As in other age groups, surgery for uncontrolled arrhythmias is associated with the least favorable prognosis. This should be considered in the preoperative evaluation, and perhaps improved by endo- and epicardial mapping.

Excellent long-term survival occurs in those patients who have aneurysm repair and in whom the indication for surgery is angina. All survivors in this group are now in N.Y.H.A. functional class I or II. There appears to be a marked male predominance of patients with ventricular aneurysm in this age group, and late thromboembolic episodes are very infrequent. In view of the shortened survival in patients with ventricular aneurysms treated medically, the long-term benefits of surgical repair (in association with coronary revascularization, if feasible) in patients 45 years and under seems strongly indicated.

References

Abrams DL, Edelist A, Luria MH, Miller AJ (1963) Ventricular aneurysm. A reappraisal based on a study of 65 consecutive autopsied cases. Circulation 27:164–169
Burton NA, Stinson EB, Oyer PE, Shumway NE (1979) Left ventricular aneurysm. Preoperative risk factors and long-term postoperative results. J Thorac Cardiovasc Surg 77:65–75

Cabin HS, Roberts WC (1980) True ventricular aneurysm and healed myocardial infarction. Clinical and necropsy observations including quantification of degrees of coronary arterial narrowing. Am J Cardiol 46:754–763

Cooley DA, Collins HA, Morris GC, Chapman DW (1958) Ventricular aneurysm after myocardial infarction: Surgical excision with use of temporary cardiopulmonary bypass. JAMA 167:557–560

Cooperman M, Stinson EB, Griepp RB, Shumway NE (1975) Survival and function after left ventricular aneurysmectomy. J Thorac Cardiovasc 69:321–328

Davis RW, Ebert PA (1972) Ventricular aneurysm. A clinical-pathologic correlation. Am J Cardiol 29:1–6

Dubnow MH, Burchell HB, Titus JL (1963) Postinfarction ventricular aneurysm. A clinico-morphologic and electrocardiographic study of 80 cases. Am Heart J 70:753–760

Hutchinson JE III, Green GG, Mekhjian HA et al. (1978) Combined left ventricular aneurysm and coronary artery bypass surgery. Arch Surg 113:1236–1249

Laks H, Kaiser GC, Bardner HB et al. (1978) Coronary revascularization under age 40 years. Risk factors and results of surgery. Am J Cardiol 41:584–589

Moran JM, Scanlon PJ, Nemickas R, Pifarre R (1976) Surgical treatment of postinfarction ventricular aneurysm. Ann Thorac Surg 21:107–113

Schlichter J, Hellerstein HK, Katz LN (1954) Aneurysm of the heart: A correlative study of 102 proven cases. Medicine (Baltimore) 33:46–86

Shaw RC, Ferguson TB, Weldon CS, Connors JP (1978) Left ventricular aneurysm resection: Indications and long-term follow-up. Ann Thorac Surg 25:336–339

Surgical Treatment of Chronic Ventricular Tachycardia After Myocardial Infarction

G. Guiraudon[1], C. Cabrol[2], G. Fontaine[3], R. Frank[3], J. Barra[2], and A. Pavie[2]

The modern surgical treatment of ventricular tachycardia (VT) after myocardial infarction (MT) is based on the mechanism of the arrhythmia and the significance of the pathological lesions [1, 2].

Chronic VT after MI may be terminated and induced by electrical stimulation [3]. This characteristic is suggestive of an underlying reentrant phenomenon. In MI, necrosis is maximal at the center of the infarcted area, which becomes fibrosed and thin walled [4]. Ventricular mapping demonstrates no electrical activity over this zone and it can therefore play no role in the genesis of arrhythmias. Around the central necrosis zone is situated a border zone consisting of ischemic and normal muscle, and fibrosis, the limits of which are difficult to delineate. Ischemic lesions are located essentially in the subendocardial layers. Endocardial fibrosis develops opposite the entire infarcted area. Therefore, the limits of the pathological area can be located by endocavitary exploration. The border of the endocardial fibrosis corresponds to the maximal extension of the lesions. Ventricular mapping demonstrates slow conduction and delayed potentials over the border zone [5–8]. This situation favors the initiation of reentry [9]. The border zone is where the arrhythmias arise, as this is where part of the reentry circuit responsible for the VT is located [9]. The epicardial site of origin of VT is situated in healthy myocardium at the edge of the border zone [7] whereas the endocardial origin of VT is situated within the limits of endocardial fibrosis [10].

However, not all MI results in localised organised scars. Some give rise to post-ischemic cardiomyopathy with dilatation.

Aneurysmectomy resects or excludes the central fibrous zone which plays no role in the genesis of arrhythmias. This operation, which only gives mediocre results, cannot be considered to be the treatment of choice VT after MI [11].

Since 1975, our team has been engaged in the development of surgical treatment adapted to the pathological lesions and to the mechanism of the arrhythmia: encircling endocardial ventriculotomy (EEV) [12], and simple ventriculotomy at the point of origin of VT determined by epicardial mapping. The latter technique is the same as that developed by our team for the treatment of nonischemic VT [13].

1 Cardiovascular and Thoracic Surgery, University Hospital, London, Ont., Canada
2 Service de Chirurgie Cardio-Vasculaires, Hôpitaux de Paris 47 et 83, boulevard de l'Hôpital, F-75651 Paris Cedex 13, France
3 Service de Cardiologie, Hôpital Jean Rostand, 91. Inry, France

Table 1. Clinical profile and angiographic data of patients treated by EEV

No.	Name	Age	Symptoms	Age of infarct	ECG site of infarct	ST segment elevation	Major coronary narrowing	Ejection fraction	Wall motion abnormality
1	BEIL	48	Syncope	1 mo	Ant.	V1 V5	RCA–LAD		Apical
2	TAVI	60		34 mo	Post.		RCA – LCA	0.35	Inferior
3	SOUV	59	Syncope	32 mo	Ant.	V1 V6	LAD–LCA	0.29	Anterior
4	CHAB	55	Angina	8 yrs	Ant.	V1 V6	LCA	0.21	Apical
5	LEPY	40		several months	Post.	D2 D3 aVF	RCA		Anteroinferior
6	MARZ	36		2 yrs	Septum		LAD–RCA	0.34	Diffuse (RAD)
7	FREM	60	Cardiac arrest	6 weeks	Septum		LAD–RCA–LCA		Posteroapical
8	PRAD	50		15 yrs	Ant.	V2 V3	LAD	0.29	Anterior
9	RUDA	66	Palpitations	5 mo	Post.		RCA	0.36	Posterior
10	DOUR	61		11 yrs	Ant.		RCA	0.27	Anterior Calcif.
11	LAVI	61		10 yrs	Ant.		RCA	0.35	Posterior False aneurysm
12	TOMA	53		13 yrs	Ant.				Anterior
13	HORE	55	Angina	1 yrs	Ant-Lat.	V2 V4	LAD–LCA	0.36	Apical
14	BEAU	52	Dizziness	?	Post.		RCA		Inferior
15	VAND	57		8 yrs	Ant.	V1 V4	LAD		Anterior
16	VANK	47		1 yrs	Ant.		LAD (traumatic)		Anterior
17	LEPE	43	Syncope	3 mo	Ant.	V2 V5	LAD	0.24	Anterior
18	ANSE	61	Syncope, cardiac arrest	10 yrs	Ant.	V2 V3	Left main stem LAD–LCA	0.46	Anterior
19	HART	42	Syncope	6 mo	Ant.		LAD		Anterior
20	THEA	59	Angor	5 mo	Post.		RCA–LAD–LCA	0.28	Inferior
21	SABA	57	Dizziness	14 mo	Ant.	V2 V4	LAD–LCA	0.49	Anterior
22	MEAU	61		2 yrs	Inf.		RCA	0.43	Inferior
23	DRUA	50		11 yrs	Post.	D3 aVF	RCA–LCA	0.10	Inferior
24	THOM	56	Congestive heart failure	1 mo	Ant.		LAD–RCA–LCA	0.22	Anterior
25	VANS	41	Low output failure	1 mo	Ant.		LAD–RCA–LCA	0.27	Anterior
26	CHEP	52	Syncope	6 mo	Ant.	V2 V4	LAD	0.35	Anterior
27	VAGN	52	Syncope	10 yrs	Ant.	V2 V4	LAD–RCA–LCA	0.37	Anterior, calcification
28	FECT	26		weeks	Ant.	V2 V6	LAD		Anterior
29	NOEL	44	Dizziness	1 yrs	Post.		LAD–LCA		Posterior

Encircling Endocardial Ventriculotomy

Materials and Methods

Our experience is based on a series of 29 patients (Table I) with an average age of
54 years (range 36 to 66 years). Recurrent syncope related to ventricular tachycardia
occurred in seven. All patients had a history of previous MI.

Serial surface electrocardiograms (ECG) showed evidence of MI. Ten patients
had posterior wall infarction, 17 anterior wall infarction, and two septal infarction.
Coronary arteriography revealed coronary arterial narrowing of more than 70% in
at least one major coronary vessel in 28 patients. One patient had no significant coronary artery narrowing, 13 had one-vessel disease, eight had two-vessel disease,
and seven patients had three-vessel disease (including two with left main stem disease).

Single plane left ventricular cineangiography was performed in the right anterior oblique projection. Left ventricular aneurysm was considered to be present
when there was a definite area of akinetic or dyskinetic myocardium. There was excellent correlation between ECG site of the previous infarction and aneurysm location.

The delay between MI and the first attack of VT ranged from 1 month to 15
years.

The surgical indication was based on the failure or troublesome side effects of
medical treatment. A last trial with Amiodarone or Aprindine was usually performed when possible before surgery.

Operative Technique

The heart is approached through a median sternotomy. A careful macroscopic examination is carried out but the limits of the ischemic zone cannot be distinguished
from the epicardial aspect. Epicardial mapping is routinely performed during sinus
rhythm to identify the zones of slow conduction and low amplitude potentials. Epi-
caridal mapping during triggered VT may lead to serious hemodynamic disturbances, in which case it is carried out under cover of normothermic cardiopulmonary bypass.

After entering the left ventricle (LV) through the thin-walled fibrotic zone, a
complete examination of the endocardial surface can be carried out. Endocardial
fibrosis, the limits of which correspond to the maximal extent of the ischemic lesions. may involve the free wall of the LV, the septum, the papillary muscles, or a
combination of these. The EEV follows the edge of endocardial fibrosis.

At the free wall of the ventricle, the ventriculotomy is a full thickness section,
sparing the epicardium and the coronary vessels. At the septum, the ventriculotomy
is deep, almost transmural.

The relationship of EEV to the coronary vessels, the papillary muscles and
the septum is as follows. The coronary vessels and the perpendicular penetrating
branches are spared. EEV may exclude a papillary muscle without impairing its
function; nine posterior papillary muscles were excluded in ten posterior scars, and

Table 2. Operative procedure and results

No.	Name	Encircling endocardial ventriculotomy					Results		Follow-up period
		Ant.wall	Inf.wall	Septum	Papillory muscle	AC bypass graft	Early	Late	
1	BEIL	+	+	+	0	RCA	S	S (CHF)	54 mo
2	TAVI	0	+	+	Post.		S	Relapse 36 mo (Pace-maker + Drugs)	56 mo
3	SOUV	+	+	+	0		S	Died of pneumonia (CHF?)	2 mo
4	CHAB	+	+	+	0		S	S	49 mo
5	LEPY	+	+	+	0		S	S Died relapse MI	24 mo
6	MARZ	+	+	+	0		VT	S Drugs discontinued 6 mo	40 mo
7	FREM	+	+	+	0		Died at operation		11 days
8	PRAD	+	+	+	0		S	Controlled by drugs died relapse MI	26 mo
9	RUDA	0	+	+	0		New configuration VT	Controlled by drugs	29 mo
10	DOUR	+	0	+	Ant. inf.		S	S	28 mo
11	LAVI	0	+	+	Post.		S Died of hypokalemia		11 days
12	TOMA	+	0	−	0		S	S	27 mo
13	Hore	+	+	+	Post.		S	S	27 mo
14	BEAU	+	+	+	Post.		S	S	22 mo
15	Vand	+	+	+	0		S	S	22 mo
16	VANK	+	+	+	0	LAD	S	S	20 mo
17	LEPE	+	0	+	0		S	S	17 mo
18	ANSE	+	+	+	0		S	S	17 mo
19	HART	+	+	+	0		S	S	16 mo
20	THEA	0	+	+	Post.	LCA	S	S	14 mo
21	SABA	+	+	+	0	LCA	S	S	14 mo
22	MEAU	0	+	+	Post.		S	S	14 mo
23	DRUA	0	+	+	Post.		S	S	13 mo
24	THOM	+	+	+	0		S		28 days
25	VANS	+	+	+	0		LOF		
26	CHEP	+	+	+	+		S	S	8 mo
27	VAGN	+	+	+	0		S	S	6 mo
28	FECT	+	+	+	0		S	S	5 mo
29	NOEL	+	+	+	+	LAD	S	S	4 mo

two papillary muscles in 17 anterior scars and no mitral valve dysfunction was observed after surgery.

The septum was involved in 28 of 29 patients. As the thickness of the septum cannot be measured accurately, "quasi transmural" ventriculotomy is performed step by step. It is transmural in some points. The depth of these points determines the depth of ventriculotomy.

EEV achieves its objective by creating a fibrous scar barrier around the diseased zone.

Results

Four patients died in the perioperative period: two at operation (unable to come off bypass), one are after discharge on the 11th postoperative day (hypokalemia) and one on the 20th postoperative day (pulmonary embolism). Three patients died during long-term follow-up, one of pneumonia and the other two of recurrent MI. None of these deaths was related to recurrence of VT.

One early relapse of VT was observed, in a patient with posterior MI involving the right ventricle. Epicardial mapping and the configuration of the VT suggested that the right ventricular scar may have been responsible for the relapse.

Late relapse of VT was observed in three cases. In the first case, VT occured 2 months after operation but it was possible to discontinue antiarrhythmic therapy after 6 months without further recurrence, with a 3 year follow-up. The other two patients relapsed at 30 and 36 months respectively. These attacks were easily controlled with low doses of antiarrhythmic therapy.

Simple Ventriculotomy

Three patients aged 66, 60 and 62 years presented with VT over 10–18 years after MI of the septal, anterior and posterior wall respectively. None of these patients had angiographic features of left ventricular aneurysm.

At operation, epicardial mapping localised the origin of VT at the presumed site of MI although there was no visible scar either on the surface of the heart or on inspection after ventriculotomy.

Simple ventriculotomy at the site of origin was carried out by an endocardial approach in the first two cases, via a limited ventriculotomy at the apex of the left ventricle. In the third case simple transmural ventriculotomy was performed on the diaphragmatic wall of the left ventricle; this patient died at surgery of low output failure, the two others have had no further attacks of VT with a 6 year and a 3 month follow-up respectively.

Discussion

Rationale of Encircling Endocardial Ventriculotomy

EEV may have three possible effects on the pathophysiology of the infarct scar:

- When located between earliest endocardial and epicardial break-through of VT it may divide the mandatory pathway joining those points so interrupting the ventricular reentrant mechanism.
- EEV may undermine the peripheral area of the border zone and so upset the critical conditions essential for the initiation of reentry.
- The clear cut fibrous scar secondary to EEV excludes the whole infarct scar preventing abnormal electrical activity from involving the ventricles. There is some evidence in favor of this concept of exclusion [14] based on studies of EEV performed in animal experiments: After EEV the conduction between excluded infarct scar and normal myocardium is extremely delayed. Periodic electrical activity over the excluded area does not involve the ventricles.

In conclusion, each of these mechanisms may be partially responsible for the effectiveness of EEV. However, the rationale of EEV is based less on how to cut, than where to cut. The surgical action must be aimed at the edge of the border zone. The encircling ventriculotomy undermines the arrhythmogenic mechanism whatever its location around the infarct scar.

Aneurysmectomy

The results of aneurysmectomy in the surgical treatment of VT are controversial [15–17]. A study by W. Sealy and Oldham [18] reported an overall success rate of 58%. In our hospital 22 aneurysmectomies were performed to interrupt resistant VT. Four patients died during the perioperative period, and nine patients relapsed after surgery. Two of nine deaths were related to the early relapse of VT. Mason et al. [19] reported 56 patients surgically treated by conventional techniques, of whom 48 patients underwent aneurysmectomy, with associated coronary artery bypass performed in 32 cases. Eight patients had coronary bypass grafting alonge, because at surgery aneurysm was not identifiable or resectable. There were 11 early deaths after surgery, nine related to VT, and ten late deaths. Of the 35 survivors 20 required continued antiarrhythmic therapy.

Most of the early deaths resulted from relapse of VT and most patients required continued antiarrhythmic drug therapy. These results suggest a need for more effective surgery. The failure of aneurysmectomy in preventing VT is due to the following reasons: (a) it resects of leaves in place only the central fibrous part of the scar which plays no role in the genesis of tachycardia: and (b) it respects the border zone which is the site of arrhythmias, so only by chance may resection or suturing involve the site of arrhythmia. Aneurysmectomy is not always feasible and can no longer be considered the procedure of choice for the surgical treatment of VT after MI.

Other Surgical Procedures

Endocardial resection (ER) after peroperative endocardial mapping was developed by A. H. Harken et al. [20] and Josephson et al. [21]. Under normothermic cardiopulmonary bypass, the left ventricle is entered through a conventional aneurysmectomy. If the VT is still inducible, endocardial mapping determines the site of earliest endocardial break-through of the tachycardia. When feasible, ER 2–3 cm around from the site of origin of VT is carried out. When ER is not feasible the procedure is not clearly defined and the resection of the site of origin of VT may be incomplete [11]. In Horowitz's series of 30 patients, there were two operative deaths and three late deaths, and three patients presented with VT after surgery. The results of ER are similar to those of EEV. However, ER is essentiallynapplicable to anterior aneurysms and is not always feasible, especially when dealing with posterior scars. Endocardial mapping of the configuration of VT is mandatory [22] and although this point is not mentioned in Horowitz's paper, patients may present with multiple configuration of VT.

The hypothesis that several configurations of VT correspond to a single arrhythmogenic zone located in the border area has not been established. In a recent case, two configurations of VT were found on epicardial and endocardial mapping to correspond to two distinct arrhythmogenic areas 6 cm apart, one situated in the septum and the orther in the free wall of the left ventricle [23].

Some of our patients had up to eight configurations of VT which could arise from different arrhythmogenic sites [23, 24]. EEV is always feasible, even in posterior scars and can be performed even when mapping is not complete or not available [25].

EEV, ER, or aneurysmectomy can be performed when a so called aneurysm exists. For most authors an aneurysm is an infarct scar which comprises a relatively large central fibrotic thin walled and dilated area which provides an easy approach to the cavity of the left ventricle. After entering the left ventricle, the limits of endocardial fibrosis determine the limits of the border zone. Endocardial fibrosis is the only reliable anatomical landmark when dealing with aneurysm and infarct scar.

Simple Ventriculotomy

The 3 patients treated by simple ventriculotomy merit discussion. They illustrate that endocardial mapping is only feasible when a large fibrous plaque is present to allow easy access to the endocardial surface of the left ventricle. Epicardial mapping is very useful when there is no visible scar as the chronology between the earliest break-through and the onset of QRS may be determined. Epicardial mapping may also show the septal origin of VT and so guide the surgical approach to the left ventricular cavity.

References

1. Arciniegas JG, Klein H, Karp RB, Kouchoukos NT, James TN, Kirklin JW, Waldo AL (1980) Surgical treatment of life-threatening ventricular tachyarrhythmias. Circulation [Suppl III] 62:137

2. Gallagher JJ, Cox JL (1979) Status of surgery for ventricular arrhythmias. Circulation 60:1440
3. Wellens HJJ, Lie KI, Durrer D (1974) Further observations on ventricular tachycardias as studied by electrical stimulation of the heart. Circulation 49:647
4. Mallory GK, White PD, Salgedo-Salgar J (1939) The speed of healing of myocardial infarction. Am Heart J 18:647
5. Boineau JP, Cox JL (1973) Slow ventricular activation in acute myocardial infarction. A source of reentrant premature ventricular contractions circulation 48:702
6. Fontaine G, Guiraudon G, Frank R, Vedel J, Coutte R, Dragodanne C, Phan-Thuc H, Grosgogeat Y (1976) Cartographies epicardiques dans 4. cas de tachycardie ventriculaire par reentree apres infarctus du myocarde. I. Origine de la tachycardie et attitude chirurgicale. Arch Mal Coieur 11:1099
7. Fontaine G, Guiraudon G, Frank R, Vedel J, Grosgogeat Y, Cabrol C, Facquet J (1977) Stimulation studies and epicardial mapping in ventricular tachycardia: Study of mechanisms and selection for surgery. In: Kulbertus H (ed) Reentrant arrhythmias. MTP, Lancaster, pp 334–350
8. Guiraudon G, Frank R, Fontaine G (1974) Interet des cartographies dans le trailement chirurgical des tachycardies ventriculaires rebelles recidivantes Nouv Presse Med 3:273
9. El-Sherif N, Gomes J, Kelen GJ, Kahn RG, Zeiler RH (1980) Electrophysiology of reentrant ventricular arrhythmias in the late myocardial infarction period. In: Bircks W, Loogen F, Schulte HD, Seipel L (eds) Medical and surgical management of tachyarrhythmias. Springer, Berlin Heidelberg New York, 2
10. Horowitz LN, Josephson ME, Kastor JA, Harken AH (1979) Intraoperative epicardial and endocardial mapping of Am J Cardiol 43:401
11. Horowitz LN, Harken AH, Kastor JA, Josephson ME (1980) Ventricular resection guided by epicardial and endocardial mapping for treatment of recurrent ventricular tachycardia. N Engl J Med 302:589
12. Guiraudon G, Fontaine G, Frank R, Escande G, Etievent P, Cabrol C (1978) Encircling endocardial ventriculotomy. A new surgical treatment for life-threatening ventricular tachycardias resistant to medical treatment following myocardial infarction. Ann Thorac Surg 26:438
13. Fontaine G, Guiraudon G, Frank R, Gerbaux A, Cousteau JP, Barillon A, Gay J, Dabrol C, Facquet J (1975) La cartographie epicardique et le traitement chirurgical par simple ventriculotomie de certaines tachycardies ventriculaires rebelles par reentree. Arch Mal Cœur 68:113
14. Ungerleider RM, Stanley TE, Williams JM, Lofland GK, Cox JL (1980) Physiologic effects of the encircling endocardial ventriculotomy (EEV) for refractory ischemic ventricular tachycardia. Circulation 62:4, 215
15. Mason JW, Stinson EB (1980) Comparison of efficacy of map-guided to blind myocardial resection for recurrent ventricular tachycardia. Circulation Suppl III 62:1007
16. Spurrell RAJ, Yates AK, Thornburn CW, Sowton GE, Deuchar DC (1975) Surgical treatment of ventricular tachycardia after epicardial mapping studies. Br Heart J 37:115
17. Witting JH Boineau JP (1975) Surgical treatment of ventricular arrhythmias using epicardial transmural and epicardial mapping. Ann Thorac Surg 20:117
18. Sealy WC, Oldham HN (1978) Surgical treatment of malignant ventricular arrhythmias by sympathectomy, coronary artery grafts and heart wall resection. In: Advances in the management of arrhythmias. Kelly DT (ed) Australia Telectronics, p 218
19. Mason JW, Buda AJ, Stinson EB, Harrison DC (1980) Surgical therapy of ventricular tachyarrhythmias in ischemic heart disease using conventional techniques. In: Bircks W, Loogen F, Schulte HD, Seipel L (eds) Medical and surgical management of tachyarrhythmias. Springer, Berlin Heidelberg New York, p 175
20. Harken AH, Josephson ME, Horowitz LN (1979) Surgical endocardial resection for the treatment of malignant ventricular tachycardia. Ann Surg 190:456
21. Josephson ME, Harken AH, Horowitz LN (1979) Endocardial excision: A new surgical technique for the treatment of recurrent ventricular tachycardia. Circulation 60:1430
22. Horowitz LN, Josephson ME, Harken AH (1980) Epicardial and endocardial activation during sustained ventricular tachycardia in man. Circulation 61:1227

23. Guiraudon G, Fontaine G, Frank R, Leandri R, Barra J, Cabrol C (to be published) Surgical treatment of ventricular tachycardia guided by ventricular mapping in 23 patients without coronary artery disease. Ann Thorac Surg
24. Guiraudon G, Fontaine G, Frank R, Pavi A, Grosgogeat Y, Cabrol C (1980) Is the reentry concept a guide to the surgical treatment of chronic ventricular tachycardia. In: Bircks W, Loogen F, Schulte HD, Seipel L (eds) Springer, Berlin Heidelberg New York, p 155
25. Guiraudon G, Fontaine G, Frank R, Grosgogeat Y, Cabrol C (1980) Encircling endocardial ventriculotomy. Late follow-up results. Circulation [Suppl III] 62:1233

Subject Index

Cardiovascular Surgery

Editors: W. Bircks, J. Ostermeyer,
H. D. Schulte
1981. 300 figures, 271 tables.
XXII, 767 pages
Cloth DM 138,–
ISBN 3-540-10929-3

Evaluation of Cardiac Function by Echocardiography

Editors: W. Bleifeld, S. Effert, P. Hanrath,
D. Mathey
1980. 160 figures, 17 tables. IX, 198 pages
Cloth DM 64,–
ISBN 3-540-10045-8

H. Ewerbeck
Differential Diagnosis in Pediatrics

A Compendium of Symptoms and Findings

Translated and revised from the German
edition by J. Remischovsky
1980. 28 tables. XVI, 471 pages
DM 38,–
ISBN 3-540-90474-3

Myocardial Biopsy

Diagnostic Significance

Editor: H.-D. Bolte
1980. 60 figures, 30 tables.
XIV, 146 pages
Cloth DM 48,–
ISBN 3-540-10063-6

Myocardial Failure

Editors: G. Riecker, A. Weber, J. Goodwin
Co-Editors: H.-D. Bolte, B. Lüderitz,
B. E. Strauer, E. Erdmann
1977. 172 figures, 52 tables. XII, 374 pages
(International Boehringer Mannheim
Symposia)
DM 48,–
ISBN 3-540-08225-5
Distribution rights for Japan:
Nankodo Co. Ltd., Tokyo

Paediatric Pathology

Editor: C. L. Berry
With contributions by numerous experts
1981. 673 figures. XI, 697 pages
Cloth DM 170,–
ISBN 3-540-10507-7
Distribution rights for Japan:
Maruzen Co. Ltd., Tokyo

Rheumatic Valvular Disease in Children

Editors: J. B. Borman, M. S. Gotsman
With contributions by numerous experts
1980. 105 figures, 43 tables. IX, 231 pages
DM 98,–
ISBN 3-540-10079-2

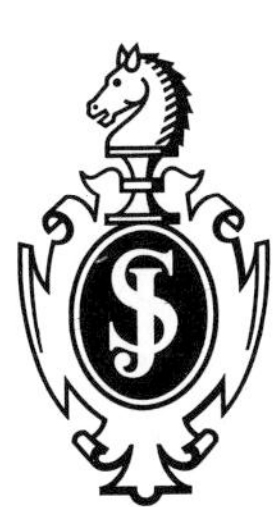

Springer-Verlag
Berlin
Heidelberg
New York

Pediatric Cardiology

ISSN 0172-0643   Title No. 246

Joint Editors: I. Carr, Chicago, IL; G. Graham, London (Managing); F. Macartney, London; R. A. Miller, Chicago, IL

Advisory Editorial Board: R. H. Anderson, R. Arcilla, L. Bargeron, A. J. Beuren, K. Bühlmeyer, A. R. Castañeda, A. Choussat, J. Edwards, J. Endrys, B. Friedli, H. Gelband, W. Gersony, I. H. Gessner, P. C. Gillette, T. Graham, Jr., P. Heintzen, J. I. E. Hoffman, F. James, J. Kachaner, J. Kamarás, M. Lev, J. R. Malm, M. Michaelsson, A. Nadas, H. Neufeld, J. Noonan, M. H. Paul, M. Quero Jiménez, W. J. Rashkind, R. D. Rowe, A. M. Rudolph, D. J. Sahn, J. Stark, N. S. Talner, C. Thorén, L. H. S. Van Mierop, R. Van Praagh, R. G. Williams

Pediatric Cardiology brings together in **one** journal advances relevant to all aspects of this and related disciplines, including cardiac surgery. Such information has in the past been scattered among journals devoted principally to adult cardiology, cardiac surgery, general pediatrics, etc.

The journal publishes original papers, lectures on "the state of the art"; editorials on topical clinical and scientific issues; special features such as unusual ECG, angiocardiographic, echocardiographic, and surgical observations; regular reviews of selected topics; book reviews; letters to the editor; and abstracts of important national, regional and international meetings.

For your order or for information on subscriptions please write to:
Springer-Verlag, Journal Promotion, P.O. Box 105 180, D-6900 Heidelberg, West-Germany

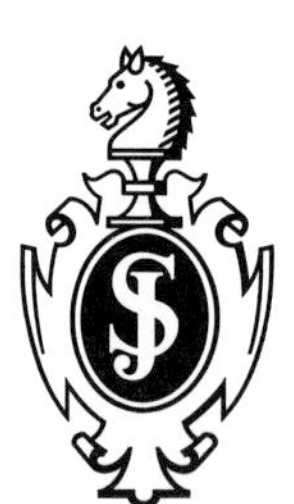

Springer-Verlag
Berlin
Heidelberg
New York